SECOND EDITION

Teaching in Nursing Practice

A Professional Model

SECOND EDITION

Teaching in Nursing Practice

A Professional Model

Nancy I. Whitman, R.N., Ph.D.
Associate Professor and Nursing Department Chair
Lynchburg College
Lynchburg, Virginia
Former Assistant Professor
University of Virginia

Barbara A. Graham, R.N., Ed.D.
Associate Professor in Nursing
University of Virginia
School of Nursing
Charlottesville, Virginia

Carol J. Gleit, R.N., Ed.D.
Associate Professor in Nursing
University of Virginia
School of Nursing
Charlottesville, Virginia

Marlyn Duncan Boyd, R.N., Ph.D., C.H.E.S.
Health Education Consultant and Adjunct Associate Professor
Department of Health Promotion and Education
School of Public Health
University of South Carolina College of Nursing
Columbia, South Carolina

APPLETON & LANGE
Norwalk, Connecticut

0-8385-8824-7

Copyright © 1992 by Appleton & Lange
Simon & Schuster Business and Professional Group
Copyright © 1986 by Appleton-Century-Crofts

94 95 96 / 10 9 8 7 6 5 4

Prentice Hall International (UK) Limited, *London*
Prentice Hall of Australia Pty. Limited, *Sydney*
Prentice Hall Canada, Inc., *Toronto*
Prentice Hall Hispanoamericana, S.A., *Mexico*
Prentice Hall of India Private Limited, *New Delhi*
Prentice Hall of Japan, Inc., *Tokyo*
Simon & Schuster Asia Pte. Ltd., *Singapore*
Editora Prentice Hall do Brasil Ltda., *Rio de Janeiro*
Prentice Hall, *Englewood Cliffs, New Jersey*

Library of Congress Cataloging-in-Publication Data

Teaching in nursing practice : a professional model / Nancy I. Whitman
    . . . [et al.]. — 2nd ed.
       p. cm.
    Includes index.
    ISBN 0-8385-8824-7
    1. Health education. 2. Nursing. I. Whitman, Nancy I.
    [DNLM: 1. Health Education—nurses' instruction. 2. Learning—
nurses' instruction. 3. Teaching—nurses' instruction. WY 105 T253]
RT90.3.T43 1992
610.73'071'1—dc20
DNLM/DLC
for Library of Congress   92-7354
                                                              CIP

Senior Editor: Barbara Norwitz
Production Editor: Sheilah Holmes
Designer: Steven Byrum

PRINTED IN THE UNITED STATES OF AMERICA

Contents

Preface

In the practice of nursing, and as nurse educators, we have engaged in a variety of health-teaching activities. We have a wide range of experience in community and inpatient settings with populations of diverse ages and health states. These have provided us with evidence of the need for health education as well as a rich background in health teaching from which to draw. We firmly believe that health teaching is an essential part of the nurse's role today; in fact, in certain practice situations, it is the main focus of that role. If nurses are expected to provide effective teaching, they must have an understanding of the teaching process and learning theory. These conditions have inspired us to prepare a comprehensive text to prepare nurses as health teachers.

While the importance of teaching as a part of the nurse's role has only escalated, many nursing programs do not provide a specific course in the process and practice of teaching in nursing. Basic nursing texts emphasize the teaching role of the nurse, but few provide more than a cursory overview of the teaching and learning process. This book provides a foundation for the process of teaching and learning. It is intended for students in undergraduate and graduate nursing programs to use as a required text or recommended reading. We believe our book will be an excellent resource for nurses who have limited exposure to such content in formal programs. Our text is unique in that it includes examples of educational activities that focus on both health promotion and teaching associated with illness. Health teaching involves individuals and groups, yet textbooks provide limited information about the group experience. We have included a chapter on group process and teaching methods. Our text also provides beginning nurses and other health professionals with the depth of information necessary to put theory into practice. Discussions focus on teaching different types of learners in a variety of health-care settings.

Since the first edition was published, teaching by nurses has continued to be an essential part of their role. With increasing knowledge about the relationship of lifestyle behaviors and certain diseases, education about health promoting and illness-preventing behaviors has become even more important. In this edition, the authors have expanded upon the role of the nurse in teaching in home health, the school setting, and occupational health. In addition, more emphasis has been placed upon AIDS education and educational strategies for the elderly. To improve the ease of using the information about the teaching process, there is a separate chapter (Chapter 10) about the teaching process itself followed by a chapter detailing general information about effective teaching strategies.

Teaching continues to be a vital part of the role of nurses. With changes in the health care delivery system it is imperative that nurses be not only effective, but efficient nurse-teachers. The authors believe that the contents of this text can foster this among nurses.

The book is organized into four units to provide ready access to certain content areas commonly associated with the teaching process. Unit I: Health Education and Professional Practice contains four chapters that explore the development and implementation of educational practice in relation to nurses and health-care delivery. Local, state, and national policies that affect these practices are also discussed. In addition, standards of practice from a variety of disciplines related to health teaching are enumerated. In Chapter 3 the teaching role of the nurse is examined by illustrating how nurses can maximize the teaching role in wellness and illness settings. Chapter 4 describes theories of learning. The authors believe that understanding theories of learning is essential to planning and implementing teaching programs.

The steps of the teaching process are delineated and specifically discussed in the remaining three units of the book. Unit II focuses on the learning environment, Unit III on the learner, and Unit IV on teaching strategies. Unit II: Teaching and Learning Variables: A Holistic Perspective contains one chapter which explores the effect of the environment upon the teaching–learning process. Specific suggestions for enhancing the environment are given. Unit III: Learner Readiness: Factors Affecting the Client as a Learner contains four chapters. The first three chapters examine factors that affect the readiness of an individual to learn and the subsequent selection of teaching–learning strategies. The last chapter discusses the assessment of a learner or potential learner. Unit IV: Strategies for Health Education, begins with a chapter on The Teaching Process. The concluding chapters provide discussions of teaching strategies for effective teaching in general, for clients of different ages, clients with different health values, and for group situations. There is also a chapter on clients with special needs related to educational, cultural, mental, and physical factors.

To aid in assessment, planning, implementation, and evaluation of teaching, specific tools and guidelines are included throughout the text. In addition, Chapter 16 contains a wealth of information about health education resources.

Nancy I. Whitman
Barbara A. Graham
Carol J. Gleit
Marlyn Duncan Boyd

Health Education and Professional Practice

In this unit the nurse is introduced to the theoretical foundations for the professional practice of health education. The professional model used to organize the content of this book encompasses four major components: the social service ideal, the client state, nursing practice strategies, and practice environment. These four concepts are discussed in detail in Chapter 1.

In Chapter 2, the legal guidelines and mandates for nurses' involvement in health education are reviewed. Although many nurses teach because they have identified a need and want to help clients, nurses must also teach because it is a legally mandated aspect of their roles as nurses.

Some of the settings in which nurses teach are discussed in Chapter 3. Industrial sites, schools, and hospitals are common teaching environments for nurses. The nurse can provide health education in virtually any setting. However, nurses must realize that although they are always the teacher, clients' needs will vary depending upon the setting.

Chapter 4 provides an in-depth discussion of theories of learning. Because nurses teach many types of concepts and skills, as well as people from many different educational, cultural, religious, and socioeconomic backgrounds, they must be aware of a variety of learning theories. Depending on the task to be learned and the unique characteristics of the learner, nurses may use cognitive, behavioral, or humanist theory as the basis for their teaching.

1

A Professional Model for Teaching in Nursing Practice

Marlyn Duncan Boyd
Barbara A. Graham
Carol J. Gleit
Nancy I. Whitman

In the late 1950s, Eleanor Lambersten, a respected leader in nursing education, defined nursing as a "dynamic, therapeutic, and educative process in meeting the health needs of society" (Lambersten, 1958, p. 80). Today, education about preventive health practices and health promotion is considered an essential component of comprehensive health care. Education is also a means of improving the health status of the American public. Nurses have a major role in this educational process. This text provides a theoretical and practical foundation for the nurse's role as a teacher of health practices and health care in today's society.

IMPORTANCE OF EDUCATION ABOUT HEALTH

The American public has access to more health information than ever before. Much of this information is disseminated through the various media. Educational programming sponsored by health-care agencies, industries, and schools have also raised the public's awareness of health matters.

Why is education about health receiving such attention? The answer to this question relates to the American people's philosophy about living, advancements in knowledge and technology, and economic factors. It is recognized that a society's most valuable resource is its people. By protecting and promoting the health of its members, the best interests of society will be served. The higher the level of health in a population, the more likely that individuals will be productive. They can share in the responsibilities of family life and they can contribute to the well-being of the communities in which they live and the country as a whole. People in good health can approach this daily living with vigor and enthusiasm. In promoting optimal health among its people, a society has the potential for improving the overall quality of life.

A more informed and health-conscious public has been evolving for some time. This can be attributed to scientific achievement, a greater sense of self-responsibility for health, and concern about the high cost of health care. Historically, knowledge of disease prevention and health promotion is quite recent. Through the 1800s, epidemics of cholera, scarlet fever, malaria, yellow fever, typhoid, and smallpox were common. Communities began to associate unfavorable environmental conditions such as polluted water, inadequate sewage disposal, crowded living conditions, and contaminated food sources with outbreaks of disease. As understanding of community sanitation improved, there were further efforts to clean up cities and promote more wholesome surroundings. The result was a dramatic reduction in morbidity and mortality (Winslow et al., 1952). Scientific advances in the field of bacteriology also led to improvements in sanitation and personal hygiene practices. Further gains are yet to be made through education of the public as new knowledge related to disease and health promotion becomes available. William Foege, former Director of the National Center for Disease Control, has noted that nearly all the gains against the once great killers came as a result of improvements in sanitation, housing, nutrition, and the prevention of disease through immunization (Pender, 1982).

Other advancements, such as the ability to synthesize substances like insulin in the laboratory, and the development of life-saving equipment, have resulted in more people surviving life-threatening events. It is now possible for victims of trauma, fragile neonates, and chronically ill individuals to survive in increasing numbers. Improvements in therapeutic and rehabilitative measures have meant that more individuals live and return to the community. Individuals and their families must learn how to manage the resulting health-care needs. Diabetics must learn diet and activity management, how to monitor their insulin requirements, and the proper technique for administering insulin. Parents of a child with a meningomyelocele repair must learn bladder and bowel training methods, techniques for aiding ambulation, the implications of mobility limitations, and strategies for coping with a handicapped child.

In addition to many technological advancements in health care, the general public is more health conscious. The quest for health information is at an all-time high. These phenomena have led some individuals to call this a time of "health-awakening" or a "health revolution." The impact of public interest in health matters and a demand for more federal legislation related to health was reflected in the passage of the National Consumer Health Information Act of 1976. The establishment of the Bureau of Health Education, the Offices of Health Information and Health Promotion, and Physical Fitness and Sports Medicine has also furthered the cause of health education (Pender, 1982). Education related to health received another boost when the National Health Planning and Resource Development Act of 1974 (Public Law 93–641) cited education of the public in health matters as one of the ten health priorities for the nation. The public health scene has changed dramatically since the turn of the century. The life expectancy of newborn infants has been increased by approximately 25 years, from 47 years to an average of 73 years today (Stamler, 1981). Emphasis on prevention rather than treatment has contributed to greater life expectancy. Furthermore, there is substantial evidence that correlates improper diet, lack of exercise, inadequate rest and relaxation, lack of attention to personal safety, and alcohol and tobacco use to the incidence of certain diseases. All of these behaviors are under individual control. The 1990 Objectives of the Nation for Promoting Health and Preventing Disease stated that "most important for today's health threats, there are activities that individuals may take voluntarily to promote healthier habits of living. . . . " (U.S. Department of Health and Human Services, 1990, p. 2). This document includes numerous references to education as a means of improving health and reducing risk factors.

Lastly, economic factors have made education related to disease prevention and health promotion very attractive. Prospective payment systems, such as that based upon the Diagnostic Related Groups (DRG) patient classifications, are placing limits on the dollars available for institutional care of health problems. Clearly, this is an economic incentive to avoid the need for prolonged or intensive hospitalization. Educational programs can effectively reduce the frequency and duration of hospitalization. In the mid-70's, Green stated "Cost–benefit analyses of alternative health services clearly favor preventive health programs and self-care programs with a major health education component" (1976, p. 57–61). Heart disease, for example, can result in a 1 to 2 week hospitalization for treatment of myocardial infarction. This may involve treatment in an intensive-care setting, which is expensive in terms of the cost of care as well as in the high cost of laboratory tests, medications, and specialists' fees. Programs to educate the public about dietary practices, exercise habits, and stress management techniques are minimal in cost by comparison.

A 1974 study found that hemophiliacs who were taught self-infusion reduced their inpatient days from 432 to 42, decreased their outpatient days from 23 to 5.5, and realized a 45 percent reduction of costs per patient (Blue Cross Association, 1974). More recent findings indicate that these benefits of patient education have continued. A California outpatient patient education program for diabetics reduced hospitalization by 73 percent and length of stay by 78 percent with a real savings of $2319.00 per patient. Similar programs in five other states have reported the hospitalization stay reductions to range from 32 to 72 percent (Hull, 1989). Numerous other studies have been conducted that show the positive effect of patient education efforts. In ensuing years, studies have shown that patient education programs have facilitated recovery from surgery, mediated the ill effects of procedures such as endoscopy and cast removal (Smith, 1989), increased self-care post surgery (Williams, et al., 1988), increased the incidence of women performing self-breast exams (Roche & Gosnell, 1989), and increased patient compliance (Kroshus & Abbott, 1989), to mention but a few.

Prevention-oriented programs may be the programs that realize the greatest impact from education efforts. Immunization programs are one of the most successful forms of primary prevention; these vaccines have drastically reduced morbidity from communicable diseases. There has not been a reportable case of smallpox in the United States since 1949, and the World Health Assembly declared global eradication of this disease in 1980 (Benenson, 1985). Unfortunately, third-party payment for health education programs is not routinely available, despite proven cost savings and lessened morbidity and mortality.

The amount spent in dollars for treatment of preventable health problems is only part of the cost. Human suffering and losses to society in terms of productivity are equally important. The consequence of many diseases is a reduced or lessened ability to fulfill social roles. If, on the other hand, there were educational programs to help individuals maintain or improve their health status, society would better conserve its human resources.

The prominence of health education in our society today is the result of expanded knowledge of disease prevention and control. Further gains have been made by individuals assuming responsibility for health-related behaviors which they control. There is also increasing awareness of the long-term economic advantages to society of health promotion and disease prevention.

NURSES' INVOLVEMENT IN HEALTH TEACHING

Health teaching is not a new role for nurses. In the 1800s Florence Nightingale wrote about sanitation, housing, care of the sick in hospitals, and health teaching. Nightingale recognized that it was not enough for people to be interested in health information, but that the test was whether they practiced it later in their homes (Bennett, 1975). Lillian Wald was another nurse who was interested in health teaching. Wald developed a settlement house in New York City in the early 1900s that was a forerunner of the community center. In her writing, Wald stressed her teaching role. She noted that for "the families who came to visit patients in the wards, [she] outlined a course of instruction in home nursing adapted to their needs, and gave it in an old building . . . " (Wald, 1915, p. 3). Wald also initiated instructional programs for new mothers, children, and invalids, who were not only taught about the health benefits of visits to the country but taken on such outings.

As Lillian Wald worked to establish a settlement house, the field of public health nursing was developing. The concept of disease prevention emerged as a principle underlying all health care and "it became impressed upon these young professional nurses . . . that if the poor people knew a little more, much suffering might be avoided" (Jensen, 1959, p. 223). The health teaching was carried out by public health nurses in homes and other community settings. During the middle of this century, outpatient departments of hospitals were also identified as sites for health-care teaching.

More recently, a broader concept of health and major achievements in health technology have enhanced the teaching role of nurses. Health is no longer viewed as merely the absence of disease, but the presence of a positive capacity to lead an energetic and productive life (Spradley, 1985, p. 8). Instead, it involves individuals seeking physical, mental, emotional, and spiritual well-being. As a result of this broadened concept, health promotion, disease prevention, and rehabilitation have become major objectives of health care, including nursing care. Comprehensive health care has led to an increased emphasis on the teaching role of the nurse.

As envisioned by our nursing leaders in the 1800s, patient education continues to be a primary component of nurses' practice outside the hospital setting. Nurses are increasingly involved in home health care and the range of knowledge and technologies that must be taught to those receiving their care at home is increasing almost on a daily basis (Barkauskas, 1990; Johnson & Jackson, 1989). Nursing homes, a once neglected practice arena, are showing a surge of patient education programs, particularly with the increase in the aged population and the need for elder care alternatives (Mezey & Lynaugh, 1989). Occupational Health Promotion programs are becoming a standard. One study found that of 5000 of the largest firms in the United States, 46 percent had wellness and/or disease prevention programs for their employees. Another 38 percent of the survey respondents indicated that they had plans to begin at least one program (Katzman & Smith, 1989). Physicians' offices are also becoming more aggressive in providing formal patient education (Hankey & Elandt, 1988). For example, physicians often provide information related to follow-up care of illnesses and instruction about possible complications; pharmacists are increasingly involved in disseminating information about drugs; nutrition and meal planning are often taught by dieticians. In fact, a 1981 survey conducted within a major medical center assessing the views of individuals from seven disciplines (physicians, nurses, health science librarians, therapists, social workers, dieticians, and pharmacists) revealed that all 631 participants felt they should have a role in health teaching (Assessment of Patient Education Programs at the University of Virginia Hospital, 1981). Clearly, many professionals from health-related disciplines see themselves involved with the educational process. In addition to those professionals more commonly identified with health care, health educators have emerged. Specialized education about program development and evaluation prepares health educators to conduct and evaluate health programs related to preventable health problems. Although a number of professionals may participate in health teaching, nurses are increasingly responsible for this role.

Nurses have unlimited opportunities to educate individuals regarding their health. Nurses are employed in hospitals, community agencies, schools, clinics, and industrial settings where they have contact with large numbers of individuals of varied ages and social backgrounds. Nurses are accepted members of the health-care team and usually spend more time with patients or clients than other team members. This contact provides the opportunity to develop rapport and build trust, to completely assess individual learning needs, and to provide continuity throughout the teaching process. Nurses are in a key position to further their role as health teachers. In addition, a nurse's educational preparation includes courses in wellness and illness, as well as human behavior. Even more important, nurse educators are placing greater emphasis on the teaching-learning process in preparing students to meet comprehensive health-care needs. The practice standards set forth by the American Nurses' Association and the Patient's Bill of Rights established by the American Hospital Association include a statement about the nurse's responsibility to teach. The Social Policy Statement (1980) developed by the American Nurses' Association states that nursing includes an array of functions including physical care, anticipatory guidance, and health teaching and counseling. A nurse's position on the health team, her contact with health-care recipients, and both educational and professional standards promote the role of the nurse as a teacher. This role is continuing to evolve and is discussed in further detail in Chapter 3.

TEACHING: A COMPONENT OF PROFESSIONAL NURSING

The importance of health teaching as a part of nursing has been recognized for years. Yet there is some evidence that perceptions about the teaching role are not consistent among nurses. For example, studies reported in the literature speak to the confusion on the part of some nurses about their preparation for teaching (Boyd & Hollander, 1988). Questions have been raised as to how committed some nurses are to the teaching role and the extent to which nurses should be involved in the teaching and learning process. Pohl, in the mid-1960s, conducted a landmark study clearly identifying nurses' lack of preparation for teaching. Others have continued to voice this concern. Ackerman (1981), Dodge (1972), Jenny (1978), and Graham and Gleit (1980) have reported inconsistency between what nurses and patients believe teaching ought to involve, as well as lack of preparation for the teaching role. If nurses are legally and professionally expected to teach and are committed to that role, they must be adequately prepared. This textbook, therefore, is specifically designed to provide a foundation for the role of teaching in nursing and to guide nurses in becoming more knowledgeable and proficient in carrying out teaching activities.

A PROFESSIONAL MODEL FOR TEACHING IN NURSING PRACTICE

While health teaching is only one aspect of nursing practice, albeit a major one, many factors influence the teaching role. For example, nurses' commitment to health teaching is closely related to their understanding of professionalism and nursing roles and the extent to which they accept accountability for their actions. The quality of health teaching is influenced by nurses' use of appropriate teaching strategies and knowledge of the teaching and learning process. Nurses understand that a teaching plan takes into account client characteristics such as risk factors and cultural background which will help to determine an individual's view of health. Nurses are also aware that various aspects of the practice environment such as physical surroundings and geographic location can facilitate or deter health-teaching efforts. The framework of this professional model provides a mechanism for organizing and describing concepts related to the teaching role.* The professional model

---

*The professional model described in this text was adapted from the conceptual framework developed by the faculty of the University of Virginia School of Nursing.

consists of four components: (1) social service ideal, (2) practice environment, (3) client state,† and (4) nursing practice strategies. Social service ideal encompasses characteristics essential to and descriptive of the nature of the nursing profession. The practice environment addresses environmental characteristics that influence the practice of nursing. The third component, client state, describes how the profession of nursing views the members of society, its clients. Nursing practice strategies, the model's fourth component, describes interventions that are unique to nursing. The professional model provides a framework for presenting concepts essential to the nurse's role as health teacher. The four units in this text are organized around these concepts.

Social Service Ideal

The social service ideal of the professional model embodies a number of characteristics generally regarded as essential to the practice of a profession. Inherent in the social service ideal is the notion that society grants members of a profession the right to practice. The members, in this case nurses, reciprocate by operating in the best interest of the public (Kellams, 1973). The public is further protected by certain professional mandates such as self-governance, codes of ethics, licensure, and standards of practice.

The social service ideal captures the spirit of a profession. It symbolizes a high level of practice. The social service ideal places emphasis on the client rather than on tasks or functions. An underlying assumption is that professional practice is based on scientific principles, for example, health teaching is accomplished by a process of assessment, planning, implementation, and evaluation.

Client advocacy is a major feature of the social service ideal. Nurses act as client advocates by correcting misinformation, assisting clients to expand their health options, and supporting them in making more informed decisions about health matters. Nurses consider health teaching to be one of their important responsibilities, while also recognizing the role of other health team members in the education process.

Professional autonomy is another important characteristic of the social service ideal. This implies some control over one's practice. In nursing, health teaching may be initiated by nurses and exemplifies the independent nature of nursing practice.

The social service ideal also includes the practice goals of the profession. The sheer number of nurses practicing in a diversity of settings, plus their contact with thousands of clients, provides an unprecedented opportunity for nurses to promote healthy life styles and self-responsibility for health in a large segment of the population. The goal of nurses' health teaching is to assist clients to achieve their wellness potential, and to ultimately improve quality of life. Table 1–1 lists examples of teaching concepts related to the social service ideal.

Further discussion of the social service ideal can be found in Chapters 2, 3, and

---

†The term *client* is used here broadly to refer to any individual the nurse is working within professional practice. In subsequent discussions, the authors distinguish between use of the terms *client* and *patient*.

TABLE 1–1. EXAMPLES OF TEACHING CONCEPTS FROM EACH OF THE FOUR COMPONENTS IN THE PROFESSIONAL NURSING MODEL

Concepts of the Professional Model Incorporated into the Teaching Role			
Social Service Ideal	*Client State*	*Practice Environment*	*Nursing Practice Strategies*
Nature of a profession	Developmental characteristics:	Facilities	Health maintenance strategies
Codes of ethics		Physical aspects	
Nursing roles	Cognitive psychomotor tasks	Organization of services	Administration, management, and leadership strategies
Standards of practice			
Advocacy	Support systems	Philosophy, policies, procedures of setting	
Accountability	Health status		Teaching skills
Nursing process	Health maintenance practices/needs	Health delivery system	Communication
	Risk factors	Community orientation and values	Assessment skills and use of tools
	Access to care		Evaluative skills
	Psychological status	Roles of other health-care providers	Group process skills
	Culture		Methods of documentation
	Belief and value system	Government intervention in health care	
		Geographic location of practice site	

Adapted from *University of Virginia School of Nursing. Self-study report. Charlottesville, Va.: University of Virginia Printing Services, 1979.*

4, in which topics such as policies and practices of nursing, legal aspects of the nurse as a teacher, the role of the nurse, and theories of learning are presented.

The Nursing Practice Environment

Every profession practices in some definable setting. The practice environment is often narrowly perceived as the physical setting in which the nurse practices. The hospital is the most commonly identified facility for this practice. Community settings such as neighborhood health clinics, schools, industrial plants, and individual homes are also common practice environments. When evaluating the practice environment in relation to teaching and learning, the adequacy of physical conditions, such as space and visual surroundings, is an important consideration. The psychological environment can also affect the teaching-learning interaction. The practice environment is composed of numerous influential characteristics other than those defined above. Characteristics of the health-care system as a whole can vastly influence the nurse's teaching practice. Policies and procedures of the system affect both the role and functions of the nurse in a particular setting. In some public health systems the nurse is independently responsible for designing and implementing a teaching plan. A hospital system may require the initiation of teaching by, or collaboration with, other health team members, especially the physician. In other settings the teaching role may be assigned to other health-care specialists. The administration and the philosophy of the system can support or impede teaching activities. Roles, functions, and personal philosophies of health-care team members also influence the nurse's role in teaching.

Community factors play a part in defining the nurse's practice environment. Here, the term *community* is used in a broad sense that includes not only the distance and terrain the nurse must traverse for interaction to take place but also demographic characteristics. The social mores of the community contribute to shaping the practice environment. Value systems of a community can provide congruence or dissonance for an individual nurse's actions. The political climate, in conjunction with existing legislation that governs nursing practice, is also an influential factor. Economics of the health-care delivery system affect the nurse's practice environment. The effects of all these community factors may interact. A nurse's teaching effectiveness may be limited by inadequate staffing patterns, lack of available teaching aids, or lack of support by the administration for time used for teaching activities. The mores and beliefs of the client's community may hinder and erode the teaching and learning, or the client may have difficulty returning for follow-up teaching.

Many factors are influential in shaping the nurse's practice environment. All environmental factors affect the teaching practice of the nurse to some degree. A detailed discussion of facilitators and barriers to teaching and learning can be found in Unit II.

Nature of the Client State

Characteristics of the client state are another component of the professional nursing model. Since the client is the focus of the nursing profession, knowledge about the client is essential for determining appropriate strategies. Here the client-learner is referred to as a patient, consumer, individual, family, group, or community. The nature of the client state requires comprehensive knowledge about human beings, derived from both the pure and applied sciences. Through the use of knowledge from the physiologic, psychological, and social sciences, nurses have an understanding of man's physiologic functioning (health state, energy level) and psychosocial state (drives, motivations, values, and beliefs). Acting upon this understanding, nurses can make appropriate decisions to optimize the teaching-learning process. Through an in-depth assessment of the client, nurses determine whether teaching is needed and if so, the nature of that teaching. They then proceed to plan, implement, and evaluate the teaching-learning process. This process is based on a holistic approach to meeting the educational needs of the client. For example, while engaging in teaching about a specific medication regimen, the nurse assesses the client's knowledge about a prescribed medication as well as its action, expected effect, possible side effects, and dosage schedule. The nurse also notes the client's degree of belief in the need for the medication and what "good" or "bad" effects the client expects from the medication. In addition, the nurse assesses the influence that family members or other significant individuals may have on the medication regimen and how the particular medication may affect or alter the client's normal pattern of living. Assessment based upon the knowledge of the client helps the nurse to plan and develop strategies for implementing teaching content. Nurses can also identify actual or potential obstacles to the success of the prescribed medication regime. Knowledge of the client facilitates effective teaching-learning interaction.

The level of health or wellness of a client may range from high-level wellness to near death. Between these two extremes the client can experience a temporary illness, a permanent or progressive illness, or multiple variations of these. When teaching clients in various states of health and illness, nurses provide health information, help to promote and maintain wellness, and assist clients to recuperate from illness. In some instances, they help prepare individuals for death.

The nature of the client state is further described in Unit III in relation to factors affecting the client as a learner.

Nursing Practice Strategies

Nursing practice strategies refer to the body of knowledge, skills, and techniques used in nursing practice. Nursing practice strategies also communicate the unique way in which nurses use information and skills acquired from other disciplines. A nurse's teaching strategies are drawn from a broad spectrum of disciplines. Through the use of this information, a nurse makes professional judgments about the most appropriate type of teaching strategy needed with a particular client.

Nurses use a broad array of knowledge and skills to carry out teaching. Following the steps of the teaching process, the nurse first gathers data about the educational needs of a specific client or client population. After collecting information from a variety of sources, a primary need is identified. In a family planning clinic, a nurse may plan and organize classes on sexuality, sexual expression, conception, and contraception. These activities require the use of educational, leadership, and management strategies. The nurse in this situation may use some of the same planning and management strategies that are taught to corporate managers and the same educational strategies used by a classroom teacher. The applications of the management and education strategies to nursing practice, however, make them unique. To continue the example, the nurse will then teach classes using communication skills derived from the psychosocial disciplines. The nursing process is completed with an evaluation of the effectiveness of the teaching session. Although the skills of the process are drawn from other disciplines, the content, client state, and practice environment differentiate teaching in nursing from that of other disciplines.

Nursing practice strategies are the active component of nursing practice. These strategies involve the use of ideas, skills, and techniques to help clients learn to manage illness and to obtain and maintain their optimal level of wellness. The strategies used by the nurse in the teaching role are discussed in Unit IV. Teaching strategies are the core of this teaching role and are chosen for a given situation based on knowledge about the social service idea, client state, and practice environment. Material addressed in Unit VI includes general strategies for teaching and specific strategies for a variety of situations. There is also emphasis on strategies for teaching populations with special needs, found in Chapter 14.

DEFINITIONS OF PRACTICE

Various disciplines often use similar terminology in different ways. The following section defines terminology used in the educational process. Different categories of learners as they are used throughout this book are also described.

Definition of the Educational Process

Although the concept of health education is not new, terminology remains inconsistent and confusing. Patient education, client education, and consumer education are heard frequently in discussions of health care. These terms provide a general idea about the nature of the content and health status of the individual receiving the health education. In some situations the term *patient education* may be used loosely (referring to anyone learning about health care or illness); in others, the term may convey a narrower definition. The following definitions clarify the authors' use of each term.

Patient education is the use of the educational process for individuals, their families, and other significant persons when dependence upon the health-care system for diagnosis, treatment, or rehabilitation is required. Although the individual may be exposed to general health information, educational content is focused primarily on the disease or condition and its implications.

Client education is the use of the educational process for individuals who are partners in the health education effort. The learner and teacher mutually identify the subject matter to be taught and then decide how the educational process will be carried out. Client education often implies an increasingly autonomous and self-directed role for the learner.

Consumer education is the use of the educational process by any individual or group of individuals who are independent decision makers. A consumer identifies the health-learning need and initiates the learning process. The teacher facilitates the learning process.

The main difference in the terminology discussed above is the learner's level of dependence. Figure 1–1 graphically represents this continuum.

Health education has a variety of interpretations. Clarification of its use is therefore important. Traditionally, the terms *health* and *illness* were interpreted as opposing states on a continuum. Good health was the absence of symptoms of a disease; bad health or illness included the symptoms and behaviors present during a disease state. Health education, then, was related to learning about maintaining good health. The term *illness education* is not used as a label for content related to illness. Definitions are continuing to evolve, however, and the term *high-level wellness* is now frequently referred to as a process of continued growth and develop-

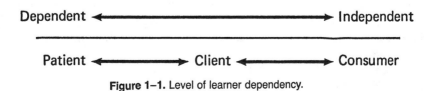

Figure 1–1. Level of learner dependency.

ment and self-actualization of the whole person (physical, mental, social, and spiritual) (Baronowski, 1981). In this context, health is identified as a state or stage, denoting one point in time. Using this view of health, the interpretation of health education is broad. The teaching content may relate to any state along the health continuum. Teaching content may include management techniques for diabetes or wellness strategies for stress reduction. Illness and wellness are not seen as mutually exclusive. It is possible that a nurse might be working with an individual learning certain aspects of both illness and wellness.

Teaching Assistance Based on Learner Need

Learners differ in the amount of teaching assistance required for making behavioral changes. For consumers, self-responsibility is usually high. The nurse-teacher can facilitate learning by making suggestions, serving as a resource person, or giving encouragement and support to ideas the individual already has for behavior change. Mutual decision making by the nurse and client help the client sort out values and attitudes toward specific health topics before attempting change. Consciousness-raising efforts may be important for all learners, but perhaps more so with patients because of their dependent role. Nurses can facilitate patient awareness of the areas of health care in which they can participate.

Nurses involved in patient education may find that the patient has little previous knowledge of the content to be learned; whereas, client teaching relies heavily on the knowledge and skills already acquired. Both patient and client education have a place in the health-care system. The hospitalized patient may not have the physical or psychological energy to be self-directing. For patients who are depleted in physical or psychological energy, it may be necessary for the nurse to teach all aspects of a specific task. The completion of the specific task may lead to an improved health status for the patient. As patients improve in their physical and emotional health they can assume a higher degree of self-responsibility for their health. A nurse is also responsible for helping individuals to make decisions about their health. Basic differences exist among individuals in the amount of assistance required from the nurse. The nurse must accurately assess the amount of learner dependence and strive through the educative process to help the individual become more self-directed. Involvement and cooperation of the individual in each phase of the learning process promotes a more autonomous learner.

SUMMARY

The teaching role of the nurse is growing in importance today. In this chapter a brief historical overview of the growth of this role was presented. It was noted that the idea of nurses participating in health teaching is not new, and that other health professions also include teaching as part of their role. Teaching is increasingly recognized as an essential component of a nurse's role in providing comprehensive health care.

The professional model, a framework for the teaching process, was introduced. This model, composed of the social service ideal, client state, practice environment, and practice strategies, provides a logical way to organize and examine various concepts that are part of the teaching process or that influence the teaching roles of the nurse. The authors believe that knowledge about these concepts is essential for one to be an effective nurse-teacher.

Terms used to identify the educational process within the health-care system were defined. These include patient education, client education, consumer education, and health education. The nurse may be involved in any part of the educational processes. These processes are influenced by professional standards as well as by legislative and regulatory policies. Chapter 2 provides the information on policies and procedures as they pertain to individuals involved in the health education process. Ethical and legal issues as well as professional standards are also considered. The teaching role of the nurse is examined in Chapter 3. Chapter 4 lays the foundation for teaching through discussion of theories of learning.

REFERENCES AND READINGS

Ackerman, A. M., Partridge, K. M., & Kalmer, H. Effective integration of health education into baccalaureate nursing curriculum. *Journal of Nursing Education*, February 1981, 37–44.

Assessment of Patient Education Programs at the University of Virginia Hospitals. Planning Subcommittee of Patient Education Committee Report, Unpublished manuscript, December 3, 1981.

Barkauskas, V. H. Home health care. *Annual Review of Nursing Research*, 1990, *8*, 103–132.

Baronowski, T. Toward the definition of concepts of health and disease, wellness and illness. *Health Values: Achieving High Level Wellness*, 1981, *5*(6), 246–256.

Benenson, A. S. (Ed.). *Control of communicable disease in man.* Washington, D.C.: American Public Health Association, 1985.

Bennett, E. R. (Ed.). *Florence Nightingale—Her wit and wisdom.* New York: Peter Pauper Press, 1975.

Boyd, M. D., & Hollander, R. Patient education: A study of registered nurses' attitudes, time spent teaching, and their administrative support. *Advances in Health Education: Current Research*, 1988, *1*(1), 101–110.

Blue Cross Association. *White paper: Patient education, health care services.* Blue Cross Association, August 1974.

Dodge, J. S. What patients should be told. *American Journal of Nursing*, October 1972, *72*(10), 1852–1854.

Graham, B., & Gleit, C. Health education: Are nurses really prepared? *Journal of Nursing Education*, October 1980, *19*(8), 4–6.

Green, L. The potential of health education includes cost effectiveness. *Hospitals JAHA*, May 1, 1976, *50*, 57–61.

Hankey, T. L., & Elandt, N. J. Collaborative approaches to patient education in the family physician's office. *Patient Education and Counseling*, 1988, *12*, 267–275.

Honan, S., Krsnak, G., Peterson, D., & Torkelson, R. The nurse as patient educator: Perceived responsibilities and factors enhancing role development. *The Journal of Continuing Education in Nursing*, 1988, *19*(1), 33–37.

Hull, M. How to set up a diabetes education program. *RN*, *52*(11), 61–64

Jenny, J. Patient teaching as a curriculum thread. *The Canadian Nurse,* February 1978, 28–29.

Jensen, D. M. *History and trends of professional nursing.* St. Louis: C. V. Mosby, 1959.

Johnson, E. A., & Jackson, J. E. Teaching the home care client. *Nursing Clinics of North America,* 1989, *24*(3), 687–693.

Katzman, M. S., & Smith, K. J. Occupational health-promotion programs: Evaluation efforts and measured cost savings. *Health Values,* 1989, *13*(2), 3–10.

Kellams, S. E. Higher education as a potential profession. *Journal of Research and Development,* Winter 1973, *6*(2), 30–41.

Kroshus, M. G., & Abbott, J. A. Quality assurance of a rheumatoid arthritis education program. *Patient Education and Counseling, 1989, 12,* 213–224.

Lambertsen, E. C. *Education for nursing leadership.* Philadelphia: Lippincott, 1958.

Lipetz, M. J., Bussigel, M. N., Bannerman, J., & Risley, B. What is wrong with patient education programs? *Nursing Outlook,* 1990, *38*(4), 184–189.

Mezey, M. D., & Lynaugh, J. E. The teaching nursing home program. *Nursing Clinics of North America,* 1989, *24*(3), 769–779.

Pender, N. J. *Health promotion in nursing practice.* Norwalk, Conn.: Appleton-Century-Crofts, 1982.

Pohl, M. L. Teaching activities of the nurse practitioner. *Nursing Research,* Winter 1965, *4*(1), 4–11.

Porter, Y. Brief: Evaluation of nursing documentation of patient teaching. *The Journal of Continuing Education in Nursing,* 1990, *21*(3), 134–137.

Roche, M., & Gosnell, D. J. Evaluation of a hospital teaching program for breast self-examination. *Patient Education and Counseling,* 1989, *13,* 31–41.

Smith, C. J. Overview of patient education: Opportunities and challenges for the twenty-first century. *Nursing Clinics of North America,* 1989, *24*(3), 583–587.

Spradley, B. W. *Community health nursing concepts and practice* (2nd ed.). Boston: Little, Brown, 1985.

Stamler, J. Disease of the cardiovascular system. In D. Clark, & B. MacMahon (Eds.), *Preventive and community medicine* (2nd ed.). Boston: Little, Brown, 1981.

U.S. Department of Health and Human Services. *Promoting health/preventing disease objectives for the nation.* Washington, D.C.: U.S. Government Printing Office, 1990.

University of Virginia, School of Nursing. *Self-study report.* Charlottesville, Va.: University of Virginia Printing Services, 1979.

Wald, L. D. *The house on Henry Street.* New York: Henry Holt, 1915.

Williams, P. D., Valderrama, M. A., Gloria, M. D., et al. Effects of preparation for mastectomy/hysterectomy on women's post-operative self-care behaviors. *International Journal of Nursing Studies,* 1988, *25*(3), 191–206.

Winslow, C. E. A., Smillie, W. G., Doull, J., & Gordon, J. E. *History of epidemiology in America.* C. V. Mosby, 1952.

2

Policies, Guidelines, and Legal Mandates for Health Teaching

Marlyn Duncan Boyd

This chapter highlights events on the national level which have played an important role in promoting the inclusion of health education throughout the health-care system. Nurses must have an understanding of what has happened within their profession that affects their practice. Likewise, they must also have an understanding of factors that affect the practice of nursing as reflected in national trends, federal legislation, and accreditating agency mandates.

Health education as a component of health care has developed slowly over more than a century. Most of the growth has occurred in the past 30 years. Health education is continuing to be refined as an art and a science within nursing and other health professions. The practice of health education as an integral aspect of comprehensive health care is now encompassed ethically and professionally by an expanding array of health-care providers.

In the past, physicians claimed the right and responsibility for patient education; however, today other health professionals also provide these services. Nursing, more so than other professions, is proving to be a leader in this aspect of health care. Nurses have accepted the fact that those professionals who have the privilege and responsibility of educating consumers must obtain the knowledge and skills to adequately perform in the health-teaching role. Moreover, if professionals are incorporating the practice of education into their existing responsibilities, they will be both professionally and legally accountable for these efforts. Nursing has accepted this challenge and responsibility and is a leader in current trends in health education.

HISTORICAL TRENDS IN HEALTH EDUCATION

Organizations
Although health education has been practiced for a century or more by both physicians and nurses (National League of Nursing Education, 1918; Bordley & Harvey,

1976), the concept of health education as an integral component of health care has only truly emerged in the last 30 years. As early as 1850 professionals acknowledged the need to teach practitioners to preserve health and prevent disease (Bordley & Harvey, 1976). This need was also readily incorporated into nursing education (National League of Nursing Education, 1918).

Several events in the 1900s promoted recognition of the importance of health education but perhaps those with the greatest impact occurred in the latter part of the century. In 1950, the Society of Public Health Education was organized to promote, encourage, and contribute to the advancement of health (Askey, 1982). In 1957, the first health education journal was published—*Health Education Monographs*. In 1958, the International Journal of Health Education began publication in Geneva, Switzerland. Between 1950 and 1963, national trends in health education reflected concern for general consumer health and public health education. Evidence that professionals were becoming involved in health education research, and sharing their knowledge with other professions was seen when in 1963 health education was listed as a subject heading in the *Index Medicus* for the first time (U.S. Department of Health, Education and Welfare, 1963). As professionals began to differentiate between health education and patient education, the *Index Medicus* listed for the first time "patient education" as a separate listing in 1966 (U.S. Dept. of HEW, 1966). By the end of 1970, the *Index Medicus* listed 220 citations for Health Education (U.S. Dept. of HEW, 1970).

The 1970s brought the establishment of the American Society for Health Manpower Education and Training (ASHET, 1970), which specifically noted patient education managers among the professionals solicited as members (Askey, 1982). Also, President Nixon appointed a Committee for Health Education and in 1973 established the Bureau of Health Education and Health Promotion within the Centers of Disease Control (Bordley & Harvey, 1976).

In the 1970s, consumers began to assert their rights in regard to health care by organizing several groups including the Patients' Rights Organization (1971), Medicine in the Public Interest (1973), and Healthright (1973) (Askey, 1982). All three groups were organized on the national level to promote consumer involvement in health care.

The years 1974 and 1975 were a particular time of growth for patient education. The American Hospital Association (AHA) issued a statement making health education a priority item. The AHA requested that hospital leadership plan, implement, and document health education programs (AHA, 1975). The Blue Cross Association approved the White Paper on Patient Health Education in 1974, and it has served as a landmark for patient education. The study emphasized that patient education programs, combined with the routine services of the hospital, offer the potential for both cost containment and improved patient care. The study recommended that the Blue Cross Association encourage hospitals to develop programs in health education and be supported financially by third-party payment (insurance) (Blue Cross Association, 1974). Reimbursement by third-party payers for health education, however, has not been a frequent method of payment in most programs.

The White Paper also included specific guidelines for the development of health education programs (Table 2–1).

In July, 1975, the AHA, in conjunction with the National Bureau of Health Education, distributed "The Hospital Inpatient Education Survey" to 5770 community hospitals. Of those hospitals surveyed, 4670 (80.9 percent) returned the questionnaire. Slightly more than half of the hospitals (57 percent) responded that they had a formal health education program of some type. Of those hospitals that indicated that they had one or more formal programs, 329 hospitals (12.75 percent) had specific hospital policies on patient education. When policy making was done by a committee, nurses were the most frequently cited professionals who made up the committees (93.7 percent). Physicians and administrators were often members of patient education committees as well. Usually the responsibility for the coordination of health education was within the department of nursing. In addition, within those hospitals that indicated that a position was allocated for directing health education, the position was filled by a registered nurse (AHA, 1977). These data seemed to indicate that, in the hospitals surveyed, nurses more so than any other group of professionals were initiating, planning, directing, and implementing formal health education.

In the private sector during the mid-1970s, the National Center for Health Education was founded. The Center's goal was to develop and encourage educa-

TABLE 2–1. GUIDELINES FOR PROGRAMS IN PATIENT EDUCATION

1. The purpose and operational objectives of the program should be clearly stated, and the techniques for meeting the objectives should be specified.
2. Patient education should be provided as an integral element of the total patient care process within a supportive organizational framework.* Existing hospital-based programs in patient education shall be reviewed by either the Joint Commission on Accreditation of Hospitals or the Bureau of Hospitals of the American Osteopathic Association.
3. Necessary and appropriate health education should be developed and financed as a routine element of the care of each patient.
4. Educational methodologies should be directed to specific case types and desired behavioral changes and the results of such interventions as to cost and quality of care should be documented. As in other expenses, continuing management evaluation of the cost effectiveness of the service should be conducted. Programs should be revised over time to reflect the results of such evaluation.

It is appropriate that the Blue Cross system encourage the development of cost-effective programs in patient education. Where patient education is properly related to the other components of the total patient care process, there is clear potential for reduction of health care costs and improvement in the quality of health care processes and outcomes. Blue Cross Plans share responsibility with those providing patient education to ensure that this potential is realized. Accordingly, the Blue Cross System should play an active part in the development, implementation, and evaluation of sound programs in patient education.

*Examples of this organizational framework are the hospital, home care program, HMO, or community health education program.
Used with permission from White Paper: Patient Health Education, *Blue Cross Association, Chicago, 1974.*

tional activities and to promote the public's understanding of what people can do to influence their own health (Lee & Garvey, 1977).

By the late 1970s, health education had attained high visibility, there were more publications in professional journals, and new journals devoted to health education began publication (U.S. Dept. of HEW, 1979). There was also new federal and accrediting agency legislation. Public Health Law 94–317, the Health Promotion–Disease Act, was passed by Congress in 1976 and helped bring to the government's attention the need for health promotion research and the empirical benefits of health education (PL 94–317, 1976). In addition, the American Hospital Association issued the 1977 publication "Professional, Accreditation, and Legal Statements Supporting Patient Education." Each of these milestones in health education served to heighten the awareness of professionals and consumers of the need for health instruction in both hospitals and communities.

In the late 1970s, professionals involved in health education began to band together. These groups varied in professional and agency make-up and their size ranged from two or more hospitals to entire regional affiliations (American Hospital Association, 1980). Their goals varied from trying to meet specific professional and institutional needs in the areas of health education to working as a lobbying force for political change in health care. By 1980, more than 40 support groups had been identified and the success of these groups was demonstrated by their rapid growth. An example of such a group is the Patient Education Consortium of Southwestern Virginia (PECOS-VA). It is a group of 15 hospital representatives who meet on a regular basis to discuss health education. The majority of the representatives are nurses who serve as patient education coordinators, but other hospital personnel involved in educating patients are also represented. In 1989 the International Council for Patient Education was formed (Redman & Bartlett, 1989).

The advent of Diagnostic Related Groups (DRGs) in the early 1980s promoted the growth of health education. Push for cost-containment measures has resulted in earlier hospital discharges and the need for home care. This has increased the demand for health education in both the hospital and the community.

In the area of professional education, the need for adequate preparation in health teaching has long been recognized by various health professionals. The Johns Hopkins University began to develop a curriculum for health education in 1979, and Dartmouth Medical School offered an elective in patient education to first and second year students (Physician's Patient Education Newsletter, 1978). In preparing nurses as health teachers, some nursing education programs may now require separate courses in health education and teaching (University of South Carolina, 1991). The quest for recognition of nurses as health teachers is not a recent phenomenon. For decades, nursing leaders have recognized that health teaching is an independent nursing function (National League of Nursing Education, 1918; 1937; American Nurses' Association, 1954; 1986) and an expected component of every nurse's duty owed to each patient as a standard of care (American Nurses' Association, 1986; Creighton, 1987). Although health education has long been recognized as a nursing function, it has traditionally been integrated into other components of nursing care and not viewed as a separate and definable part of quality care.

In just 30 years, health education has come from an almost unknown concept for many health professionals to an issue of prominence to consumers, professionals, and governing and accreditating agencies.

POLICIES AND MANDATES AFFECTING HEALTH EDUCATION

Mandates for health education from the federal government came in the mid-1960s. With the passage of the Comprehensive Health Planning Act (Public Health Law 89–97, 1965) and the establishment of Medicare and Medicaid, the federal government noted the importance of preventive and rehabilitative aspects of health care. Under P.L. 89–97, to qualify for Medicare payments a hospital has to show evidence that patient education has been a part of patient care. "The patient has the right to communicate with those responsible for his care, and receive from them adequate information concerning the nature and extent of his medical problem. . . . In addition, he has a right to expect adequate instruction in self-care in the interim between visits to the hospital or to the physician. The final progress note should include any instructions given to the patient and family. (Joint Commission for the Accreditation of Hospitals, 1979, p. 24, recently renamed Joint Commission for the Accreditation of Hospital Organizations [JCAHO]).

The 1981 (JCAH) *Accreditation Manual for Hospitals* mandated the following accreditation requirements for hospital-based patient education:

> The following information shall be documented in each patient's medical record . . . patient disposition and any pertinent instructions given to the patient and/or family for follow-up care (p. 68). . . . Patient education and patient/family knowledge of self-care shall be given special consideration in the nursing plan. The instructions and counseling given to the patient must be consistent with that of the reasonable medical practitioner. The plan of care must be documented and should reflect current standards of nursing practice. The plans shall include . . . patient/family education . . . (pp. 118, 119)

The manual spoke specifically to the nurse's role in health education: "The instruction of the patient or of the appropriate nursing department/service personnel who advise the patient, verbally or in writing, on the importance and correct use of medication to be taken following discharge in the interest of assuring safe and correct self-administration, when such instruction is requested by the responsible practitioner or as provided by written medical staff policy. . . . " (p. 142). Referring to the documentation of patient education, the manual states that "personnel . . . shall document the written instructions given to the patient and/or family concerning appropriate care after discharge from the hospital . . . " (p. 191). These standards supported the need for hospitals to develop patient education programs and materials which would adequately educate patients. Failure to meet the above standards could result in increased mortality for patients and malpractice suits against hospitals and health-care professionals. The JCAH Accreditation Manual for Hospitals also mandates the evidence of health education prior to a hospital's

TABLE 2–2. A PATIENT'S BILL OF RIGHTS

The American Hospital Association presents a Patient's Bill of Rights with the expectation that observance of these rights will contribute to more effective patient care and greater satisfaction for the patient, his physician, and the hospital organization. Further, the Association presents these rights in the expectation that they will be supported by the hospital on behalf of its patients, as an integral part of the healing process. It is recognized that a personal relationship between the physician and the patient is essential for the provision of proper medical care. The traditional physician–patient relationship takes on a new dimension when care is rendered within an organizational structure. Legal precedent has established that the institution itself also has a responsibility to the patient. It is in recognition of these factors that these rights are affirmed.

1. The patient has the right to considerate and respectful care.
2. The patient has the right to obtain from his physician complete current information concerning his diagnosis, treatment, and prognosis in terms the patient can be reasonably expected to understand. When it is not medically advisable to give such information to the patient, the information should be made available to an appropriate person in his behalf. He has the right to know by name the physician responsible for coordinating his care.
3. The patient has the right to receive from his physician information necessary to give informed consent prior to the start of any procedure and/or treatment. Except in emergencies, such information for informed consent should include but not necessarily be limited to the specific procedure and/or treatment, the medically significant risks involved, and the probable duration of incapacitation. Where medically significant alternatives for care or treatment exist, or when the patient requests information concerning medical alternatives, the patient has the right to such information. The patient also has the right to know the name of the person responsible for the procedures and/or treatment.
4. The patient has the right to refuse treatment to the extent permitted by law, and to be informed of the medical consequences of his action.
5. The patient has the right to every consideration of his privacy concerning his own medical care program. Case discussion, consultation, examination, and treatment are confidential and should be conducted discreetly. Those not directly involved in his care must have the permission of the patient to be present.
6. The patient has the right to expect that all communications and records pertaining to his care should be treated as confidential.
7. The patient has the right to expect that within its capacity a hospital must make reasonable response to the request of a patient for services. The hospital must provide evaluation, service, and/or referral as indicated by the urgency of the case. When medically permissible, a patient may be transferred to another locality only after he has received complete information and explanation concerning the needs for and alternatives to such a transfer. The institution to which the patient is to be transferred must first have accepted the patient for transfer.
8. The patient has the right to obtain information as to any relationship of his hospital to other health care and educational institutions insofar as his care is concerned. The patient has the right to obtain information as to the existence of any professional relationships among individuals, by name, who are treating him.
9. The patient has the right to be advised if the hospital proposes to engage in or perform human experimentation affecting his care or treatment. The patient has the right to refuse to participate in such research projects.
10. The patient has the right to expect reasonable continuity of care. He has the right to know in advance what appointment times and physicians are available and where. The patient has the right to expect that the hospital will provide a mechanism whereby he is informed by his physician or a delegate of the physician of the patient's continuing health care requirements following discharge.

TABLE 2-2. (*Continued*)

11. The patient has the right to examine and receive an explanation of his bill regardless of source of payment.
12. The patient has the right to know what hospital rules and regulations apply to his conduct as a patient.

No catalogue of rights can guarantee for the patient the kind of treatment he has a right to expect. A hospital has many functions to perform, including the prevention and treatment of disease, the education of both health professionals and patients, and the conduct of clinical research. All these activities must be conducted with an overriding concern for the patient and, above all, the recognition of his dignity as a human being. Success in achieving this recognition assures success in the defense of the rights of the patient.

Reprinted with permission by the American Hospital Association, copyright 1972.

inclusion in Medicare and Medicaid programs. These initial efforts by JCAH to give credibility and legitimacy to health education have been strengthened in future statements (JCAH, 1986).

Perhaps the most well-known health education document to both patients and professionals is "A Patient's Bill of Rights" (Table 2–2). This statement by the AHA in 1973 was made with the "expectation that observance of these rights will contribute to more effective patient care and greater satisfaction for the patient, his physician, and the hospital organization" (AHA, Statement on a Patient's Bill of Rights, 1973, p. 1). The statement has been adopted in its original form by many hospitals, and others have developed similar statements of their own. Some states have mandated that hospitals adopt the bill. Patients' rights have gained further support by the Health Care Financing Administration, which proposed that hospitals be required to have written policies stating the rights of patients before they can qualify for inclusion in Medicare and Medicaid programs (AHA, 1973).

NURSING, THE LAW, AND HEALTH EDUCATION

The nurse's accountability in health education is governed by laws and ethical standards of practice. Nurses, as professionals, are autonomous and are legally responsible for acts of commission or omission; although nurses may share teaching responsibilities with other health professionals they are solely accountable for the outcomes of their own practice decisions.

Nurses' practice of health education is guided and governed by several professional bodies. On the national level, there is the American Nurses' Association, which has a 22-volume series of standards for a wide scope of nursing specialty areas. Nursing specialty areas themselves, such as the Association of Operating Room Nurses, Critical Care Nurses Association, and Emergency Room Nurses Association, further delineate these standards for their practitioners. The Joint Commission on the Accreditation of Hospitals provides Nursing Service Standards to guide hospitals in providing quality nursing care. At the state level, the Nurse Practice Acts are the legal authority that governs practice. Finally, there are institutional policies such as procedure and policy manuals that guide provision of care. These cannot circumvent the Nurse Practice Act that, again, legally defines practice standards for nurses of a given state (Creighton, 1987).

The Nurse Practice Acts contain the strongest legal mandates for nurses' involvement in health education. All 50 states have Nurse Practice Acts designed to define the functions of nurses and establish licensing mechanisms. These definitions are not static but change as the role and scope of nursing change. An example of a model Nurse Practice Act is shown in Table 2–3. Although some similarities exist among practice acts, it is important for each nurse to be aware of the legal boundaries under which he or she practices. In addition, the explicitness of mandates for health education for nurses varies among nurse practice acts. For example, the "Interpretation of the Legal Definitions of Nursing Practice" of the North Carolina Board of Nursing states: "The RN is accountable for: determining and counseling/teaching needs of patients and their families; designing a plan for counseling/teaching the patient, including selection of the most competent staff and most appropriate resources and schedules; initiating the plan; and evaluating the plan and making changes as needed" (North Carolina Board of Nursing, 1977, p. 2). Clearly, the nurse in North Carolina is legally responsible for health education!

In support of the accepted role of the nurse as an educator, the National League of Nursing, in its publication *Nursing's Role in Patients' Rights*, stated that patients have the right to information—in terms they and their families can easily understand. Patients also have the right to appropriate instruction so they can pursue an optimal level of wellness and understand their basic health needs (National League of Nursing, 1977).

As public awareness of patients' rights increases and as health education becomes more strongly mandated by governing bodies and accreditating agencies, the question of liability becomes a special concern to nurses. The level of acceptable performance is the same for health education as in any other aspect of nursing practice. Coupled with this is the increasing use of "custom" by courts to establish standards of care (Annas, 1975); which is to say, what is the customary or standard practice in a given locality or situation? For example, is preoperative teaching an

---

TABLE 2–3. MODEL NURSE PRACTICE ACT

Model Act
Section II
B. Practice of Nursing by a Registered Nurse. The practice of nursing as performed by a registered nurse is a process in which substantial specialized knowledge derived from the biological, physical, and behavioral sciences is applied to the care, treatment, counsel, and health teaching of persons who are experiencing changes in the normal health processes; or who require assistance in the maintenance of health or other management of illness, injury, and infirmity or in the achievement of a dignified death; and such additional acts as are recognized by the nursing profession as proper to be performed by a registered nurse.

Excerpted from Model Practice Act. American Nurses' Association. Kansas City, Mo., 1976. Used with permission.

expected standard of care before surgery? Is making sure a diabetic has injected insulin properly before discharge a customary practice?

The risk of liability is increasing for nurses who do not provide adequate health education (Creighton, 1985; 1987; 1988). Liability presents itself in two basic forms: negligence and malpractice. Negligence has been defined as the omission to do something that a reasonable person, guided by ordinary considerations which ordinarily regulate human affairs, would do. Or, doing something that a reasonable and prudent person would not do. To establish that a nurse has been negligent, a plaintiff must show: (1) evidence that establishes that the nurse should have performed the act and the standard of care applicable to the situation; (2) breach of that duty and the existence of a resulting injury; and (3) that the violation of practice was the proximate cause of the injury (Creighton, 1981). In other words, if a nurse failed to provide the required patient education and the patient could show that an injury resulted from a lack of that information or instruction, the nurse could be sued for negligence. An example of this can be found in Bass v. Barksdale. A patient sued a nurse and two physicians for treatment allegedly resulting in blindness. Mrs. Bass testified that Nurse Barksdale did not tell her about symptoms to expect from medications, did not tell her she should have her vision checked on a prescribed basis, and did not give her any written material for review. Nurse Barksdale testified that she had taught the patient. The jury found evidence in the record to establish the failure of Nurse Barksdale to properly inform Mrs. Bass of the drug's side effects (lack of documentation) (Creighton, 1988). Another case involving a nurse's alleged failure to provide information and lack of documentation is found in Kaiser v. Suburban Transportation System. A passenger sued to recover damages resulting from a bus wreck caused by the driver losing consciousness. The driver had been taking pyribenzamine. At the trial, the bus driver testified that neither the doctor nor the nurse gave him any instructions about the possible side effects of the drug. Evidence was also found in the chart to support his testimony (lack of documentation) (Creighton, 1985). Nurses frequently provide medication instruction to patients. The potential for nurses to be named as plaintiffs in resulting malpractice cases is a real one. These are not isolated cases but two of many that support that the public and the legal profession view nurses as accountable for the teaching or the lack thereof (Creighton, 1985; 1986; 1987; 1988).

Malpractice has been defined as any professional misconduct involving unreasonable lack of skill or fidelity in professional or judiciary duties, evil practice, or illegal or immoral conduct (Fiesta, 1983). This breach of professional conduct primarily deals with performing treatments or procedures on a patient that are not ordered or indicated, or the practicing of poor nursing judgment or skill. Traditional examples of malpractice in nursing include a nurse improperly giving an injection resulting in damage to a patient's sciatic nerve or when a nurse fails to notify a physician in sufficient time to deliver an infant and there are resulting complications. Given the definition of malpractice above, is it unreasonable for nurses to expect to be named in malpractice suits involving poor teaching (no assessment, improper strategies, no evaluation), lack of teaching, or lack of documentation of teaching and its measurable outcomes? The lack of using the teaching process to guide teaching and a lack of sufficient knowledge and skills to teach and promote learning *can* result in a patient's decreased health status.

In recent years, nurses have been increasingly named as defendants in malpractice cases. This increase may be accounted for in part by the growing recognition of nursing as a profession and the expanded role of the nurse (Fiesta, 1983). Nurses must therefore be aware of their responsibilities in the area of health teaching. Even the most conscientious nurse can be sued. To weather such a suit, the nurse needs to have used prudent nursing judgment, documented so that a jury can easily establish the quality of her health teaching and objective patient outcomes, and have adequate malpractice insurance to cover lawyer and court costs, lost wages during the trial, and perhaps a settlement.

DOCUMENTATION OF HEALTH TEACHING

Documentation of health teaching serves several very important functions. Charting serves as an important communication medium among an ever growing number of health professionals involved in patient care. Charting helps to communicate plans, treatments, procedures, results of health care actions, and patients' responses. It is a permanent record of the patient's voyage through the health-care system and his or her experiences and responses. The chart and its documentation also serves as a key piece of evidence in a malpractice or negligence suit. Proper documentation can be an essential part of a nurse's defense in a court of law. Descriptive and objective documentation can also be a great asset because cases may take months or years before they are settled. Memories may become vague and witnesses may be difficult to locate, but a well-written description of teaching and the patient's response does not change.

Documentation of health teaching is often the exception rather than the rule. For example, Porter found that nurses only documented patient teaching 15 percent of the time and Boyd (unpublished data) found that nurses' documentation of teaching was sporadic and sparse at best. Nurses give several reasons for not documenting health teaching, perhaps, the most common reason is lack of time, including patient workload, type of patient, and length of hospital stay. Others include not knowing how, no rewards or reprimands, and no administrative mandates. Researchers have found that there are some factors that increase documentation of health teaching. These factors include making health teaching an explicit part of job descriptions; merit raise and promotion criteria; part of quality assurance audits; administrative emphasis on documentation; the use of checklists, flow sheets, and teaching plans; and staff development emphasis (Porter, 1990; Boyd, unpublished; ASHET, 1985). Porter found that by implementing the use of a teaching plan and administrative emphasis documentation improved 75 percent! Boyd (unpublished) found that, by providing staff inservice on legal implications of documentation and techniques of effective documentation of health teaching in conjunction with an administrative emphasis on health teaching, documentation steadily increased over a 1-year period.

It is imperative that nurses keep in mind that from a legal perspective *if it is not documented, it did not happen* (Creighton, 1987). So much of nurses' teaching is incidental and is given at the "teachable moment"; therefore, nurses may not document this spontaneous teaching as they would something more formal. Sound documentation of health teaching should adhere to guidelines for other charting, including that it be:

1. Accurate and concise. Detail enough of the teaching content so that there is no ambiguity about what you taught. If the content is a standard within the profession (how to self-inject insulin, for example) or generally accepted information (signs and symptoms of hypo- or hyperglycemia, how the heart works, or the effect digoxin has on the heart), you do not need to write it out word for word.

2. Objective. Use descriptive words that convey a detailed picture/account of what occurred and the patient's response. Cliche terms like "doing well," "appears to be," "seems to be," "understands," "no problems" will not stand up in court (Creighton, 1987). It is essential that you communicate actions—"self-injected insulin as taught with 100 percent accuracy," "gave appropriate responses to what she would do if home alone and began to experience angina," "80 percent correct responses to questions on test, Life Saving Tips for Diabetics" (in chart).

3. Charted promptly. Time dulls recall—of the nurse! Make every effort to chart as soon as possible after teaching. Never wait for more than a few hours after your shift to chart. What you taught or did not teach can affect the patient's response to treatments, procedures, medications, and how other health professionals approach the patient.

4. Charted legibly and use only standard abbreviations. Again, how well your charting communicates to a jury can affect its decision (Creighton, 1987). Likewise, it is extremely frustrating and time consuming for other health professionals to try to decipher your teaching documentation.

5. A part of the permanent record. Health-teaching checklist, teaching plans, and flow sheets as well as progress notes and anecdotal notes must remain a part of the permanent chart. They cannot serve just as a communication medium between staff members. Their legal significance will not permit them to be throw-away items.

INFORMED CONSENT

Perhaps the biggest legal issue in health education at this time is that of informed consent. No other single issue of patient care has received as much publicity and legal action. The nurse's role in informed consent is an area of confusion for many practitioners.

Justice Benjamin N. Cardozo in 1914 established the legal basis for informed consent. He noted that every human being of adult years and sound mind has a right to determine what shall be done with his or her own body. (Schloendorff v. Society of New York Hospitals, 1914). Individual autonomy was not a new concept, even in 1914. The freedom of an individual to make decisions about one's own body is a fundamental right in American common law. This right is carried over into health-care settings and has been protected and encouraged by ethical and professional codes of practice, legislation, and policies of governing and accreditating agencies.

In discussing informed consent, bear in mind that any procedure performed on a person without a formal, voluntarily signed consent constitutes battery (O'Connor, 1981; Creighton, 1986). Informed consent serves several functions: to promote patient autonomy and decision making; to meet legal directives; and to protect physicians from litigation. There are two basic standards in the United States for informed consent. First, patients have the right to receive that amount of information or disclosure which is customarily given by their local medical community. This standard is the norm in most states (O'Connor, 1981; Creighton, 1986). The second, a more liberal approach, is that patients have the right to receive information that an average, reasonable patient would consider to be necessary to make informed decisions (O'Connor, 1981; Rothman & Rothman, 1981; Stewart & Ufford, 1981; Creighton, 1986).

The nurse's obligation in informed consent is often hazy to many practitioners. It is not a nurse's responsibility or function to obtain a signed consent form, nor should a nurse be responsible for explaining a medical procedure or any concomitant risks. Explaining medical procedures and obtaining a signed consent is the physician's responsibility. Informed consent consists of two distinct components: the disclosure and the consent. From a legal perspective, the nurse's role in informed consent should be minimal. The nurse cannot act in the physician's behalf and provide disclosure. Disclosure is a right and a responsibility of the physician. If the nurse becomes involved in disclosure, she may be interfering with the physician–patient relationship (Creighton, 1986). Purists may even see nurses' involvement in disclosure as practicing medicine. Consent involves witnessing a signature. Nurses are often asked to witness the consent form, in which case they verify that the patient was mentally competent and also signed the form voluntarily without any form of coercion. By witnessing the consent, the nurse is not endorsing the quality or scope of the medical explanations.

Nurses are responsible for informing the physician of a patient's potential limitations for giving informed consent, such as being illiterate or needing glasses or a hearing aid. A nurse is responsible for informing the attending physician immediately if a patient changes his mind or wants to withdraw from a procedure or treatment once it has begun (Rankin & Duffy, 1983; Rothman & Rothman, 1981).

To date, informed consent has been confined to medical procedures. If and when it becomes necessary for patients to give informed consent to nursing procedures, the nurse will then carry the responsibility of adequately informing the patient. Even without the legal boundaries set by a signed consent form, nurses need to inform patients of routine procedures, how their bodies function or dysfunction and what medications or treatments are being used and what effect they will have

All of these activities are within the realm of health education and support the patient's right to know.

Health education as an independent nursing function may not always be readily accepted by other health-care professionals. Should conflicts arise, the use of diplomacy and proper administrative channels may help to defuse any conflict. At other times, nurses may need to decide whether to jeopardize their positions or careers to meet the educational needs of a patient. In regard to patient education, "her primary responsibility is to the patient and her profession and . . . she is secondarily responsible to the physician and the institution. . . . " (Rankin & Duffy, 1983, p. 101).

SUMMARY

A growing emphasis on health education has been evident over the past 30 years. This emphasis has been found within the nursing profession as well as within other health-care disciplines.

It seems that our nation has become more health conscious. State and federal legislation has promoted health education through the initiation of the National Center for Health Education, the Centers for Disease Control, and Medicare and Medicaid programs. Health professional groups have passed supportive statements about health education, and consumer groups have become active in promoting consumers' rights in health care.

The nurse's involvement in health education is an outgrowth of moral and ethical values as well as the result of professional mandates. Such mandates include the Nurse Practice Acts, which define the legal parameters of nursing practice. Some state nurse practice acts have more explicit expectations for nurses' involvement in health education than others.

Nurse practice acts require nurses to teach individuals about health matters. It follows that nurses are legally responsible for their actions as health teachers. Nurses must also be aware of their responsibilities in the area of informed consent for medical procedures.

REFERENCES AND READINGS

American Hospital Association. Statement on patient education. *Health Education.* Chicago: American Hospital Association, July/August 1972, 32, 22.

American Hospital Association. *Statement on a patient's bill of rights.* Chicago: American Hospital Association, 1973.

American Hospital Association. *Statement on health education: Role and responsibility of health care institutions.* Chicago: American Hospital Association, 1975.

American Hospital Association. *The hospital inpatient education survey.* Chicago: American Hospital Association, 1977.

American Hospital Association. *Patient health education association meeting summary.* Chicago: American Hospital Association, 1980.

American Hospital Association. *Policy and statement on the hospital's responsibility for patient education services.* Chicago: American Hospital Association, 1981.

American Nurses' Association. *Model nurse practice act.* Kansas City: American Nurses' Association, 1976.

American Nurses' Association, ANA Nursing Standards, Kansas City, MO, summer, 1986.

American Society for Health, Education, and Training, Center for Health Promotion. Patient education conversation by mail, 1985.

Annas, G. J. *The rights of hospitalized patients.* New York: Discussion 1975.

Askey, D. (Ed.). *Encyclopedia of associations* (16th ed.) (Vol. 1). Detroit: Gale Research, 1982.

Barnett v. Hawk Pharmacy, Inc. 220 Kan. 318, 552 P2d1002, 1976.

Blue Cross Association. *White paper: Patient education, health care services.* Blue Cross Association, August 1974.

Bordley, J., & Harvey, A. M. *Two centuries of American medicine.* Philadelphia: Saunders, 1976.

Boyd, M. D. Public health nurses response to staff development intervention to improve patient teaching. Unpublished research, 1991.

College of Nursing, University of South Carolina, Columbia, SC, 1991.

Creighton, H. Informed consent. *Nursing Management,* 1986, *17*(10), 11–13.

Creighton, H. Legal significance of charting—Part 1. *Nursing Management,* 1987, *18*(9), 17, 20, 22.

Creighton, H. Legal significance of Charting—Part 2. *Nursing Management,* 1987, *18*(10), 14–15.

Creighton, H. Legal implications of policy and procedure manual—Part 1. *Nursing Management,* 1987, *18*(4), 22–24, 28.

Creighton, H. Legal problems of home care nurses. *Nursing Management,* 1988, *19*(11), 23–26.

Creighton, H. Legal implications of policy and procedure manuals—Part 2. *Nursing Management,* 1987, *18*(5), 16, 18.

Creighton, H. *Law every nurse should know* (4th ed.). Philadelphia: Saunders, 1981.

Creighton, H. Patient teaching. *Nursing Management,* 1985, *16*(1), 12, 16, 18.

Fiesta, J. *The law & liability: A guide for nurses.* New York: Wiley, 1983.

Green, L., Krueter, M. W., Deeds, S., & Partridge, K. *Health education planning: A diagnostic approach.* Palo Alto, Calif.: Mayfield, 1980.

JCAH Accreditation Manual for Hospitals. JCAH, Chicago, IL, 1986.

Porter, Y. Brief: Evaluation of nurses' documentation of patient teaching. *The Journal of Continuing Education in Nursing,* 1990, *21*(3), 134–137.

Redman, B. L., & Bartlett, E. E. The International Patient Education Council: A step forward for patient education research and practice. *Patient Education and Counseling,* 1989, *13*, 1–2.

3

Teaching in Selected Settings

Barbara A. Graham
Carol J. Gleit

More nurses are employed in different practice settings than ever before. In whatever setting or population served, health teaching is an essential component of nursing practice. The expanding scope of practice and a changing health-care environment have strengthened nursing's role and responsibility for health teaching. A major change, is the way hospitals are reimbursed for services that has led to a decline in hospital lengths of stay. The dramatic growth in the home health-care industry in the past ten (10) years attests to the need of many patients and families for follow-up teaching and therapies in the home.

While chronic diseases and conditions continue to be the leading causes of morbidity and mortality, the HIV-AIDS epidemic is a serious threat to the health of large segments of the population (Leviton, et al., 1990). The World Health Organization (WHO) recently projected continued expansion of the AIDS epidemic worldwide. WHO estimates that there are 1.3 million cases of AIDS worldwide now, and projects that by the turn of the century there will be up to 30 million people infected: 15 to 20 million adults and 10 million infants and children. If infection rates speed up, these projections will have to be revised upward (Nation's Health, 1991). Many of the health concerns facing society today might be prevented or ameliorated were there more concerted efforts in health education. As key providers of health/patient education, nurses must take the lead in preventive and control measures.

Nursing practice encompasses a broad spectrum of service settings that include public health, hospitals, homes, physicians' offices, schools, industries, clinics, extended care facilities, adult homes, penal institutions, the military, etc.

This chapter addresses the teaching role in community and inpatient settings. Equal emphasis is placed on each. The first section begins with a discussion of school health, occupational health, and home health. The next section presents patient teaching and discharge planning teaching.

SCHOOL HEALTH

Historically, school systems in this country have played a major role in health education efforts but it was not until 1850 when tax-supported public schools came into existence that health education began as an organized national effort (Creswell & Newman, 1989).

In large cities, physicians were hired to inspect school children with contagious diseases. As public school attendance grew, diseases spread quickly among children, often out of control. By 1902, many children with contagious diseases were absent from school. Lillian Wald, a nurse from the Henry Street Settlement, persuaded the New York City Board of Health to allow one of her nurses to be sent to four schools to demonstrate through home visits that teaching proper hygiene and other measures might prevent the spread of disease. The demonstration was so successful that subsequently the Board of Health employed 12 more nurses for the New York City Schools. What followed was a dramatic decline in school absenteeism (Buhler-Wilkerson, 1988). Visiting nurses also helped to control communicable diseases through preventive programs to halt the spread of tuberculosis in infants, mothers, and school children. It is clear even from these early efforts that nurses considered health education and prevention to be priorities within their practice.

Today, public school systems continue to be a major purveyor of health education. Schools are mandated to provide health education beginning in the primary grades and continuing through high school. There is, however, much variation in what is taught and who teaches it. Many schools have access to a school nurse, others do not. The employers of school nurses may be either boards of education or there may be a contractual agreement between schools and public health departments to provide nursing services. It is not unusual for school nurses to provide services to more than one school population.

HEALTH EDUCATION

Certain areas of health education continue to be controversial. State Boards of Education and local school boards have varying degrees of control over subject matter in health education. Parental views of what should be taught may be in conflict with those of teachers and school officials. For example, family life education including sex education continues to be controversial in some areas. In certain school districts, parents have organized to develop their own version of family life education and offer it as an alternative to that taught in public schools. As active participants in health education efforts, school nurses must be fully apprised of school policies and regulations within their school district and state.

School nurses may teach formal classes in health education, and/or serve as a resource to teachers who are responsible for the health curriculum. School nurses are advisors and consultants to the schools curriculum committee regarding health education subject matter. Nurses access health education materials and they assist in identifying experts in the health field who can contribute to the school health program. A basic health education curriculum includes:

nutrition	safety and accident prevention
personal health	growth and development
consumer health	prevention and control of disease
environmental health	substance use and abuse

(Creswell & Newman, 1989)

Schools also educate students in the prevention of diseases and conditions to which they are most vulnerable. The severity of the current HIV-AIDS epidemic and its future consequences requires preventive education. The United States Surgeon General and others have advocated that HIV-AIDS education be implemented for all students at each grade level so that children will grow up knowing how to protect themselves from this disease. In 1988, the Centers for Disease Control (CDC) established a Division of Adolescent and School Health within the Center for Chronic Disease Prevention and Health Promotion to assist in this effort (Seffin, 1990). The CDC receives government support to assist schools nationwide to implement effective HIV education. A major factor to consider in HIV-AIDS education is that the epidemic has generated a great deal of fear and misinformation. There has also been discrimination against school children with HIV. In several states, amidst much media attention, children with HIV have been excluded from school. Despite public education efforts, misconceptions about the disease have been difficult to overcome. School nurses play a vital role in meeting the challenge of this epidemic from both a health education and policy perspective. AIDS, a severe, life-threatening clinical condition, was first recognized as a syndrome in 1981. This syndrome is the late clinical stage of infection with the human immunodeficiency virus (HIV). It most often results in progressive damage to the immune and other organ systems, especially the central nervous system (Benenson, 1990). Appropriate terminology must be used in HIV-AIDS education. The President's Commission on the Human Immunodeficiency Virus Epidemic stated that the term AIDS is obsolete and that HIV Infection more correctly defines the problem. It recommended that public health officials, the health-care community and others focus on the full course of HIV infection rather than concentrating on later stages of the disease (Kerr, 1990).

As a result of the HIV-AIDS epidemic, school health programs, as well as policies and procedures, are receiving more attention. Schools are being required to develop and implement HIV-AIDS education, and to establish procedures to assure confidentiality (Brainerd, 1989). Schools must also update policies on communicable disease control and develop protocols for handling body fluids in HIV cases. These events have fueled more aggressive efforts to promote sexuality education in school curricula (Johnson, 1991). A recent survey of 26 public school districts in this country showed that only 33 percent of sexually active respondents reported always using condoms. The remaining respondents reported sporadic use or no use at all. Obviously, unprotected sexual behavior puts teens at an increased risk for HIV infection (Jones, Ellis, et al., 1991). Nurses must be sure this issue is addressed in school curricula on HIV prevention.

In Kansas, school nurses and health teachers worked together to develop an HIV-AIDS curriculum. A Task Force was formed to review publications and videotapes to determine the most appropriate education for elementary school children. School nurses expanded the existing growth and development curriculum for sixth grade students to include HIV-AIDS education. In describing the efforts of the Task Force, Nauman (1989), emphasized the value of school nurses working closely with health teachers and others to integrate HIV-AIDS in the school curriculum.

As schools look for effective methods for teaching HIV-AIDS education, Walsh, et al. (1990), suggest such efforts be developmentally based beginning in the elementary school years. A developmental framework could be structured around ways children of different ages understand the definition of cause, treatment, and consequences of AIDS. They suggest that young children cannot conceptualize body organs therefore it makes little sense to teach them causes of the disease or preventive behavior. In young children, fear of disease is the greatest concern and can be dealt with best by reassurances from authority figures. For example, "Teachers, mothers, fathers, physicians, nurses, and other adults are assumed to be 'all-wise bearers of the truth'" (Ibid). Older children, however, must be given specific information about preventive measures. AIDS information should be factual and presented in a way that is readily understandable. Older children can comprehend that the disease is to be avoided and develop a "healthy fear" of its consequences.

A wide range of HIV-AIDS education materials are available. Two examples are: (1) Guidelines for Effective School Health Education, developed by the Centers for Disease Control of the United States Public Health Service, and (2) AIDS Education: Curriculum and Health Policy, prepared by Yarber (1987), Indiana University.

It is important that school health programs include education to prevent premature development of chronic conditions such as cardiovascular diseases. Since these are the so-called man-made diseases, health education should emphasize primary prevention in the form of health promotion in nutrition, exercise, and stress management. The development of social skills to enable students to resist peer pressure and learning effective decision making must also be encouraged. The challenge to school nurses, teachers and others, is to provide the best possible foundation on which children can build their health knowledge and practices (Creswell & Newman, 1989).

To promote nutritional health, the *Citizens' Commission on School Nutrition* developed a program for improving school lunches. Because it is difficult to change children's food preferences, the Commission recommended making changes in two stages, the first to be accomplished by 1995 and the second by the year 2000. The Commission recommended that school lunch nutrition standards be consistent with current dietary standards. Other recommendations are as follows:

	Stage 1	**Stage 2**
FAT:	Reduce total fat to 35 percent of calories, with no more than a third from saturated fat.	Reduce fat to 30 percent of calories.
FIBER:	Increase consumption of high-fiber foods, providing at least eight (8) servings a month.	Fifteen high-fiber servings a month. Half of all bread and grain servings should be 100 percent whole grains.
SODIUM:	Average sodium content of lunch, 1000 milligrams.	Average sodium content, 800 milligrams.
NON-NUTRITIOUS FOODS:	Ban sale of non-nutritious foods at school.	
CHOLESTEROL:	Reduce average cholesterol content of meals to 100 milligrams or less.	
SUGAR:	No more than 20 percent sugar by weight in school breakfast cereals.	Avoid sugary, high-fat desserts.
ADDITIVES:	Eliminate or reduce acesulfame-K, asparatame, BHA, BHT, caffeine, monosodium glutamate, saccharin, sodium nitrite, sulfite, yellow dye No. 5.	
MILK:	Standard beverage should be milk with two (2) percent fat; whole milk should not be required.	Standard beverage should be milk with one (1) percent fat or less.
MONEY:	Increase funds for lunches. Increase financing for Nutrition Education and Training program to $25 million by 1993.	Financing beyond 1994 should be tied to inflation.

Obviously, today's school nurses are faced with many challenges. Children with chronic diseases and conditions have been mainstreamed into public schools. They have special needs for advocacy and health monitoring. Teenage pregnancy rates are rising and many school children are sexually abused.

School budgets around the country have been reduced and in some instances school nurses have been replaced with health clerks and school health assistants (Whited & Starke, 1989). Oda (1991) has described school nursing as the "invisible nursing practice" and suggests that to change this perception nurses must be more educationally prepared, influence health policy, and conduct research that shows the outcome of nursing interventions. Nurses must work toward a more positive image of the profession, one that is indispensable to the health of school children.

OCCUPATIONAL HEALTH

In 1888, the first industrial nurse was hired by a group of Pennsylvania coal miners. Betty Moulder's work required that she visit coal miners' homes and care for those who were ailing (Pinkham, 1988). But the nurse who is generally considered the matriarch of industrial nursing was Ada Mayo Stewart who began working for the Vermont Marble Company in 1895. When making home visits her duties ranged from teaching good health habits to bathing infants. She also dressed wounds, dealt with emergencies, and assisted doctors. The number of industries employing nurses grew from 60 in 1914 to 871 by 1918. There were two factors responsible for the dramatic growth during this period. The first was World War I during which the federal government required health services for defense contract workers (Ibid). The second factor was the high rates of tuberculosis among workers. Mary Louise Brown, a Certified Occupational Health Nurse, author of two books on occupational health nursing and considered to be an authority in the field, was quoted as saying that "tuberculosis was almost as serious as we think AIDS is today" (Ibid). In 1977, the American Association of Industrial Nurses (AAIN) changed its name to the more comprehensive American Association of Occupational Health Nursing (AAOHN). It is estimated that 20,000 to 30,000 nurses are employed in the field, 11,000 of whom are members of AAOHN (Ibid).

Occupational health nurses comprise the largest health specialty group employed in industry. Because an occupational health nurse has contact with virtually all employees at one time or another, there are many opportunities to initiate health teaching and other health promotion activities. With the exception of school children, no other population is more accessible nor has more potential for making health gains than the millions of working adults in this country. Even if the employee–nurse ratio is quite high, which is usually the case, nurses can contribute greatly to an employee health promotion program.

Nurses employed in occupational health must work closely with both management and production personnel. In some instances, management's perceptions of the nurse's role may be quite narrow. Management may view care of the ill or injured worker, or responsibility for workmen's compensation to be the nurse's major contribution to the industrial scene. Management may not be aware of the benefits derived from an employee health promotion program. One way to help "sell" this idea is to design an exercise or nutrition program for management personnel. Keeping current with advances in occupational health and sharing information about innovative health programs are other ways to obtain management support. In contract negotiations with organized unions, nurses may act as employee advocates by seeking to obtain health promotion benefits.

Health Education/Health Promotion

There is much concern in the industrial world over escalating health-care costs that have increased at a greater rate than all other consumable goods and services. American businesses are absorbing the direct costs of insurance premiums as well as the indirect costs of absenteeism and retraining. Corporations and insurance companies are placing greater emphasis on controllable risk factors among their personnel. The extent of body weight, exercise level, smoking, alcohol intake, seat belt use, etc. determines a given company's risk level and the cost of insurance premiums (Chenoweth, March 1988). Many companies are recognizing that their employees are their greatest resource and have adopted worksite health promotion programs. It has been predicted that in the 1990s, worksite health promotion programs will be a standard tool for maximizing employee productivity. Such a program would:

1. be accountable for results;
2. facilitate development of a health-promoting work environment;
3. obtain high rates of participation including high-risk employees;
4. effectively reach employees and retirees wherever they work and live;
5. incorporate the best current scientific information and behavior change techniques.

(Chen, Jr., 1989)

The current fiscal climate offers many opportunities to promote employee health. The national initiative for the Year 2000, Objectives for the Nation include at least 30 statements related to worksite health. Excerpts of the objectives are as follows:

- Objective 2.13: Increase the proportion of worksites offering employer-sponsored fitness programs . . . (according to the size of the employee work force). . . .
- Objective 3.1: Reduce cigarette smoking . . . among blue collar employees: 22 percent.
- Objective 4.17: Extend adoption of alcohol- and drug-free work environment policies to at least 40 percent of worksites. . . .
- Objective 9.18: Increase to at least 70 percent the proportion of worksites . . . that have implemented occupational health programs for disease prevention and health promotion.
- Objective 9.25: Increase . . . the proportion of worksites . . . that provide programs to reduce employee stress.
- Objective 15.22: Increase . . . the proportion of worksites . . . that offer activities in high blood pressure education and control.
- Objective 15.23: Increase . . . the proportion of worksites . . . that offer activities in cholesterol education and control to their employees.
- Objective 20.15: Increase . . . the proportion of workplaces . . . that offer a health promotion program in which 20 percent or more of the employees participate regularly. . . .

- Objective 20.16: Increase . . . the proportion of hourly workers who participate regularly in health promotion activities in the workplace.

Commentaries to most of these objectives are printed in the draft copy of Promoting Health/Preventive Disease: Year 2000 Objectives for the Nation (1989). Occupational nurses focusing on worksite health promotion have never had such a large and visible national agenda for action.

The first step in planning a health promotion program is to assess the needs and interests of the employee population. Topics such as weight reduction, physical fitness, stress management, smoking cessation, and retirement planning are often noted as areas of concern. Based on the assessment, a series of health education presentations could be implemented.

Another approach to employee health assessment is the use of a risk factor or health appraisal questionnaire. The health appraisal forms could be displayed with other health literature where it is readily accessible. Once the employee has completed the appraisal questionnaire, it is important for the nurse to discuss areas of concern and approaches to risk reduction.

The nurse's clinic provides an avenue for disseminating health information. There is an abundance of printed health information available, often free of charge. These publications should be readily accessible. Health information materials could be selected according to age, sex, and risk factors in the employee population. These materials can stimulate questions and follow-up teaching by the nurse.

The impact of the HIV-AIDS epidemic is being felt across all segments of society. The workplace is no exception. A survey of 67 corporations in 1987 revealed that 66 of the 67 corporations had at least one employee with AIDS. The number of cases and background of the infected employees tended to reflect the experience of the surrounding community. The largest number of cases, 56, were reported among 68,000 employees of one corporation, many of whom resided on the West Coast (Schneider, 1989). The work setting provides an opportune setting for (HIV-AIDS) education. In order to reach all employees, educational activities must be offered several times during the day and evening. Small group discussions are useful in allaying fear of the disease and correcting misinformation. Educational sessions provide accurate up-to-date information about the disease, and are tailored to the needs of the specific work setting. Information regarding community resources and availability of HIV testing must be included. Confidentiality of all medical/health records must be assured.

Several corporations have established formal and informal health and education policies for employees with HIV-AIDS and their coworkers. These include Bank of America, AT&T, C&P, etc. The U.S. Office of Personnel Management has drafted a formal written policy that addresses AIDS in the workplace. Copies of the new policy can be obtained by calling or writing the Office of Employee and Labor Relations, U.S. Office of Personnel Management, 1900 E Street NW, Room 7635, Washington, DC 20415; (202) 653–8551 (Friddle et al., 1988). The Centers for Disease Control have also drafted HIV-AIDS recommendations.

Occupational health nurses use their knowledge of community resources and organizations to provide speakers and other services to the employee population. Local health departments and other agencies may assist in large-scale screening of employees for hypertension and cholesterol levels. There may be schools of nursing in the area that wish to have students gain health teaching experience with an adult population. The use of undergraduate and graduate nursing students as health teachers is an excellent way to contribute to nursing education programs, provide valuable learning experiences for students, and at the same time benefit employees.

In addition to health education, nurses in occupational settings have a captive audience for the dissemination of health information. Colorful, eye-catching bulletin boards can be set up in well-traveled areas such as the cafeteria or main corridors. Information about a particular health topic could be featured on a monthly or biweekly basis. A suggestion box for future health topics could also be provided. Another method of disseminating health information is through an employee newsletter. Health tips and information about seasonal health hazards as well as preventive health activities would provide the basis for a regular publication about health. Again, suggestions for topics could be solicited.

Nurses in occupational settings must evaluate their health programs and publish the results. There is a great need for research to support nursing's contribution to employee health. Occupational health nurses have a unique advantage in that they have a well, relatively stable population to work with over time. What better opportunity to study the effects of employee health programs?

The current cost-conscious climate in the business world has been building for some years. It presents the estimated 20,000 to 30,000 occupational health nurses in this country with rich opportunities to take the lead in establishing and managing worksite health promotion programs. At the least, occupational health nurses must play a key role in their company's wellness program. In a number of publications describing worksite programs, however, the author found no mention of nursing involvement. Are nurses' contributions not being recognized? Occupational nurses promote the health of employees on a daily basis and have been for years. Nurses must share these experiences with others in publications and at conferences. Clearly, worksite health promotion requires the expertise of a number of health disciplines, but the core of such programs is employee health, the basis for occupational health nursing.

HOME HEALTH CARE

The recent growth in home health care has given greater visibility to nurses who provide these services; and has called attention to home health as a specialty area within nursing practice (Graham, 1989). With the aging population and the probability of an increasing number of individuals with functional deficits, the need for home care services will continue to increase. In 1989, there were 8105 home health agencies operating nationwide; this was a 12 percent increase over 1988, and 53 percent more than were in business at the end of 1986. These data were reported from a national survey that also showed that the majority of patients are referred for home health care from acute care hospitals (Marion Laboratories, 1989). Advances in technology and changes in reimbursement mechanisms have fueled the growth in home health care. Nurses are providing high-tech care to home-bound clients and teaching them and their families how to perform procedures that heretofore were considered in the professional's domain. Clients and families are often required to modify their diet and food preparation as well as manage their medication regimens and other therapies. Nurses must understand regulations that govern reimbursement for home care services. Medicare accounted for 56 percent of home health agency revenues in 1988, followed by Medicaid at 13.5 percent and private insurance at 9.6 percent (Marion Laboratories, 1989). Under Medicare, a skilled nursing service is defined as a service that requires the skills of a registered nurse or a licensed practical nurse under the supervision of a registered nurse. The service must be reasonable and necessary to the treatment of the beneficiary's illness or injury. Nurses must understand what teaching/training activities constitute a skilled care service and therefore reimbursable under Medicare. Teaching and training that require the skills of a licensed nurse include, but *are not limited to,* the following:

1. Teaching the self-administration of injectable medications, or a complex range of medications;
2. Teaching a newly diagnosed diabetic or caregiver all aspects of diabetes management, including how to prepare and to administer insulin injections, to prepare and follow a diabetic diet, to observe foot-care precautions, and to observe for and understand signs of hyperglycemia and hypoglycemia;
3. Teaching self-administration of medical gases;
4. Teaching wound care where the complexity of the wound, the overall condition of the beneficiary, or the ability of the caregiver makes teaching necessary;
5. Teaching care for a recent ostomy or where reinforcement of ostomy care is needed;
6. Teaching self-catheterization;
7. Teaching self-administration of gastrostomy or enteral feedings;
8. Teaching care for and maintenance of peripheral and central venous lines and administration of intravenous medications through such lines;
9. Teaching bowel or bladder training when bowl or bladder dysfunction exists;
10. Teaching how to perform the activities of daily living when the beneficiary or caregiver must use special techniques and adaptive devices due to a loss of function;
11. Teaching transfer techniques, e.g., from bed to chair, which are needed for safe transfer.
12. Teaching proper body alignment and positioning, and timing techniques of a bed-bound beneficiary;
13. Teaching ambulation with prescribed assistive devices (such as crutches, walker, cane, etc.) that are needed due to a recent functional loss;

14. Teaching prosthesis care and gait training;
15. Teaching the use and care of braces, splints, and orthotics and associated skin care;
16. Teaching the proper care and application of any specialized dressings or skin treatments (for example, dressings or treatments needed by beneficiaries with severe or widespread fungal infections, active and severe psoriasis or eczema, or due to skin deterioration from radiation treatments);
17. Teaching the preparation and maintenance of a therapeutic diet; and
18. Teaching proper administration of oral medication, including signs of side effects and avoidance of interaction with other medications and food.

(United States Department of Health and Human Services, 1989).

Clients referred for home care may already know how to manage certain aspects of their care. However, due to shorter hospital stays, higher acuity levels, and other factors, they still must learn how to adapt to the home environment. Individuals in need of home health services have not necessarily been hospitalized, prior to referral for home care. Often the main objective of home care is client/family education. It is not unusual for the home health nurse to have little or no information about a client's learning needs when making the first home contact. Even if a client/family have been taught aspects of self-care it is the client/family who will ultimately assume care responsibilities. An assessment of learning needs at an early stage of care is essential to ensure quality care and cost-effectiveness (Keating & Kelman, 1988).

The home health nurse identifies the main caregivers and involves them in all phases of the teaching plan. (Johnson & Jackson, 1989). While teaching in home care usually revolves around the prescribed plan of care, the home care nurse first identifies the nursing diagnoses related to the referral, the medical diagnosis, and/or health problem(s). The nurse, together with the client/family, decide on the nursing diagnoses in order of priority (Keating & Kelman, 1988). Educational needs of the home care client must be determined in relation to the three domains of learning. A client may need to learn a diabetic medication regimen (cognitive domain), a skill to self-inject insulin (psychomotor domain), and to understand the need to learn management of the diabetic condition (affective domain). In addition to learning self-care measures, clients also need to be informed about available resources both financial and personal (DeMuth, 1989). Nurses must keep abreast of available community resources, know how to access them and be advocates when the health care system is not responsive to client needs.

Judicious use of time is a significant factor in home health care because reimbursement mechanisms are usually based on number of visits within a specified time. Third-party reimbursers may minimize the importance of client education. A strategy for nurses is to educate policymakers of third-party payors as to the value of client and family teaching (Shannon, 1989). Medicare reimbursement requires full documentation of teaching activities and the client's response to these efforts. Client/family education is the foundation for home care services. Administrative personnel of home care agencies must understand and value the importance of client teaching as well. This could be demonstrated by providing in-service education offerings and including client/family teaching criteria in evaluating staff performance.

THE TEACHING ROLE IN A SHELTERED WORKSHOP

Another group that can benefit from health teaching is the mentally retarded. Many communities have sheltered workshops where these individuals are employed to perform a particular task and are paid for their work. For example, local industries may opt to pay workshop employees to do certain repetitive production tasks. The benefits are twofold. The employees learn how to perform a skill and are paid for their work, both of which promote a positive self-concept and independence. The industry benefits by having repetitive production tasks done well and by contributing to community productivity. Some of these handicapped adults may have poor personal hygiene, may be overweight, and have poor dietary habits. They may also lead very sedentary lives. Such a group is in great need of health teaching. Nurses who provide health teaching to these groups often find that workshop administrators recognize the need for improved health practices and are agreeable to teaching activities being held during the workday. Teaching these adults requires patience and much reinforcement. The teaching may include how to prepare nutritious low-cost meals or how to shop for food. Improving personal hygiene practices means that these individuals may be more readily accepted by others. Personal activities such as bathing, shampooing hair, and brushing teeth must be reinforced. Teaching a health promotion activity such as physical exercise offers the handicapped a sense of accomplishment and improved fitness as well. Nurses who teach these groups can also support local Special Olympic Games for the handicapped and encourage these clients to enter the contests. Win or lose, the boost to their confidence and morale is obvious.

HOSPITALIZED PATIENTS AND TEACHING

Within the last several years, there has become more of a blur between hospital and home teaching as to what content is taught where. The advent of DRGs has drastically shortened hospital stays, and thus new ways of delivering teaching have developed involving cross-overs of hospitals and homecare referrals of health teaching. Some clients are being directly discharged from intensive care units (Bauknecht, 1985). This means that some of the teaching that was formerly done in hospitals is now taking place in the community. Hospitals are taking on what once was a community-based prerogative in that offering health teaching in the community in the areas of risk appraisal and risk reduction has become more popular.

Organizing Teaching Services

There are different ways in which teaching efforts in hospitals can be organized. One is called unit-based. In some instances, nurses and other health professionals assigned to surgical or cardiac units provide the teaching. In this case the teaching is performed by the nurse as part of the nursing care given. In other situations, there may be specialists such as ostomate nurses on a cancer surgery unit, who would teach all patients on the unit who have had ostomy surgery. In this situation, the particular unit is the central place for the teaching. Another way of organizing hospital patient teaching is a hospital-wide system operating out of a patient education department. In this situation, there may be nurses or other professionals whose major assignment is to carry out the patient teaching throughout the hospital, going onto various units to provide the teaching. There may also be closed circuit television at each patient's bedside for viewing sessions such as preoperative teaching. For hospitals having patient education departments, there may be one or more nurses that do not themselves provide the patient teaching, but rather work with nurses on the hospital units in the content and process of teaching, so that the nurse engages in teaching those patients assigned to her care with the assistance of the patient education department.

Whether patient teaching is organized on a unit-based or hospital-wide system, there may be other health professionals involved. Physical and occupational therapists and dietitians also teach, so an interdisciplinary approach may be used. For example, on a rehabilitation unit, often a multidisciplinary team meets to plan for teaching and other care activities. Physicians, according to medical practice acts, have the ultimate responsibility for deciding which individuals need teaching and what content is necessary. Nurses who are delegated teaching responsibilities in this way would be operating in a dependent role. In this dependent role, the extent and content of what is taught would vary from specific detailed instructions to a broad approach of "teach patient diabetic care." The latter would offer the nurse flexibility, and in some cases would involve collaboration with others. Interdependent functioning occurs when there is collaboration among health professionals in the decision making for the assessment, planning, intervention, and evaluation of teaching. Within the hospital setting, nurses also can engage in independent functioning, whereby the nurse initiates the teaching and carries it through to the evaluation phase. There can be role blurring involved, to the extent that if many professionals teach, overlapping or gaps can occur. There also has been a long-standing dispute among physicians and nurses, dietitians, physical therapists, as to where the basis for decision making should occur.

More recently some hospitals, both community hospitals and large teaching hospitals, have begun to offer health teaching programs to residents in the community. These may be nutrition awareness sessions, physical fitness, and stress management sessions. They may be offered on a continual basis or more sporadically. Jogging clubs for postmyocardial infarction victims are an example.

We are beginning to see alternative sites for patient teaching. Shortened lengths of hospital stays or no presurgical admission have opened outpatient surgical units for prehospital teaching, informed consent signing, and preparation for discharge. At the University of Virginia Medical Center, an increasing amount of presurgical teaching and physical assessment are done at the outpatient level by nurses, and the department is doubling in size in under a year. Nurses stationed in these departments are reimbursable by third-party payers. Earlier discharges do not mean, however, that patient recoveries are faster, so it is imperative that services needed are planned for and carefully implemented.

Toon (1990) points out that there also is a movement afoot toward more outpatient radiation, outpatient chemotherapy, and home pain control. Because the hospital is the most expensive place for receiving health and illness care, more and better communication among health team members will be needed to bridge the gap between hospital and home care.

Types of Teaching Services

Within the hospital setting there are many varieties of teaching. There are different topics and age groups of individuals with different levels of illness.

DiMateo (1991, p. 347), as well as McHatton (1985), points out that there are different demands placed on an individual at different illness stages. In the first illness stage, survival, the patients' chances to live depend on moment-to-moment or day-to-day interventions. If the patient has had a heart attack, immediate treatments must be efficient and effective for the short term and influencing for the long term. If surgery is performed for breast cancer removal, additional interventions to prevent metastases will be necessary. Focusing on the life-threatening nature of illness and the treatments will consume most psychological and physical energy available. Choices made in this stage can have a long-lasting impact of the quality of long-term survival, thus the import of quality decisions. Teaching goals at this stage often are in the areas of decreasing anxiety, informing the patient about procedures and equipment, and teaching survival skills. In addition, many patients at this level of illness are in a dependent role and may look to health professionals for decision-making assistance. For those requiring intermediate care, therapeutic and preventive health teaching is in order, such as "the reasons for coughing and deep breathing, the need for support stockings and ambulating frequently, the use of medications, exercise, special diets, the level of risk of future illness and hospitalization, how to overcome setbacks during recovery, and/or how to cope with depression" (Rankin & Stallings, 1990, p. 307). During the rehabilitation phase, a bedridden person who has been taken care of must learn to resume his/her health status at as independent a level of functioning as possible. Much time and effort will be expended in learning to react to the term cancer, to walk, to talk coherently, or to brush his own teeth, or lift a fork to his mouth. Learning to adjust to a new body image will be part of the needed teaching. Hopefully, rehabilitation will lead to full recovery. When this is not possible, accepting and learning to live with chronic disability will be steps of learning. Terminal illness may be another possibility. Learning to deal with pain, disfigurement, and loss of energy as the illness progresses may help the individual and family comes to terms with the prospect of death. Thus, a wide range of learning opportunities exists in hospitalized patients. For outpatient settings, emphasis is on maintenance needs such as medication, regimens, dietary schedules, and prevention of further complications.

Many hospitals, regardless of their type, size, and location, have incorporated patient education programs, especially since JCAHO has required patient education documentation for some areas since 1979. Cardiac rehabilitation teaching and discharge planning can be found in most hospitals.

Cardiac rehabilitation has for many years been incorporated in treatment plans of patients have a myocardial infarction in an attempt to effect behavioral change. Educational content such as anxiety reduction sessions, explanation of procedures and events, knowledge of myocardial infarction and its treatment, diet, medications, risk factors, activity levels, and prevention of symptoms often begins in the cardiac care unit and continues in the postcoronary care units. Educational sessions can be a mixture of individual and group programs. Contact is usually continued after the patient returns home, and sessions with families are frequently included. Raleigh and Oltohan (1987) studied the effects of a structured inpatient teaching program for cardiac patients. Planned individualized nursing instructions about heart disease risk factors, rehabilitation, resumption of normal activities, and activity programs were carried out. Results indicated that the experimental group was more knowledgeable about the disease and less anxious about discharge home; at a 2-month follow-up, the experimental group had achieved a statistically significant activity increase over the control group. Meloche (1985), as well as Speers (1989) in another study, found that a Cardiac Club had a positive influence on patient behaviors. This type of postdischarge teaching programs provides an open forum for learning more about cardiac diagnoses, developing effective coping mechanisms, and choosing more healthy life styles.

There are ranges of educational interventions being tests at hospitals and other health-care institutions that provide active educational opportunities for patients to discuss and make decisions about their hospitalizations in a warm home-like environment. Giloth (1990) writes of two model hospital programs that have achieved patient involvement in a comprehensive way. The first, located at New York University, is the Cooperative Care Model, having 104 beds, that has been successfully operating for 10 years. The other, a smaller unit and more recent, is Planetree, managed by the University of Washington. Major aspects of these two hospital programs include stress reduction, increased access to educational resources, 24-hour visiting, patients wearing their own clothes, and many other ideas that "give control" to the patients. Both institutions view their use of primary nursing as crucial to success. As yet there are not many structural settings that would easily accommodate this approach. Both of these institutions renovated space to provide a soothing, home-like environment.

Lindeman (1988) has summarized much of the major published nursing research on patient education. Although nurses are more or less at a beginning stage, many categories are presented and the reader is referred to this source for more details. Target populations were categorized as maternal–infant, surgical, cardiovascular, chronic illness, psychiatric–mental health, and diagnostic procedures. All of these groupings represented patients who responded to patient education, and

Lindeman concluded that patient education does make a difference in learning. Redman (1985) mentioned psychiatric patient education as an opportunity for nurses to become involved with the advent of special geriatric rehabilitation and assessment units in hospitals for preventing institutionalization of elderly. Additionally, Redman (1985) pointed out that most developments in patient education occur within disease-specific areas of cure such as Lindeman categorized.

SUMMARY

One variable that Lindeman (1988) looked at in her review of patient education research was the effect of the health-care setting on learning. A generalization made was that the organizational structure of the health-care setting was less important than the value of patient education as perceived by staff and administration. Additionally, Lindeman found that regardless of setting, patients viewed education as important. Contradictory to Lindeman's conclusions, Lipetz et al in a 1990 article concluded from their survey that a number of impediments exist in preventing successful patient teaching in hospitals.

The benefits of patient education have usually been reported in short-term gains (Kruger, 1988). Long-term benefits that can be translated into healthier people and resulting cost-effective interventions need documentation. Lindeman (1988), Scalzi, Burke, and Greenland (1980), Steele & Ruziki (1987), in evaluating effectiveness of cardiac teaching during hospitalization, found effectiveness for the short term, and that hospital educational experiences are not of sufficient length to induce long-term changes. Concern is expressed about impact of DRGs and early discharge with some teaching being moved from hospital to home settings. Wood (1989) reported on research involving 39 adult day care centers that suggests heavier care clienteles in community-based long-term care agencies since the advent of DRGs; could it happen that the less sick will not have needed access to care? We are in the midst of change so results are uncertain.

A strength of teaching is that regardless of the setting, it is the nurse who maintains the continued contact with the recipient of health care. If nurses perceive themselves in a teaching role, there will be a commitment to teach and a desire to influence others to teach.

REFERENCES AND READINGS

Anderson, D. M., & Christenson, G. M. Ethnic breakdown of AIDS related knowledge and attitudes from the National Adolescent Student Health Survey. *Journal of Health Education*, January-February 1991, *22*(1).

Bauknecht, V. L. Testimony cites impact of DRG system. *American Nurse*, 1985, *17*, 3–3.

Benenson, A. S. *Control of communicable diseases in man*. Washington, D.C., The American Public Health Association, 1990.

Brainerd, E. J. HIV in the school setting: The school nurses' role. *Journal of School Health*, September 1989, *59*(7).

Buhler-Wilkerson, K. Public health nursing: In sickness and health. In E. T. Anderson & J. M. McFarlane (Eds.), *Community as client.* St. Louis, Mo.: J. B. Lippincott Company, 1988.

Chen, Moon S. The most important influences in worksite health promotion: Conclusion of the panel discussion. *Health Education,* December 1989, *20*(7).

Chenoweth, David. Health promotion programs examined through cost-effectiveness analysis. *Occupational Health and Safety,* January 1990.

Chenoweth, David. Occupational health management must deal with a myriad of issues. *Occupational Health and Safety,* March 1988.

Collis, June L., & Dukes, Carol A. Toward some principles of school nursing. *Journal of School Health,* March 1989, *59*(3).

Conroy, Carol. Suicide in the workplace: Incidence, victim characteristics, and external cause of death. *Journal of Occupational Medicine,* October 1989, *31*(10).

Creswell, W. H., & Newman, I. M. Times, mirror. *School Health Practice.* St. Louis, Mo.: Mosby Publishing Company, 1989.

Daley, R. *Patient teaching manual I, II.* Springhouse, Pa., Keith Lassner Publisher, 1987.

DeMuth, J. S. Patient teaching in ambulatory settings. *Nursing Clinics of North America,* September 1989, *24*(3).

DiMateo, M. R. The psychology of health, illness, and medical care. Brooks/Cole Publishing Co, Pacific Grove, CA, 1991.

Drew, L. A., Biordi, D., & Gillies, G. A. How discharge planners and home health nurses view their patients. *Nursing management,* 1990, *12*(8), 66–70.

Duryea, Elias J. Doubling: Enhancing the role play technique in schools. *Journal of School Health,* March 1990, *60*-(3).

Frank, Jeanne. Epilepsy: The school nurses dilemma. *Journal of School Health,* January 1990, *60*(1).

Friddle, J., McElroy, M., Gordon, J., & Pinkham, J. How companies can ease the burden of AIDS at work. *Occupational Health and Safety,* July 1988.

Gerson, Shari. Coors program proves that wellness means more than physical fitness. *Occupational Health and Safety,* June 1990.

Giloth, B. E. Promoting patient involvement: Educational, organizational, and environmental strategies. *Patient Education and Counseling,* 1990, *15,* 29–38.

Goerth, Charles R. Serious legal issues leads OHNS to step out of clinic into courtroom. *Occupational Health and Safety,* June 1988.

Graham, B. A. Preparing case managers. *Caring,* February 1989.

Hataway, D. Effect of preoperative instruction on postoperative outcomes: A meta analysis. *Nursing Research,* 1986, *35*(5), 269–281.

Honan, S., Krsnak, G., Petersen, D., et al. The nurse as patient educator: Perceived responsibilities and factors enhancing role development. *Patient Education,* 1989, *19*(5), 33–37.

Hopp, J. W., & Hills, R. Determining patient education needs. *Respiratory Therapy,* November-December 1985, 38–43.

Humphrey, Carol J. *Home Care Nursing Handbook.* Norwalk, Ct.: Appleton-Century-Crofts Publishers, 1986.

Jackson, Janet E., & Johnson, Elizabeth A. *Patient Education in Home Care.* Rockville, Md.: Aspen Publication, 1988.

Joachin, Gloria. The school nurse as case manager for chronically ill children. *Journal of School Health,* November 1989, *59*(9).

Johnson, E. A., & Jackson, J. E. Teaching the home care client. *Nursing Clinics of North America,* September 1989, *24*(3).

Johnson, L. Beyond knowledge and practice: A challenge in health education. *Journal of Health Education,* January/February 1991, *22*(1).

Johnson, S. L., & Morse, J. M. Regaining control: A process of adjustment after myocardial infarction. *Heart and Lung,* 1990, *19*(2), 126–135.

Jones, H., Ellis, N., Tappe, M., & Lindsay, G. HIV related beliefs, knowledge and behaviors of ninth and tenth grade public school students. *Journal of Health Education,* January/February 1991, *22*(1).

Keating, S. B., Kelman, G. B. *Home health care nursing concepts and practice.* Philadelphia, Pa.: J.B. Lippincott Company, 1988.

Kerr, D. L. HIV vs. AIDS. *Journal of School Health,* October 1990, *60*(8).

Kruger, S. A review of patient education in nursing. *Journal of Nursing Staff Development,* March/April 1990, 71–75.

Leviton, L. C., Hegedus, A. M., & Kubnin, A. Evaluating aids prevention: Contributions of multiple disciplines. *Jossey-Bass, Inc.,* Summer 1990, *46.*

Lindeman, C. A. Patient education. In J. J. Fitzgerald, R. L. Taunton, & J. Q. Benoliel, (Eds.), *Annual Review of Nursing Research.* Philadelphia, Pa.: Springer Publishing Co. 1988, *6,* 29–60.

Lindeman, C. A. Patient education: Part II. In J. J. Fitzgerald, R. L. Taunton, & J. Q. Benoliel, (Eds.), *Annual Review of Nursing Research.* Philadelphia, Pa.: Springer Publishing Co., 1989, *7,* 200–212.

Lipetz, M. J., Bussigel, M. N., Bannerman, J. et al. What is wrong with patient education progress? *Nursing Outlook,* 1990, *38*(4), 184–189.

Mann, Jonathan M. Global AIDS: Status of the pandemic. *Journal of Health Education,* January-February 1991, *22*(1).

Marion Laboratories, Inc. *Marion long-term care digest.* Home Health Care Edition. Kansas City, Mo., 1989.

Martinson, I. M., & Widmer, A. *Home Health Care Nursing.* Philadelphia, Pa.: W. B. Saunders Company, 1989.

Mayer, et al. Empowering families of the clinically ill: A partnership experience in a hospital setting. *Social Work in Health Care,* 1989, *14*(4), 73–89.

McHatton, M. A theory for timely teaching. *American Journal of Nursing,* July 1985, 798–800.

Meloche, A. T. Patient education in cardiac care. *Canadian Critical Care Nursing Journal,* 1985, *2,* 24–26.

Miller, J. M., Wikoff, M., McMahon M. et al. Influence of a nursing intervention on regimen adherence and societal adjustments postmyocardial infarction. *Nursing Research,* 1988, *37*(5), 297–301.

Myers, D. *Client teaching guides for home health care.* Rockville, MD, Aspen Publishers, 1989.

Nation's Health, American Public Health Association, January 1991.

Nauman, L. A. School nursing and AIDS education. *Journal of School Health,* September 1989, *59*(7).

Oda, D. S. The invisible nursing practice. *Nursing Outlook,* January/February 1990, *39*(1).

Pinkham, J. One hundred years of industrial nursing has vastly improved workplace safety. *Occupational Health and Safety,* April 1988.

Raleigh, E. H., & Odtohan, B. C. The effect of a cardiac teaching program on patient rehabilitation. *Heart and Lung,* 1987, *16*(3), 311–316.

Rankin, S. H., & Stallings, K. D. *Patient education: Issues, principles, practices* (2nd ed) 1990. Philadelphia, PA: Lippincott Publishing Co.

Redman, B. K. New areas of theory development and practice in patient education. *Journal of Advanced Nursing*, 1985, *10*, 425–428.

Rosoff, J. I. Sex education in the schools: Policies and practices. *Family Planning Perspective*, March-April 1989, *2*(2).

Samways, Margaret C. Functionally illiterate worker also has right to understand. *Occupational Health and Safety*, January 1988.

Scalzi, C. C., Burke, L. E., & Greenland, S. Evaluation of an inpatient educational program for coronary patients and families. *Heart and Lung*, 1980, *5*(9), 846–853.

Schneider, W. J. AIDS in the workplace. *Journal of Occupational Medicine*, October 1989, *31*(10).

Seffin, John R. The comprehensive school health curriculum. Closing the gap between state-of-the-practice. *Journal of School Health*, April 1990, *60*(4).

Shannon, M. D. Skills in family teaching. In I. M. Martinson, & A. Widmer (Eds.), *Home health care nursing*. Philadelphia: W. B. Saunders Company, 1989.

Speers, A. T. Patient education: Theory and practice. *Journal of Nursing Staff Development*, May/June 1989, 121–126.

Steele, J. M., & Ruzicki, D. An evaluation of the effectiveness of cardiac teaching during hospitalization. *Heart and Lung*, 1987, *3*(16), 306–310.

Swindle, J. E. The nurse's role in giving pre-operative information to reduce anxiety in patients admitted to hospital for elective minor surgery. *Journal of Advanced Nursing*, 1989, *14*, 899–905.

Taylor, Mary E., Wang, Min Qi, Leonard, Jack (Jr), & Adame, Daniel D. Effects of contraceptive education on adolescent male contraceptive behavior and attitudes. *Health Education*, April-May 1989.

Toon, Steve. Meet Jackie Birmingham. *Continuing Care*, January 1990, 21–24.

United States Department of Health and Human Services, Health Care Financing Administration. *Home health agency manual* (Publication 11), 1989.

Walsh, M. E., & Bibace, R. Developmentally-based AIDS-HIV education. *Journal of School Health*, August 1990, *60*(6).

Whited, F., & Starke, T. School nurses: An endangered species. *Journal of School Health*, December 1989, *59*(10).

Wood, J. B. The emergence of adult day care centers as post-acute care agencies. *Journal of Aging and Health*, 1989, *4*(1), 521–540.

4

Theories of Learning

Carol J. Gleit

The purpose of this chapter is to provide an organized description of varying theoretical perspectives that may guide nurse–teachers in their teaching. Nurses practice in widely diverse settings, from acute intensive care units to public health departments to community health agencies. They interact with clients of all ages, exhibiting a variety of health states. Health education content includes a variety of topic areas in the cognitive, affective, and psychomotor domains. The cognitive domain deals with the intellectual or knowledge area. The affective domain consists of attitudes, feelings, and interests one has toward a given topic, while the psychomotor domain encompasses physical skills or sensory motor activities,. It is therefore important for nurses to have a repertoire of teaching approaches based on how individuals learn. Even if a nurse teaches in one setting, such as a kidney dialysis unit, or family planning clinic, no one single approach would be adequate. This chapter is not a survey of learning theories, but an attempt to categorize approaches for basing appropriate teaching on individualistic considerations. The reader is referred to Joyce and Weil (1986), Lafrancois (1988), Bigge (1982), Knox (1986) for other approaches and more detailed treatment than can be included in one chapter.

Many theories of learning exist, developed by learning psychologists, educators, and psychotherapists. Of the available theoretical perspectives, many contradict one another. Before the 1950s several grand theories of learning were purported. From the 1950s to the present, research in learning theories has concentrated more on smaller, narrower scopes of theory building, rather than one grand theory of learning (Bigge, 1982; Joyce & Weil, 1986; and Lafrancois 1988). From these narrow theories there could evolve more generalized theories. There is a tendency to use an increasingly eclectic approach as well, with the idea that certain theoretical approaches will work with some clients, and other approaches with others. The nature of the type of learning also calls for different approaches. Theorists of today differ not so much in their views about the nature of learning as in their opinions on areas of study and methods used. There is some interest now in combining several models to combat multifaceted health problems.

Based on the assumption that nurse–teachers use many types of theoretical bases, this chapter incorporates many viewpoints. It espouses the idea that no one approach will succeed with all clients or can reach all learning goals. Joyce and Weil (1986) have identified 80 different learning theories, some with similarities but each with separate and distinct features. There is no common classification system in evidence, but it is necessary to group theories in some comprehensible manner. Many diverse groupings exist.

The definition of learning identified in Chapter 1 stated that learning involves a persistent change in behavior as the result of experience. From this definition it is evident that the foundation for learning theories is behavior change. Three types of theories about the behavior change that occurs as the result of learning can be identified. These are cognitive theories, behavioral theories, and humanist theories. The perspectives of these theories are not mutually exclusive in all respects, but the main purpose of each differs from one another. Categorization is not simple because some theories do not neatly fit into any category. The views represented in this chapter are the work of a large number of theorists over time.

THREE MAJOR PERSPECTIVES OF LEARNING THEORY

How one theorizes about learning is consistent with one's personal definition of learning. Some theorists or interpreters claim that there is much basic disagreement in definitions of learning. What is agreed upon is that experience is the source of learning and that to learn is to change. Common to discrepant viewpoints is the following definition: Learning is a change in the individual, caused by the person's interaction with the environment, whereby he or she is more capable of dealing (adequately) with the environment. In health teaching, health beliefs, attitudes, and behaviors are the targets of this change.

Behaviorists believe that learning has taken place when changes in behavior can be observed, when new habits of behavior are shaped by events in the environment. Cognitive theorists believe that learning is an internal process, not necessarily observable, in which information is integrated or internalized into one's cognitive (intellectual) structure. Humanists stress the incorporation of the affective realm (attitude, feeling, interest) as well as the cognitive in self-directed learning.

In the next section, each of the three categories of theories will be described. Beginning teachers might want to rehearse several of the illustrations in short teaching episodes.

BEHAVIORIST PERSPECTIVE

To behaviorists, learning is the result of conditioning. Conditioning is defined as the attachment of a particular response to a particular stimulus (DiMatteo, 1991, p. 103). Conditioning has a long history, dating back to Pavlov's experience with salivating dogs and Thorndike's classic work of the 1930s. Many modifications have resulted since these early times. There are numerous variations of behaviorism, and among behavioral theorists there are sharp disagreements as to the use of the common terms *response* (reinforcer), and *consequences*. Some use an approach that intermixes various stimulus and response patterns. In addition, several terms are subsumed under the behaviorist approach, including *operant conditioning, behavior modification, social learning theory,* and *behavioral therapy.* The key feature of the behaviorist perspective is that the behavior can be overtly observed. Internal events such as thinking, forgetting, or wanting are not part of this viewpoint. Behaviorists place heavy reliance on empirical data collected by careful observation. They focus on the environment and what the person is engaging in "here and now." A primary consideration is that what a person does is a function of his environment.

Although there are many behavioral theorists, B. F. Skinner is frequently regarded as the prototype of one general category, operant conditioning. The main premise of operant conditioning is that a reinforcing stimulus (reward) which follows a response increases the likelihood that the response will be repeated. The stimulus producing the response in the first place is not centrally involved in the learning process. The original response is the result of a stimulus, but the nature of this stimulus is not relevant to operant conditioning (Bigge, 1982). The operants are the learned patterns, and the role of reinforcement is stressed. The essential feature is the relationship between the response and reinforcing stimuli. If reinforcement is presented only when the response occurs it is called contingent. Contingency management, then, is systematic control of reinforcing stimuli.

Joyce and Weil (1986, p. 342) list the procedures to set up a contingency management program as: (1) specifying the final performance, (2) assessing entering behavior (establishing baseline), (3) formulating a contingency management program, (4) instituting the program, and (5) evaluating the program. In Chapter 19 of their text, these authors provide a detailed background and further breakdown of the steps used in setting up a contingency management program.

The important terminology of behaviorism stems from defining learning as behavior change resulting from conditioning. Conditioning is the formation of a stimulus-response sequential relation resulting in an enduring change in either the pattern of behavior or the likelihood of a response of the individual (Bigge, 1982). A stimulus is "any condition, event, or change in the environment of an individual which produces a change in behavior, and may be verbal or physical" (Joyce & Weil, 1986, p. 313). A response is "a unit of overt or covert behavior, the basic unit upon which complex performances or response repertoires are built" (Joyce & Weil, 1986, p. 313). The objective is to increase the frequency of the desired response. This is done by using reinforcement.

Reinforcement

Reinforcement is the core of the behaviorist approach. The ultimately desired behavior is gradually reached through reinforcement. Effective reinforcement immediately follows a response. A reinforcer increases the frequency of a response on which it is contingent. The term *contingency* refers to reinforcement that only takes place with the desired behavior. Reinforcers may be positive or negative. Positive reinforcement (rewards) are powerful techniques in shaping and maintaining the desired behavior. Individuals can choose different things as rewards or positive reinforcers. Depending on the individual, food, money, or social rewards such as hugs, praise, smiles may be reinforcing. Psychomotor activity such as needle work for an adult, or play for a child, may be chosen. For learning more complex behavior, as learning is occurring the incomplete responses or those close to the desired behavior initially may be rewarded when the learner's repertoire is close to or approximates the desired response. Rewards are gradually restricted to those behaviors more and more similar to the desired end behavior as the change approaches and finally reaches the desired response. This gradual formation of a desired response is called shaping.

Shaping

Shaping can be used to gradually change pattern characteristics, strengthen the pattern, or lengthen the time in which the pattern is carried out. For example, those who overeat can shape their behavior pattern by putting the fork down between each bite, placing smaller portions on a salad size plate, scheduling eating only in the kitchen and not in front of the television, scheduling time to eat and time to not eat. Positive reinforcers can substitute acceptable for undesirable behavior, for example, substituting carrot or celery sticks for cigarettes or muscle relaxation for anxiety.

Shaping requires a number of skills on the part of the teacher. First, behaviors that must precede or accompany that which is to be learned, need to be identified. Then it is necessary to find and establish a unit of secondary reinforcement that will effectively mold the learner's behavior into the desired pattern. Once the learning is established the teacher gradually decreases participation with reinforcers. The pattern of reinforcement is important. Continuous reinforcement, in every instance of desirable behavior, is useful when a behavior to be learned is first introduced. Once a desired behavior is established, intermittent reinforcement maintains the behavior, by either a fixed or variable schedule. Fixed time reinforcement refers to reinforcing the behavior at set intervals, such as the second and fourth tries out of five attempts. Reinforcement results from the act—a consequence—never in advance. For example, a new sweater, or book, or movie, as a reward for jogging would not be purchased until the jogging experience itself was completed, not the promise of jogging. Intermittent reinforcers are then used, and come farther and farther apart, until the client behavior occurs without assistance from the teacher. The instructor has "faded" out. Fading is the technique of gradually withdrawing participation in the client's desired activity (learning). Ambulation is an area of patient teaching where shaping techniques can be used effectively. Each step, from sitting with balance, then standing, then walking has several minor steps or behaviors needing reinforcement before the final goal of walking is reached. Putting feet on the floor and standing erect may call for careful reinforcement. Self-feeding behavior in a stroke patient can be encouraged through shaping. Usually in patient education shaping is used with fairly complex behaviors, as in learning complicated medication schedules.

In the last 25 to 35 years, techniques of using positive rewards have been refined. The importance of the speed of the reward, of using rewards at appropriate times and for small portions of behavior or for approximations of the desired behavior have been further developed. The importance of regularly and consistently rewarding desired behavior immediately and plainly and not rewarding undesirable behavior is crucial to the success of a behaviorist approach to learning. This means that the behavior is studied very closely and in detail, so that sequences of behaviors can be broken down into small parts and taught separately. Although Joyce and Weil (1986) note that research literature on the role of self-awareness is inconclusive, the importance of cognition is increasingly seen as important. Many teachers prefer the learner alert to the desired behavior, such as, "I like the way you pulled back on the syringe when you injected your insulin this morning." Another example might be "I like the way you used your arms on the trapeze when you lifted yourself up in bed." The importance of success and encouragement to learn more are stressed.

Extinction

When there is no reinforcement, extinction occurs. If there are no rewards, the behavior will become less frequent and finally disappear. The behavior is likely to decrease over time, because one tends to repeat a behavior that has been previously rewarded. The disappearance of the behavior is called extinction. The key, then, is to reward only desirable behavior patterns. For example, a nurse may teach a mother to ignore temper tantrums of her 2-year-old child rather than reward them by attention, because even negative attention such as scolding may be rewarding to some children.

Implications for Learning

Behaviorists give attention to the behavior that is to be learned, the reinforcers which may be used, and the scheduling of reinforcers. To promote learning, then, the teacher, in conjunction with the learner when possible:

1. Identifies very specifically the behavior that is to be learned.
2. Identifies the behaviors that make up the desired end behavior. The whole is divided into a large number of small steps, and reinforcement is contingent on accomplishment of each step.
3. Identifies appropriate reinforcers and presents them consistently each time the appropriate behavior ensues, shaping the behavior for each step in the sequence until the behavior is shaped to the desired goal. Uses fading once the behavior is established.
4. Ignores undesirable behaviors using extinction.

The ultimate goal is the transferability of the behaviors to new situations. The idea is for the adapted behaviors to be incorporated into the individual's repertoire by being under his own control and monitoring.

SELF-CONTROL IN BEHAVIORISM

It is possible for an individual to be in control of his own behavior modification program. Exercising and establishing more assertive behavior are examples that fit well under self-management. Joyce and Weil (1986) detail an explanation of a self-control model summarized as follows: Problems with self-control usually deal with short-term positive gratification and long-term negative consequences. Smokers do not perceive the lung damaging effects as much as the short-term satisfaction of one cigarette. A first step is to raise the level of awareness of the short- and long-term response consequences that maintain the health-damaging behaviors.

Deliberately arranging better environmental conditions is another crucial factor in eliminating self-defeating behavior. For example, someone who is drinking coffee and wants a cigarette could switch beverages or plan to drink coffee only when cigarettes are not available. Overweight people can sabotage themselves by arranging their environments with tempting foods and a lot of time spent around the kitchen. Covert thoughts as "Just one small piece of cake won't hurt," "I just cannot give up smoking," "It always happens to me" can also be rearranged to more positive stimuli in our mental and emotional environments. Shaping is important in self-control programs, and setting realistic goals will assist in positive reinforcement. Small goals over short time-frames will generally lead to success. In other words, self-control is not an all or nothing response. It is a set of skills that can be learned and developed through practice.

DiMatteo (1991) describes the process of self-regulation as having three stages: (1) self-monitoring or self-observation, (2) self-education, and (3) self-evaluation. In the first stage, self-monitoring, the individual very deliberately and carefully attends to the details of his behavior. The person may choose to keep records of what he eats or his smoking behavior, exactly, with quantities and locations. Trigger events and feelings might also be recorded. By determining patterns that exist, behaviors can be changed. During the second phase, the identified behaviors are compared against recommended criteria, for example, the recommended speed, distance, and time for walking. During the last phase, self-reinforcement, the individual rewards him/herself for behavior approximating the goal. Purchasing a new sweater for an identified time of not smoking is a successful reinforcement, instead of an item that might sabotage the treatment endeavor. By facilitating learner awareness of current behaviors and ways of changing, the patient educator can assist a learner to successful behavioral self-regulation. Later in this chapter, the reader will find a section on self-efficacy, which deals with how clients think about action. Self-regulation deals with how clients go about acting.

Modeling

A variation on "strict" behavioral approach is the theory of modeling. The client observes a model enacting a specific behavior, sees the consequences of the model's behavior, and then attempts to match the behavior in order to obtain the same reward. The modeled behavior is the overt behavior that is acted out, not the spoken words. Bandura (1965) is credited with a great deal of the extensive research completed on modeling and has named it the social learning model. He suggests that people choose what and whom they will model, although the imitation may be conscious or unconscious. Not all behavior of the model is reproduced, but certain aspects of behavior are selected out and interwoven into a person's behavior, ultimately resulting in a unique behavior pattern. Unlike operant conditioning, the individual is not interacting directly with the environment, but observing behaviors of others and then modeling their behavior. For example, many model the behavior of more experienced individuals when first confronted with a new situation.

Bandura (1965) identifies four processes involved in modeling: (1) attention, (2) retention (remembering), (3) reproduction, and (4) reinforcement. In these processes the learner pays attention to what the model is doing, then remembers what the model has done in order to repeat it; next the learner repeats the behavior. The timing for repeating the behavior is important. Usually repeating the behavior soon leads to more accuracy. The learner must be physically capable and motivated to reproduce the behavior. In order to reproduce the behavior, it is broken down into steps and practiced. The way the learner remembers the behavior can have varying degrees of accuracy. The learner concentrates on relevant cues and ignores the irrelevant. If the individual generalizes and stores information accurately, the modeling may be true to form, but if the learner's intellectual processing system is not at a high level it may be hard to reproduce the behavior precisely. Generally, it is considered better to encourage an individual to use his or her own way or style of remembering, so that use of the behavior will more likely be correct for reinforcement and for incorporating the behavior into one's repertoire. The learner needs to accept and want to engage in the behavior that was reinforced in the model (vicarious reinforcement). Obviously, modeling is not the random copying of behaviors.

Modeling has been studied extensively, especially with children. In their early years, children are more likely to imitate adults than other children. As the child grows into a teenager, there is more of a tendency to imitate peers (Bandura, 1971).

The use of modeling is quite extensive in health education. The idea that nurses and other health professionals must serve as role models for clients has long existed and been drummed into many students' heads over the years. On the other hand, some educators take an opposing view, that is, that role modeling is not a necessary component of health education and that an educator can use his or her own flaws to motivate behavior change in clients. From their research, Gobble and Mullen (1983) concluded that although the health education faculty in one institution were indeed "well," they were not successful in having students role model a wellness life style. At this point, there is a "healthy" debate over the merits of role modeling as a way of learning. What is needed now is a more deliberative use of the model, especially the zeroing in on the importance of accuracy in remembering and generalizing the information and positive reinforcement of the behavior. Observation followed by guided practice is considered better than observation alone. Exercising assertiveness and psychomotor skills can be learned through modeling from either a demonstration or films, and then practicing under the guidance of a teacher. Reach to Recovery volunteers for mastectomy patients, and ostomate clubs are further successful examples of models. Green (1970) states that positive health (wellness) practices must be made visible to reinforce the practice of these behaviors in clients. This means that if health teachers want to be perceived as models, positive, conscious efforts must be taken to ensure that modeling occurs.

Behavior theory approaches are frequently in evidence in health teaching today. Many of the well-known weight loss, smoking cessation, assertiveness training, anxiety reduction, and relaxation programs are examples. They are frequently referred to as behavior modification because they emphasize changing the visible behavior of the learner rather than the underlying and unobservable behavior.

COGNITIVE PERSPECTIVE

Cognitive approaches to learning have been the mainstay of patient and client education. Unfortunately, "telling people what to do or transmitting information" has been and is what many health professionals consider the totality of this approach toward health teaching. Cognitive viewpoints of learning can be much more complex than this and offer several perspectives as to how people think. The cognitive approach can be used to help persons improve their thinking abilities.

Although this perspective encompasses a wide range of viewpoints, the main idea is that learning deals with the internal structuring and processing of information. Since this is an internal process, observable evidence may be limited. This is different from the behavioristic approach necessitating overt behavior as evidence of learning.

There is no single prototype representing the view of the cognitive approach, but Gagné, Bruner, Piaget, and Ausubel are familiar names associated with this school. These theorists share a similar orientation toward information-processing capability and ways in which individuals can improve their ability to master information. Information or cognitive processing refers to ways people take in environmental stimuli, organize data, sense problems, generate concepts and solutions to problems, and employ verbal and nonverbal symbols. Some theorists emphasize productive thinking by means of problem solving, while others are concerned with general intellectual ability and acquiring information through interaction with data, principles, and generalizations. In other words, there is concern both with the structure of the material to be learned and with the structure of the cognitive processing of the material. This is different from the behaviorist approach, which deals with external, not internal change.

From the cognitive viewpoint, structure of knowledge is important. Approaches to cognitive skills acquisition can be illustrated using a hierarchical type of format. This shows the structure of knowledge from factual data through increasing abstraction, proceeding from the base to the top. Figure 4–1 illustrates this concept.

Bruner (1966) and Gagné (1974) have developed models dealing with intellectual skills in the use of information, each developing a model of learning incorporating hierarchical levels. Each level builds upon the previous, simpler form. At the base of these models are facts, foundation knowledge, or skills necessary for undergirding concept formation and generalizability. In order to move into the higher levels, data must first be available for use. Once the factual base is acquired, simple discriminations can be formed, that is, the idea of how things and objects are similar and different from one another. The attempt is to sort and classify, differentiate, and

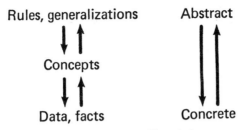

Figure 4–1. Structure of knowledge.

discriminate—in other words, to build concepts. Having concrete experiences with data and facts is considered critical to concept attainment. *Knowing* a concept means distinguishing examples from nonexamples, generating new examples of the concept, and articulating notions about the concepts.

Gagné (1974) gives eight types of learning in ascending order: (1) signal, similar to classical conditioning, (2) stimulus–response; (3) chaining, involving at least two stimulus–response connections; (4) verbal association, involving assembling verbal chains from a previously learned repertoire; (5) multiple discrimination, involving differentiated responses to varied stimuli; (6) concept, involving identifying and responding to a class of objects that have served as stimuli; (7) principle, involving applying a principle that consists of at least one chain of two or more concepts; and (8) problem solving, involving processing of at least two previously acquired principles to produce a higher level principle. The words *discriminations, concepts, rules,* and *higher order rules* are prominent in Gagné's model. Bruner's model is similar, although different terms from Gagné's are used, such as *categorizing, ordering, relating classes,* and *decision alternatives.* Refer to Gagné (1974) for a thorough description of his eight types of learning.

Bloom's taxonomy of educational objectives in the cognitive domain is another example of a hierarchical arrangement of levels of learning, consistent with Gagné and Bruner's approach. Operating cognitively, the learner would achieve objectives ranging from simple recall of material learned to highly original ways of combining and synthesizing new ideas and materials. The hierarchical structure developed by Bloom (1956) is listed in Table 4–1.

Recall
According to Bloom, at the lowest level is recall in which remembering is the major process. The client is expected to store information for later recall. Retention and retrieval are phases of learning directly concerned with memory. Memory consists of short-term memory, which holds information long enough for processing, and long-term memory, in which information is permanently stored. Rehearsal and coding are important elements in short-term memory; organization and meaning and context are important elements in long-term memory. Interference in retention or retrieval is a major cause of forgetting; for example, material may not be structured adequately or the process not rehearsed sufficiently.

TABLE 4–1. COGNITIVE DOMAIN

1.00 Knowledge

Knowledge, as defined here, involves recall or remembering of information.

1.10 Knowledge of specifics

1.11 Knowledge of terminology

1.12 Knowledge of specific facts

1.20 Knowledge of ways and means of dealing with specifics

1.21 Knowledge of conventions (characteristic ways of treating and presenting ideas and phenomena)

1.22 Knowledge of trends and sequences

1.23 Knowledge of classifications and categories

1.24 Knowledge of criteria

1.25 Knowledge of methodology

1.30 Knowledge of the universals and abstractions in a field

1.31 Knowledge of principles and generalizations

1.32 Knowledge of theories and structures

2.00 Comprehension

This represents the lowest level of understanding. It refers to a type of understanding . . . such that the individual knows what is being communicated and can make use of the material or idea being communicated without necessarily relating it to other materials or seeing its fullest implications.

2.10 Translation

Comprehension as evidenced by the care and accuracy with which the communication is paraphrased or rendered from one language or form of communication to another. Translation is judged on the basis of faithfulness and accuracy, that is, on the extent to which the material in the original communication is preserved although the form of the communication has been altered.

2.20 Interpretation

The explanation or summarization of a communication. Whereas translation involves an objective part-for-part rendering of a communication, interpretation involves a reordering, rearrangement, or new view of the material.

2.30 Extrapolation

The extension of trends or tendencies beyond the given data to determine implications, consequences, corollaries, effects, and so forth which are in accordance with the conditions described in the original communication.

3.00 Application

The use of abstractions in particular and concrete situations. The abstractions may be in the form of general ideas, rules of procedures, or generalized methods. The abstractions may also be technical principles, ideas, and theories, which must be remembered and applied.

4.00 Analysis

The breakdown of a communication into its constituent elements or parts such that the relative hierarchy of ideas is made clear or the relations between the ideas expressed are made explicit or both. Such analyses are intended to clarify the communication, to indicate how the communication is organized and the way in which it manages to convey its effects, as well as to indicate its basis and arrangement.

4.10 Analysis of elements

Identification of the elements included in a communication.

4.20 Analysis of relationships

Identification of the connections and interactions between elements and parts of a communication.

TABLE 4–1. (*Continued*)

4.30 Analysis of organizational principles
Identification of the organization, systematic arrangement, and structure which hold the communication together. This includes the "explicit" as well as "implicit" structure. It includes the bases, necessary arrangement, and mechanics which makes the communication a unit.

5.00 Synthesis
The putting together of elements and parts to form a whole. This involves the process of working with pieces, parts, elements, and so forth and arranging and combining them in such a way so as to constitute a pattern or structure not clearly present before.

5.10 Production of a unique communication
The development of a communication in which the writer or speaker attempts to convey ideas, feelings, or experiences or all three to others.

5.20 Production of a plan, or proposed set of operations
The development of a plan of work or the proposal of a plan of operations. The plan should satisfy the requirements of a task that may be given to the student or that he may develop for himself.

5.30 Derivation of a set of abstract relations
The development of a set of abstract relations either to classify or explain particular data or phenomena, or the deduction of propositions and relations from a set of basic propositions or symbolic representations.

6.00 Evaluation
Judgments about the value of material and methods for given purposes: quantitative and qualitative judgments about the extent to which material and methods satisfy criteria; use of a standard of appraisal. The criteria may be determined by the student or given to him.

6.10 Judgments in terms of internal evidence
Evaluation of the accuracy of a communication from such evidence as logical accuracy, consistency, and other internal criteria.

6.20 Judgments in terms of external criteria
Evaluation of material with reference to selected or remembered criteria.

Adapted from Bloom, B. S. (Ed.). Taxonomy of educational objectives: The classification of educational goals. Handbook I: Cognitive Domain, New York: Copyright © 1956 by Longman, Inc., pp. 201–207. Reprinted by permission.

In aiding retention and retrieval, learners need to process the information, code it, and place it in context. Aids to memory include:

1. Summarizing major meanings and the structure of what is to be remembered.
2. Deciding how the information relates to that already known.
3. Dividing what must be learned into small sets of logical subdivisions.

Because short-term memory can hold only limited amounts of material at any given time, a moderate pacing of material interspersed with concrete examples will promote retention. Information can be learned in a format showing relationships among ideas. There relationships can serve as interlocking cues for later retrieval. If the ideas relate well to each other and provide a context for each other, learners have a greater likelihood of remembering total meaning.

Comprehension

Comprehension is a step above memory/recall. It involves transferring ideas into a parallel form or restating the same ideas with different words. Intricate relationships, implications, or subtle meanings are not included. Organization of data and some analysis is used to translate and relate concepts. Interpretation is a higher step in the structure of process, requiring the examination of relationships and generalizing from known data. The operative word is to *relate* facts, concepts, and skills. This involves seeing relationships between and among ideas.

Higher Cognitive Levels

The application level requires use of the previously acquired knowledge in a new situation. The application process gives the client practice in the transfer of knowledge. Analysis, synthesis, and evaluation are similar to Gagné's and Bruner's use of generalizing a process.

Another way of describing concept formation is by Carnevali (1981), who views concepts as vehicles of thought, enabling the conceptualizer to:

- Notice and identify objects, behavior, ideas, feelings, events, and phenomena.
- Recognize commonalities, relationships, and dynamics.
- Predict outcomes and options.
- Decide on actions that are appropriate.
- Set criteria for evaluating client response to intervention (1981, p. 208).

Carnevali's example of infection as a vehicle of thought, although designed for student nurse learning, also is appropriate for client learning:

- Recognize risks for infection present in a person or situation.
- Identify cues that suggest the presence of actual infection in the person.
- Suggest strategies for preventing spread of infection and management of it either by direct action or referral.
- Seek data on values and norms of the person and his or her society that influence participation in prevention and treatment of infection and/or relationships to persons who have the infection.
- Predict areas of activities and patterns of daily living where the pathophysiology or its treatment will require change of life style.
- Develop criteria for observing and evaluating response to nursing management (p. 208).

The interaction with the environment that provides the base for more complex learning influences one's ability to distinguish a causal relationship from chance. "We appear to go from what we can feel and manipulate to what we can see and hear, to what we can think about" (Moursund, 1976, p. 119). The higher levels involve the use of that part of problem solving that involves hypothesis generating and testing. The ability to be effective at this level is dependent upon the individual having successfully passed through the earlier and simpler levels. Ross and Mico (1980) have classified problem-solving approaches as (1) trial and error, (2) gradual analysis, and (3) insight processes. In the first approach, attempts may be haphazard, so that approaches may be unrelated to the extent that the individual may not be able to duplicate them in the future. Ross and Mico view gradual analysis as a rational systematic step-by-step process. Insight is suddenly realizing a solution.

Ross and Mico (1980) list the following difficulties many people have in their problem-solving abilities:

1. Inability to define a problem clearly enough to work on it effectively.
2. Adopting mistaken attitudes and assumptions that limit information and tend to be self-perpetuating.
3. Oversimplifying by either overlooking or ignoring key elements.
4. Accommodating a rigid mental set by failing to look at a problem in other than one highly particularized way.
5. Adopting a defensive orientation in which the desire to prove one's point, rationalize errors, or protect one's feelings obstructs a clear view of the problem.
6. Allowing emotion or stress to distort rational thought processes.

Gagné (1974) has also developed a hierarchical model of learning in which each level builds on earlier, more simple learning. He views these eight types of learning as types all people engage in throughout life. As one ascends the hierarchy, there is growth from a more simple to a more complex type of learning.

These levels are interrelated in that concepts continue to grow and one's ideas are never complete but interweave with one another both horizontally and vertically. This means that the individual can "think" along one level by relating what were diverse concepts or generalizations, but can also move into higher learning levels.

Ausubel: Advance Organizer

Ausubel (1968) has contributed another dimension to the information-processing model. Ausubel maintains that a person's existing cognitive structure is the most important factor governing whether new material is potentially meaningful and how well it can be acquired and retained. He believes that before we can effectively present new material, prior knowledge must be stabilized and clarified. To facilitate learning Ausubel uses what he calls the advance organizer, which he says becomes the "intellectual scaffolding," a structure on which the learner bases ideas and facts. The advance organizer is described by Ausubel as introductory material presented before the learning task and is at a higher level of abstraction and inclusiveness than the learning task itself. It is an idea itself. In this way the material to be learned is explained, integrated, and interrelated with previously learned material. Advance organizers are generally based on major concepts, rules, and generalizations of the overall topic. For example, before learning a specific exercise regime, an explanation of physiology of the cardiovascular system, psychological changes, and types of activities would be introduced. Ausubel further describes two types of advance organizers—expository, for introducing new material, and comparative, for introducing familiar material. The advance organizer is at a higher level of abstraction and is broader than the material to be learned. This model is especially useful when indepth, extended commitment to the understanding of key ideas is necessary. Adjustments to chronic illness, such as diabetes mellitus and arthritis, are situations in which this approach could be used. Although this model has been in use over a long time frame, much recent research on the topic concludes that it is useful for providing learners cognitive structures for comprehending materials. The reader is referred to Joyce & Weil (1986) for details of implementation.

Similarities of Cognitive Structuring Among Theorists

Bruner, Gagné, and Bloom, as well as Piaget, all worked with children. All point out that the child's learning is related to language development (see further description in Chapter 8). This means that until certain developmental stages are reached, thought processes do not advance in the hierarchy. It is not until age 2 or 3 that much language development occurs, so that the earliest learnings would not involve thought processes but sensorimotor techniques. It is not until preadolescence that problem-solving experience is regularized and that hypotheses-generating and testing stages are more than rudimentary. Knox (1986), in working with adults, points out the importance of assessing where the adult learner is with respect to knowledge base, cognitive complexity, and flexibility. It is possible for an adult to need more facts about a given situation, or some aspects important to the adult's relating to facts may be missing, and assistance is then needed to fill in these basic gaps. Assistance may be needed to gain a more adequate cognitive structure or a positive approach to learning may be necessary.

Knox (1986) points out that in many instances the lower levels of learning have been acquired, so that the adult can concentrate on concepts, principles, and problem solving. Some adults have a high need for structure. Knox relates that research evidence on adults and problem solving indicates that adults tend to enlarge their repertoire of prepared solutions for problems over the years. The solution process then consists mainly of searching the repertoire, rather than generating new approaches. This can result in more effective problem solving with age even when one considers that some learning requires new solutions. Knox admits there may be less cognitive flexibility with age. Kogan's (1974) research on conceptualizing styles of younger and older adults revealed that on the whole, aging persons are not marked by conceptual deficits or loss of cognitive functioning.

Skill Learning

Some authors (Magill, 1989; Schmidt, 1988; Rosenbaum, 1991) have placed skill learning under an information-processing or cognitive model. It has been agreed for years that there is a lack of a unified orientation. The basic thesis seems to be that a great deal of information processing goes on when people attempt to learn complex motor activities, many of which are under personal control. Fitts (1965) theorized that skill learning can be divided into three phases: (1) the cognitive phase; (2) the fixation phase; and (3) the autonomic phase. Although Fitts died an untimely death in 1965, he laid the basis for skill learning, and continues to be cited as a conceptualization of the skill learning process (Salmon, 1987; Rosenbaum 1991).

Cognitive Phase. In the first or cognitive phase, the learner understands the broad picture of what the task or skill calls for and the sequence of the movement. Demonstrations are useful to the learner for assisting in what is to be learned. Additionally, a teacher may describe the act or use movies. During the initial phase, visual perceptions are heavily relied upon. In using visual perception the person organizes and interprets information through the sense of sight. One person watching a demonstration may not perceive what another learner sees. Individuals attend to different stimuli, but all sort out relevant from irrelevant cues. The learner then practices the motor skill according to how the sequence routines were perceived. The length of time it takes to complete this first phase varies according to the complexity of the task. The most important point of this phase is that the learner understands what is to be done; the learner need not do it until the second phase, the practice phase.

Hall (1985) additionally proposed that those with imagery ability can increase success resulting from mental practice. Magill (1989) agrees that mental practice is crucial.

Fixation Stage. Practice is important to fix the performance sequence. Fitts (1965) termed the practice period *fixation phase.* The amount of practice needed, again, varies with task complexity, the capabilities or physical limitations, and past experiences of the learner. The skill level the learner sets will determine how long and how hard he or she will practice. Persons of different ages seem to approach this phase differently. Children practice to see what they can do, often motivated by curiosity. Most children love to practice. Adults tend to want to see results quickly and some desire achievement quickly without much effort (Robb, 1972). It is easier for adults to lose interest and momentum when an aspect of the skill requires much practice or success is long in coming.

Fitts' work is considered to have a great deal of generality, holding for adults and children, retarded and "normal," (Schmidt, 1988, p. 273), and for feet, arms, fingers, underwater, small and large movement.

The selection and processing of stimulus information is important in this stage also. Demonstrations can be used during this stage to refine performance and correct errors. Auditory cues and verbal directions may be more useful than visual stimuli. Time necessary to complete the skill varies with the degree of accuracy or precision needed. If there is a high degree of precision needed, more frequent rest periods are needed. Learning to give oneself an injection will probably take many practice periods whether by an adult or an older child; self-catheterization may also take a child several practice periods. Having several practice periods (distributing the practice) may be chosen when parts can be practiced independently of other parts, for example wrist action for self-injection.

Whether the physical skill is learned as a whole or part by part depends on its complexity. The teacher would analyze the task as to how dependent on each other the various subtasks are. Independent parts may be practiced separately. When one is to take one's own blood pressure, learning mastery of the equipment is involved, including letting the air out of the manometer slowly before practicing applying the cuff, as well as hearing the sounds. Each of these can be practiced as a separate activity, then combined with reading the manometer at the appropriate sounds. It is possible to complicate task completion by separating parts that are dependent on one another. When learning crutch walking, the client may wish to practice the whole sequence before breaking the task into parts. During practice, feedback as to correctness of performance is crucial. Self-analysis tends to be difficult, if not inaccurate, so the teacher's feedback is absolutely necessary for error information. Further modification of responses depends on knowledge of errors made in this phase.

Autonomic Phase. The third phase involves the client's gaining increasing comfort and ease in performing the task and decreasing stress and anxiety. He is quick and consistent with little conscious involvement. Fitts (1965) calls this phase the autonomic phase. The learner no longer needs to put full concentration on performance. Once this phase is reached, few modifications are made. This phase involves a gradual period of time, perhaps years.

A long-standing and important assumption characterizing motor skill learning is that as skills become more and more practiced, they can be performed "automatically." This implies that skills can then be performed without conscious attention. However, current thinking and research has raised the issue of how attention free can motor skills be or is it that there is another process going on here? (Magill, 1989, p. 209).

Cognitive Styles

People approach learning in a variety of ways. Cognitive style refers to the manner in which an individual perceives the world and processes information according to that person's capabilities (Knox, 1986; Arndt & Underwood, 1990). Some people learn best through interacting with other people while some people learn better alone. Some learn a psychomotor skill best by manipulating objects, some by watching, some by listening, and some by reading an instruction manual. Some approach learning tasks methodically, and others use a more intuitive approach. This does not mean that a person only has one cognitive style. Many authors offer detailed explanations of cognitive style dimensions. In fact, there is a large research base. The vast majority of this research has involved children as subjects. Some of the dimensions mentioned in these studies include: (1) impulsivity—reflectiveness, wherein an impulsive responder has quick responses and a reflective responder a more deliberate, slower response. In this situation the impulsive person is quicker but makes more errors; (2) tolerance for incongruous or unrealistic experiences in which some people are more willing than others to vary from conventional experience. Intolerance is revealed by the need for more data before the unusual is accepted; and (3) broad—narrow, in which some people prefer a broad categorization of concepts rather than narrow categories containing few items. Partridge (1984), Cross (1977), Smith & Associates (1990) and Knox (1986) offer detailed descriptions of 9 to 11 different cognitive dimensions. Despite a long history of research, it is not well understood how an individual acquires his or her own unique pattern of styles.

Partridge (1984) describes Kolb's integrated model of learning style, which was developed to measure differences in learning styles along abstract—concrete and action—reflection dimensions. From Kolb's research, four prevalent learning styles were identified. These include (1) the convergers, who prefer abstract conceptualization and active experimentation, are relatively unemotional, and like to deal with things rather than people; (2) the divergers, who are good at generating ideas, tend to be people oriented and emotional, and whose preferences are concrete experiences and reflective observation; (3) the assimilators, who prefer abstract conceptualization and reflective observation, and excel at assimilating diverse items into an integrated whole. They are primarily concerned with abstract concepts and therefore tend to be less concerned with people and the practical application of ideas; and (4) the accommodators, who prefer concrete experiences and active experimentation, are risk takers, are intuitive, and often solve problems through trial and error. It can be seen that individuals with differing styles would be affected by a particular teaching strategy. More recently, Arndt and Underwood (1990) confirmed the usefulness of this categorization.

Knox (1986) points out that some adults with open and flexible approaches achieve better results with discussion, while others with more rigid and structured personality characteristics and learning styles achieve better results with lectures. The range of individual differences in reasoning, problem solving, and cognitive styles tends to increase throughout adulthood. Knox states that although there is not much tested knowledge about adult learning styles, there is some evidence that some adults experience a decrease in deductive reasoning ability beginning in their fifties, but that others achieve outstanding performance. Endorf and McNeff (1991) postulate five types of adult learners, each perceiving his/her role in learning as different.

It is important to note that rates of learning also vary, whether the learner is a child or adult. One patient undergoing preoperative teaching for gall bladder surgery may take much more or less time than another individual having the very same procedure.

Another aspect that bears consideration is the learning-to-learn process. We need to become aware of ourselves as learners. Hammond (1990) describes Maudsley's principles underlying a learning-to-learn activity. The objective is that learners become aware of and take increasing control over previously internalized processes of perception, inquiry, learning, and growth. Effective facilitation of the objective involves: (1) providing a framework for learner search for new meanings; (2) challenging learners by illuminating where current rules, assumptions, and perceptions may be inaccurate and/or dysfunctional; (3) creating opportunities to "reorganize" selves via new self-identified rules; (4) interactive learning situation where the teacher acts as a coach; (5) training in general thinking skills of self-criticisms as well as task-specific skills; and (6) instruction aimed to increasing self-confidence. Other strategies concentrate on (1) memory strategies—for remembering lists, items, vocabulary, etc.; (2) study strategies for specific types of reading, e.g., how to generate questions and summarize while reading; (3) problem-solving skills; and (4) affective support strategies (p. 153).

Several authors point out the importance of strengthening foundations for learning-to-learn as including awareness and understanding of self as learner, the ability to monitor his/her own learning process and to reflect, and, finally, ability to access and use a wide variety of modes, resources, and strategies for learning (Tibbetts, 1991; Kreitlow, 1991). In learning health- or illness-related content, it is helpful if the individual has worked through a general process of learning to learn. More often than not, current effectiveness of people in "learning to learn" is at a beginning point. This means the patient educator may need to build in more general experience before targeting specific health education. Just as smokers need to see themselves as nonsmokers and as sedentary people need to see themselves as active before successful change can occur, patients must see themselves as having the ability to learn.

Implications of Cognitive Structuring for Health Teaching

The implications for nurses in knowing how abstracting develops include the idea that dealing with the concrete before the abstract is crucial. Nurses may present new material in concrete form to facilitate higher abstraction at a later time. The support for this approach is the idea that learners perform better in abstract reasoning tasks when they are thoroughly familiar and comfortable with the factual knowledge needed for that reasoning. The raw materials of facts and data with which to form our conceptualizations are necessary. It follows that in order for thorough conceptualization to occur, memorization of facts or rote learning is required. At the conceptual level, clients often need assistance in seeing relationships among concepts and with comparing and contrasting. For those individuals who have had experience with conceptual learning, transfer to health and illness concepts is easier.

In young children, a factual base may be relatively new, so that material presented should be given in a well-organized manner, slowly, and often repetitiously. In this way the storage of new information is more lasting and more accessible for retrieval. There is a caution, however, in regard to presenting clear and unambiguous information. Clarity is usually helpful in the short run, but it may be better to have some "fuzziness" for the long term. This forces the learner to be more active; it provides experience in selecting important elements. This may put the learner in a better position for generalizing the learning to other situations. Both children and adults can find themselves in situations where they do not know all the relevant facts. Either the information was not stored when first encountered or, although stored, it was not easily retrieved. Obviously, there is a need for an awareness that additional data are needed as well as knowledge of how to seek information.

Better conceptual growth tends to occur when a wide variety of experiences is provided. This means that any single method used exclusively will not be as beneficial as use of different strategies and varied ways of practicing the learning. It is helpful for the teacher to guide the learning. There needs to be a balance between too few demands on the learner and too many. If there are too few, one is not forced into showing oneself what one can do; if there are too many, there is the risk of over structuring or forcing the person into repeated failure. In other words, practice—leading the individual to discovery through concept building and increasing abstraction—is not sufficient by itself. Familiar techniques already mastered can be used initially, then, through explanation, new or higher-level ways of proceeding can speed the rate of learners exploring new and more advanced problem-solving techniques.

Nurses must identify the learning style characteristics of clients and adapt a style appropriate to the specific learner in order to facilitate learning. For example, if a patient prefers learning only the fundamentals and then to be told what to do, but the nurse wants the patient to read extensively and ask questions, there may not be much success in the learning outcome.

HUMANIST PERSPECTIVE

Humanists, although concerned with the mechanics of the cognitive learning process, place more emphasis on the development of selfhood. Learning is viewed as a function of the whole person; "real" learning cannot take place unless both the cognitive and affective areas are involved. Motivation for learning is seen as intrinsic to the individual. Learning is self-initiated, self-evaluated, and, as contrasted with the behavioristic school, not fully subject to environmental controls. There is a focus on self and interpersonal awareness in personal development, as well as creative problem solving and effective information-processing capability.

Central to the consideration of most humanists is the concept of personal autonomy, that is, the individual's capacity for self-determination. Freedom to make choices is a very important consideration. Behavior, then, is largely a consequence of one's own choices, and there is freedom to decide how to react to the environmental stimuli encountered. In other words, individual freedom is cultivated. Words such as self-actualization, self-consistency, self-awareness, self-enhancement, self-acceptance, self-image, self-esteem, self-confidence, self-concept, congruent self, authentic self, and fully functioning self are common in the vocabulary of theorists with this perspective.

The self is seen as the sum total of everything that is distinctively the person: the body, memories, attitudes, potentialities, aspirations, feelings, experiences, and values—whatever distinguishes this person from anyone else. The person is not just seen as a collection of parts, but as the interrelationship of these qualities, characteristics, and experiences that make up this individual human being. The emphasis on the self does not mean selfishness or self-centeredness in the sense of exclusive preoccupation with one's own welfare without consideration for others, but it does mean that the self is at the heart of the person's universe. Self-concept is the personal, subjective impression of who he or she is, and includes feelings about, attitudes toward, and evaluation of oneself, one's ideas, and how one fits into one's world. This perception influences learning. For example, if someone believes he is not smart enough to learn how to inject insulin, it will probably be difficult. If one considers himself capable and loved, behavior change can be facilitated without a prior change in feelings about oneself.

There is not just one humanistic perspective. The names Carl Rogers, Abraham Maslow, Arthur Combs, Victor Frankl, Sidney Jourard, John Dewey, Sidney Simon, Howard Kirschenbaum, and Louis Raths are all names associated with this perspective. But there are some differences among them, as was true with the behaviorist and information-processing theorists.

Lafrancois (1988) has summarized the main purposes of humanistic education as emphasizing:

> Healthy social and personal development, and at the same time deemphasizing rigorous performance-oriented, test-dominated approaches to subject matter . . . providing students with experiences of success rather than failure, orientation toward discovery rather than receptive learning. The humanistic view of human functioning accepts individuals for what they are, respects their feelings and aspirations and holds that every individual has the right to self-determination (p. 130).

There is a commitment on the part of the teacher that one is free to learn what one wants to, when one wants to, because one wants to, and a trust in the capacity for developing one's own potential.

To transfer this to health and illness care settings, there is the self-care education perspective, which derives from the client's perceived needs and preferences, regardless of whether they conform to the professional's perceptions of client needs. Both the content and process assist in shifting control in health decision making from the professional to the clients. Independence and self-responsibility are fostered, that is, there is more foundation and more responsibility. Illich (1976) and Pelletier (1979) are two powerful writers on the importance of self-responsibility for health. The most important component of Ardell's high-level wellness model is self-responsibility.

There are various self-concept models available to help put the individual in touch with feelings and values so as to become self-directing. Self-concept development involves both discovering what the person values and how he or she can live in a manner consistently reflecting those values.

The values clarification model facilitates the ability to clarify values, that to a humanist, are integral to the self-concept. The basic elements of this model originated with John Dewey in the 1940s in *How We Think*. During the 1960s, Simon, Raths, and Kirschenbaum, as well as others, developed a method that can be used in health learning. In the past 15 years, there have been many applications of this model. This approach focuses on processes used by clients to arrive at value judgments consistent with their own intellectual, moral, and social structure. It is not concerned with the value judgment itself, but with clarification of an individual's own moral, ethical, or social relationships, leading to more self-understanding and clarity. Briefly, learners indicate whether they chose the value freely, considered alternatives, considered consequences, whether they prized or cherished the choice, affirmed the choice to others, acted on the choice, and whether the choice was incorporated into their life style. The appropriate use of values clarification results in increased self-responsibility with the teacher as facilitator. A more detailed description of this model is given in Chapter 7.

Kirschenbaum (1976) has a slightly different, but compatible, way of looking at the valuing process. He includes five components: thinking, feeling, choosing and decision making, communication, and acting. The thinking component involves all activities that promote more effective reasoning. The feeling component involves learning to deal with feelings and developing a stronger self-concept. Choosing and decision making include skills in setting goals, gathering information, generating and considering possibilities and their consequences. The communication component involves the ability to send clear messages, listen actively, and resolve conflict. The acting component includes behaving consistently and skillfully on the basis of values. Ford, Trygstad-Durland, and Nelms (1979) have cited ten research studies supporting the usefulness of values clarification in leading to greater self-esteem, self-direction, cognitive achievement, and decision making. In summary, although individual values differ, it is possible for each person to be clear about them, and to respect values held by others.

Psychologist Carl Rogers' (1951) self-directed model can also be used in client teaching. The nondirective model was developed from the work of Rogers and others advocating nondirective counseling. The primary goal involves client reorganization of the inner self for greater personal integration, effectiveness, and realistic self-appraisal. For this to happen, the learning environment must be one of warmth, openness, acceptance, and trust. With this environment, opportunities for learning can be facilitated and freedom enhanced. Clients assume responsibility for their own learning. In this process, values are reexamined. It is not necessary for learners to change, but to understand that personal values are important so that clients can direct their own learning. A facilitator believes that the client who sees relevant problems will want to learn, to grow, to discover, to create, to become self-disciplined.

One of the fathers of the human potential movement and the use of the affective realm in learning, Carl Rogers is well known for the idea that the learner is the only person who can define goals for learning and take responsibility for them. He stated: "It seems to me that anything that can be taught to another is relatively inconsequential, and has little or no significant influence on behavior . . . I have come to feel that the only learning which significantly influences behavior is self-discovered, self-appropriated learning" (1961, p. 276).

Rogers' ideas include a rationale for self-directed learning. He sees the goals of self-directed learning as a "fully functioning person," which he describes as a person in touch and open with his feelings and inner being:

> Such a person experiences in the present with immediacy. He is able to live in his feelings and reactions of the moment. He is not bound by the structure of his past learnings but these are a resource for him insofar as they relate to the experience of

the moment. He lives freely, subjectively, in an existential confrontation with this movement in life. . . . It seems to me that the clients who have moved most significantly in therapy live more intimately with their feelings of pain, but also more vividly with their feelings of ecstasy; that anger is more clearly felt, but so also is life; that fear is an experience that they know more deeply, but so is courage; and the reason they can live more fully in a wider range is that they have this underlying confidence in themselves as trustworthy instruments for encountering life . . . (Rogers, 1962, p. 31)

Rogers sees fully functioning people as those:

. . . who are able to take a self-initiated action to be responsible for those actions; who are capable of intelligent choice and self-direction, who are critical learners, able to evaluate the contributions made by others; who have acquired knowledge relevant to the solution of problems; who, even more importantly, are able to adapt flexibly and intelligently to new problem situations; who have internalized an adaptive mode of approach to problems, utilizing all pertinent experience freely and creatively; who are able to cooperate effectively with others in these various activities; who work, not for the approach of others, but in terms of their own socialized purposes. (Rogers, 1951, pp. 387–388)

Rogers' view of self-directed learning involves two basic steps. The first step is for the teacher–facilitator to create a climate of trust and openness in which self-direction can occur. The second step is for the individual or group to work out a self-directed plan. He sees this approach as useful for both children and adults. The teacher does not dominate or control the teaching situation but lets unfolding occur. With the teacher having "realness," respect for each person, and "empathy," the overall learning climate will be set.

More recently, Bille (1987) advocates using the humanistic model for patient and family education. This author values patients and families as co-participants in the decision-making process throughout their hospital stays. Their feelings of self-worth are maintained, their self system is enhanced, and patient and family education becomes more cost effective and cost efficient (p. 65). Thus Bille is promoting a humanistic approach for shared decision making and generating reciprocal respect for individual dignity. Koontz, Cox, and Hastings (1991) have wonderfully illustrated how they incorporate a humanistic approach to patient and family psychoeducation. This is done by enabling the nursing staff to participate more fully in patient treatment and discharge planning. Johnson and Morse (1990) found in their study of patient adjustment experiences postmyocardial infarction that regaining a sense of personal control can be aided through health providers' use of a humanistic approach.

SELF-CARE AND SELF-EFFICACY THEORISTS

Self-care means care performed by oneself for oneself, upon reaching a state of maturity whereby he/she can take consistent control in health situations. The central idea is that self-care is a learned behavior that can purposely regulate one's functioning. Patient teaching is the primary intervention used by nurses to promote self-care (Oberst, 1989). Orem's (1985) self-care model is particularly relevant to patient teaching.

Woods (1989) analyzed the major conceptual orientations underlying the empirical work published on self-care from 1980 to 1988. She points out that although self-care has been a part of family life since very early times and that the term at first glance seems simple and straightforward, it is complex.

Orem's (1980, 1985) model proposes three types of self-care: universal, developmental, and health deviation self-care. Universal self-care is associated with life processes and maintenance of the integrity of human structures, functions, and general well-being. Developmental processes are conditions and events that occur at various stages of the life cycle. Health deviation self-care arises from genetic and constitutional defects and human structural and functional deviations and their effects. As well, Orem introduced the concept of self-care agency, which means the extent to which the individual can provide his/her own self-care. Agency means the decisions and actions needed to carry out self-care. Orem herself related self-care requisites, agency, and deficits to three types of nursing systems. One of these systems promotes the development of self-care skills. Patient and client teaching are included here and are based on the client's control over his health situation and choices inherent in this control. The nursing role is to help the patient/client decrease his dependency by encouraging self-care activities. Frey and Denyes (1989) tested Orem's theory with a group of adolescents with diabetes mellitus, concluding there was support for relationships among universal and health deviation self-care concepts. Gast et al (1989) reviewed several instruments that have been developed to measure self-care agency, finding that most instrument development is at an early developmental stage. These authors profile those individuals engaging in self-care as: mobile with sufficient energy and knowledge to participate in self-care, having a repertoire of self-care skills, and the ability to reason, solve problems, and make decisions about self-care. These individuals must value health and be motivated to engage in self-care (1989, p. 37). Conn (1991) examined self-care behaviors of 160 older adults regarding their beliefs of care when ill with influenza or colds. Many of these elderly were found to engage in high levels of self-responsibility.

Self-care and self-efficacy are related terms. Self-efficacy is the belief that one can respond effectively to a situation by using available skills, and the belief that he/she can actually implement a skill. The more capable and confident the individual feels about performing health-related activity—the more likely the individual will proceed with behavior change. Redman (1985) now believes that self-efficacy theory may be a useful fresh approach for improving learning outcomes. As Egan (1990) says, self-efficacy is the opposite of passivity. Bandura (1977) has suggested that persons' expectations of themselves have much to do with their willingness to put forth effort for changing behavior. According to Bandura (1977), the primary resources needed for goal accomplishment result from past personal experience in mastering a skill, modeling behavior, persuasion, and physiological state.

These four sources all have implications in patient education. The first, physiological states, involves judging capability or strength for participating in behavioral change, very high anxiety, fatigue, and pain often indicate physical inefficacy.

In illness states, coping styles often provide clues to illness reactions. For example, initial adjustment carried on too long can immobilize patients. Various physiological and psychosocial interventions can be used to reduce high intensity feeling states so that self-care activities can be initiated.

Verbal persuasion involves influencing patients to believe in their capabilities to achieve the behavior change. How verbal persuasion is used would vary with the teaching situation, ranging from little to a great deal.

Vicarious experience involves observing others. Some relate that people, who have little information on which to base their rating of self-efficacy competence, stand to gain the most from vicarious experience. For patients in ICUs, seeing other patients improve and be discharged may increase self-efficacy (Merritt, 1989). Performance attainment is actively experiencing mastering a learning task. Simpler tasks would be achieved first; changes in self-efficacy would then be assessed, and expectations increased, and the cycle repeated.

A self-efficacy framework has been tested in several recent studies in diverse ways, for many individual and groups for life style changes. Merritt (1989) illustrates how a self-efficacy framework can be used in intensive care units. Utz (1990) describes a rating scale developed by the author for use in assessing self-efficacy features. Utz et al. (1990) use a self-efficacy framework in looking at body image and health in a sample of mitral valve prolapse patients.

Empowerment

Empowerment is a word that has come into common usage in the 1990s; a term that fits well with self-efficacy and self-care. Empowerment is an interactive process of cultivating the power in others through the sharing of knowledge, expertise, and resources (Funnell, 1990, p. 41). The term is consistent with the teaching process as described throughout this book—that involving mutual decision making at many points. The philosophy is that patients are active partners in their care. Girdano (1987) phrases the definition of empowerment slightly differently by saying that empowerment is knowing who you are and what you can do. It is self-awareness, self-understanding, self-efficacy, self-esteem, self-regard, self-love, and self-respect all rolled into a self-concept leading to self-actualization or a fully functioning person (p. 17). The idea is that one cannot empower someone else. Some see this concept as akin to internal locus of control. Anderson and Genthner (1990) identified five levels of self-responsibility in a guide for use in assessing the level of self-responsibility in a patient. The levels range from the lowest level whereby patients are overwhelmed by their disease (e.g., diabetes) and perceive themselves as hopeless and helpless victims, on up to the highest level, where patients accept their diabetes (disease) as a fact of life and take responsibility for their psychological and behavioral responses (p. 270). More details about the levels can be found in the article.

Girdano (1987) mentions the tremendous usefulness of empowerment experimental programs for alcoholics, drug dependents, battered women, abused children, and overweight individuals (p. 17). In these programs, problem-solving and risk-taking activities are delved into, as well as postactivity processing. The postactivity process is very important for internalizing what was learned about the self. Miller (1983) purports that empowerment strategies are specific to the individual, while listing broad types of strategies used, such as (1) modifying the environment, (2) helping patients set realistic goals, (3) increasing patient knowledge, (4) increased sensitivity of health team members and significant others to the imposed powerlessness, and (5) encouraging verbalization of feelings (p. 273). Noah (1990) describes a patient-controlled analgesia (PCA) program in which patients felt less helpless, a feeling of well-being, and using up to a third less medication than patients receiving intramuscular medications.

In summary, empowerment strategies can encompass the cognitive, affective, and psychomotor learning domains. Patient education designed to empower clients is far different from patient education meant to enhance compliance treatment goals. Finally, Smith and Associates (1990) say that no comprehensive program of learning can be complete if it fails to address issues of personal empowerment, including limitations imposed by society on such empowerment (p. 51).

Through empowerment, patients gain mastery over their overall health.

IMPLICATIONS OF THEORETICAL VIEW

These three schools of theories are not mutually exclusive although each represents a distinctive approach to learning, and debates may ensue as to the advantages of one approach over another. It is not necessary to adopt one theory to the exclusion of another, appropriate for different times and circumstances. It is possible to select elements of each theory useful in client teaching. All clients grow with success and do better when achievements are recognized and reinforced. Learning can be encouraged by respecting the "whole client" in a supportive learning environment. Learning can also be fostered through structuring content and its presentation into meaningful segments with appropriate feedback.

As far as what is now known, clients learn in different ways, at various rates, and with differing degrees of accuracy. Combinations of factors such as age, developmental level, intelligence, adaptability, creativity, motivation, locus of control, interpretative skills, and general personality contribute to configurations of learning styles so that no two people learn in exactly the same way. No knowledge base is presently available for using one or another learning theory for specific categories of clients, though very few clients can profit from only one way. What is important is that some clients will be more productive in learning in some environments than others, and the nurse needs to consider varied factors. Knowledge of the characteristics by which clients learn provides a nurse with the basis for identifying approaches with which clients are most or least comfortable. Teaching can increase the likelihood that the client will change in certain ways.

Behavioral changes for promotion of health, prevention of illness, or those required by illness itself can range from very specific procedures to major life changes, including changed self-concepts. Individuals differ in the amount of self-direction apparent for making the changes that affect their health. Once theoretical

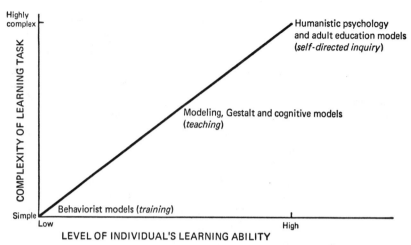

Figure 4–2. Relationship between teaching models and the learning situation. *(From Knowles, M. The adult learner: A neglected species. Copyright © 1973 by Gulf Publishing Company, Houston, Tex. Used with permission. All rights reserved.)*

viewpoints are considered, teaching can progress much further than information giving, which might be quite narrow in scope.

Knowles' (1973) model of the relationship among the three theoretical viewpoints nicely summarizes the idea that different theories of learning are appropriate for different kinds of learning. The level of complexity of the learning task, as well as the individual's learning ability, interact for determining the appropriateness of each approach. Knowles' model (Fig. 4–2) indicates that for simple learning/training, a behaviorist model may be appropriate; with a more complex learning task, a cognitive model would work more appropriately, and that a highly complex learning situation would call for a humanist/self-directed approach. Hill (1971) points out that the various learning theories have two chief values. One is in providing us with a vocabulary and conceptual framework for interpreting the examples of learning that we observe. These are valuable for anyone who is alert to the surrounding world. The other, closely related, is in suggesting where to look for solutions to practical problems. The theories do not give us solutions, but they do direct our attention to those variables that are crucial in finding solutions.

Theorists from differing perspectives at times criticize each other. Humanism has been accused by behaviorists of assuming that all clients are eager to learn, when the behaviorist does not view this as true. Behaviorists have been criticized for ignoring the motivation provided by curiosity and by removing the objectives of learning from the learner. Rogers and Skinner specifically have admitted they do not see eye to eye in most of their learning assumptions. (Rogers, 1969; chap. 18; Skinner, 1973).

TABLE 4–2. COMPARISON OF TRADITIONAL AND EMPOWERING EDUCATIONAL MODELS

Traditional Medical Model	Empowering Person-Centered Model
1. Diabetes is a physical illness.	1. Diabetes is a biopsychosocial illness.
2. Relationship of provider and patient is authoritarian based on provider expertise.	2. Relationship of provider and patient is democratic and based on shared expertise.
3. Problems and learning needs are usually identified by professional.	3. Problems and learning needs are usually identified by patient.
4. Professional is viewed as problem solver and caregiver, i.e., professional responsible for diagnosis, treatment, and outcome.	4. Patient is viewed as problem solver and caregiver, i.e., professional acts as a resource and both share responsibility for treatment and outcome.
5. Goal is compliance with recommendations. Behavioral strategies are used to increase compliance with recommended treatment. A lack of compliance is viewed as a failure of patient and provider.	5. Goal is to enable patients to make informed choices. Behavioral strategies are used to help patients change behaviors of their choosing. A lack of goal achievement is viewed as feedback and used to modify goals and strategies.
6. Behavior changes are externally motivated.	6. Behavior changes are internally motivated.
7. Patient is powerless, professional is powerful.	7. Patient and professional are powerful.

Funnell, M. M., Anderson, R. M., Arnold, M. S., et al. Empowerment: An idea whose time has come in diabetes education. The Diabetes Educator, *1990, 17 (1), 37–41.*

SUMMARY

The teaching perspectives identified in this chapter can be viewed from three points of view, reflecting different attitudes toward learning. There are situations in health teaching appropriate for transmission of relevant knowledge with the teacher initiating and directing learning. Other situations require teaching problem-solving skills, and others the process of valuing. For a nurse to use the different purposes of teaching, she must understand the different classes of theories of learning. Table 4–2 shows a comparison of two models of patient teaching. The remainder of the chapters in this unit relate to application strategies.

REFERENCES AND READINGS

Anderson, R. M., & Genthner, R. W. A guide for assessing a patient's level of personal responsibility for diabetes management. *Patient Education and Counseling,* 1990, *16,* 269–279.

Ardell, D. A. *High level wellness.* Emmaus, Pa: Rodale Press, 1978.

Arndt, M. S., & Underwood, B. Learning style theory and patient education. *The Journal of Continuing Education in Nursing*, 1990, *21*(1), 28–31.

Ausubel, D. Educational psychology: A cognitive view. New York: Holt, Rinehart and Winston, 1968.

Bandura, A. Influence of model's reinforcement contingencies on the acquisition of initiative responses. *Journal of Personality and Social Psychology.* 1965, *1*, 589–595.

Bandura, A. Analysis of modeling processes. In A. Bandura (Ed.), *Psychological modeling.* Chicago: Adline 1971.

Bandura, A. The self and mechanisms of agency. In Jerry Suls (Ed.). Psychological perspective on the self. Lawrence Eribaum Assoc., Hillsdale, MD: 1982, 3–39.

Bandura, A. Self-efficacy mechanism in human agency. *American Psychologist*, 1982, 37.

Bandura, A., & Adams, N. E. Analysis of self-efficacy theory of behavioral change. *Cognitive Therapy and Research*, 1977, *1*, 287–308.

Bigge, M. L. *Learning theories of teachers* (4th ed.). New York: Harper & Row, 1982.

Bille, D. A. Locus of Decision Making in Patient and Family Education: Its effect on promoting wellness. *Nursing Administration Quarterly* Spring 1987, 62–65.

Bloom, B. S. *Taxonomy of education objectives: Handbook I: Cognitive domain.* New York: Longman, Green, 1956.

Bruner, J. S. On cognitive growth. II. In J. S. Bruner, P. Oliver, and P. Greenfield (Eds.), *Studies in cognitive growth.* New York: Wiley, 1966.

Carnevali, D. L. Conceptualizing: Storage of knowledge for diagnosis and management. In P. H. Mitchell, & A. Loustaue, (Eds.), *Concepts basic to nursing* (3rd ed.), New York: McGraw-Hill, 1981, pp. 207–219.

Claxton, C. S., & Ralston, Y. *Learning styles: Their impact on teaching and administration.* AAHE/ERIC Higher Education Research Report No. 10, American Association for Higher Education, Washington, D.C., 1978.

Conn, V. Self-care action taken by older adults for influenza and colds. *Nursing Research*, 1991, *40*, 3, 176–181.

Cross, K. O. *Accent on learning.* San Francisco: Jossey-Bass, 1977.

DiMateo, M. R. *The psychology of health, illness, and medical care.* Pacific Grove, CA: Brooks/Cole Publishing Co., 1991.

Egan, G. *The skilled helper.* (4th Ed.). Pacific Grove, CA: Brooks/Cole Publishing Co, 1990.

Endorf, F. M., & McNoff, M. The adult learner: Five types. *Adult Learning*, May 1991, 20.

Fitts, P. M. Factors in complex skill training. In R. Glasser (Ed), *Training research and education.* New York: Wiley, 1965, pp. 177–197.

Ford, J. G. Trystad-Durland, L. N., & Nelms, B. C. *Applied decision making for nurses.* St. Louis: C. V. Mosby, 1979.

Frey, M. A., & Denyes, M. J. Health and illness self-care in adolescents with IDDM: A test of Orem's theory. *Advances in Nursing Science*, 1989, *12*, 1, 67–75.

Funnell, M. M., Anderson, R. M., Arnold, M. S. et al. Empowerment: An idea whose time has come in diabetes education. *The Diabetes Educator*, 1990, *17*, 1, 37–41.

Gagné, R. M. *Essentials of learning of instruction.* Hinsdale, Ill.: Dryden Press, 1974.

Gast, H. L., Denyes, M. J., Campbell, J. C. et al. Self-care agency: Conceptualizations and Operationalizations. *Advances in Nursing Science*, 1989, *12*, 1, 26–28.

Girdano, D. A., & Dusek, D. E. *Changing health behavior.* Scottsdale, Arizona: Gorsuch Scarisbrick Publishers, 1987.

Gobble, D., & Mullen, K. Relationships between wellness role modeling and professional training in health education. *Journal of High Level Wellness,* May/June 1983, *7*(3), 19–24.

Green, L. W. Should health education abandon attitude change strategies? Perspectives from recent research. *Health Education Monographs,* 1970, *30,* 25–48.

Hall, C. A. Pongrac, J., & Bucholz, E. The measurement of imagery ability. *Human Movement Science,* 1985, *4,* 107–118.

Hammond, D. Designing and facilitating learning to learn activities. In Smith R. M. Assoc., *Learning to learn across the life span.* San Francisco: Jossey-Bass Publisher, 1990.

Hill, W. F. *Learning: A survey of psychological interpretations.* Scranton: Chandler Publishing Co., 1971.

Huckabay, L. M. D. *Conditions of learning and instruction in learning.* St. Louis: C. V. Mosby, 1980.

Illich, I. *Medical nemesis.* New York: Bantam Books, 1976.

Johnson, S. L., & Morse, J. M. Regaining control: A process of adjustment after myocardial infarction. *Heart and Lung,* 1990, *19*(2), 126–135.

Joyce, B., & Weil, M. *Models of teaching* (3rd ed.). Englewood Cliff, N.J.: Prentice-Hall, 1986.

Kirschenbaum, H. Clarifying values clarification: Some theoretical issues, a review of research. *Group and Organizational Studies,* 1976, *1,* (99, 100), 102–114.

Knowles, M. *The adult learner: A neglected species.* Houston: Gulf Publishing Co., 1973.

Knox, A. B. *Helping adults learn.* San Francisco: Jossey-Bass, 1986.

Kogan, N. Categorizing and conceptualizing styles in younger and older adults. *Human Development,* 1974, *7,* 218–230.

Kolesnick, W. B. *Humanism and/or behaviorism in the classroom.* Boston: Allyn & Bacon, 1975.

Koontz, E., Cox, D., and Hastings, S. Implementing a Short-Term Family Support Group. *Journal of Psychosocial Nursing,* 1991, 29, *5,* 5–9.

Kreitlow, B. Adult learners. *Adult Learning,* May 1991, 7.

Lafrancois, G. R. *Psychology for teaching* (6th ed.). Wadsworth Publishing Co., Belmont, Calif: 1988.

Magill, R. A. *Motor learning: concepts and applications* (3rd ed.). Dubuque, Iowa: William Brown Publishing, 1989.

McKibbin, M., Weil, M., & Joyce, B. *Teaching and learning: Demonstration of alternatives.* Washington, D.C.: Association of Teacher Educators, 1977.

Melton, A. W. *Categories of human learning.* New York: Academic Press, 1964.

Merritt, S. L. Patient self-efficacy: A framework for designing patient education. *Focus on Critical Care,* 1989, *16*(1), 68–73.

Miller, J. F. *Coping with chronic illness: Overcoming powerlessness.* Philadelphia: F. A. Davis Publishing Company, 1983.

Moursund, J. P. *Learning and the learner.* Monterey, Calif: Brooks/Cole Publishing Co., 1976.

Mulhollan, F., & Forisha, B. E. *Skinner to Rogers: Contrasting approaches to education.* Lincoln, Neb.: Professional Educators Publication, 1972.

Noah, V. A. Pre-op teaching is the key to PCA success. *RN,* March 1990, 60–64.

Obersk, M. T. Perspectives in Research in Patient Teaching. *Nursing Clinics of North America.* 1989 24(*3*) 621–627.

O'Leary, A. Self-efficacy and health. *Behavior Research Theory,* 1985, *23,* 437–451.

O'Neil, H. F., & Spielberg, C. D. *Cognitive and affective learning strategies.* New York: Academic Press, 1979.

Orem, D. E. Nursing: Concepts of practice (2nd Ed.). New York: McGraw Hill Publishing Co., 1980.

Orem, D. E. *Nursing: Concepts of practice* (3rd Ed.). New York: McGraw-Hill Publishing Co., 1985.

Partridge, R. Learning styles: A review of selected models. In R. deTornyay (Ed.), *Successful methods of teaching for the nurse educator.* Thorogore, N.J.: Charles B. Slack, 1984, pp. 3–9.

Pellitier, K. R. *Holistic medicine.* New York: Dell Publishing Co., 1979.

Redman, B. K. New areas of theory development and practice in patient education. *Journal of Advanced Nursing,* 1985, *10,* 425–428.

Robb, M. D. *The dynamics of motor skill acquisition.* Englewood Cliffs: N.J.: Prentice-Hall, 1972.

Rogers, C. R. *Client centered therapy.* Boston: Houghton Mifflin, 1951.

Rogers, C. R. *On becoming a person.* Boston: Houghton Mifflin, 1961.

Rogers, C. R. Toward becoming a fully functioning person. *Perceiving, behaving, becoming.* Association for supervision and Curriculum Development Yearbook. Washington, D.C.: National Educational Association, 1962.

Rogers, C. R. *Freedom to learn.* Columbus, Ohio: Chas. E. Merrill, 1969.

Rosenbaum, D. A. *Human motor control.* San Diego: Academic Press, Inc., The Harcourt Brace—Jovanovich, 1991.

Ross, H. S., & Mico, P. R. Theory and Practice in health education. Palo Alto, Calif: Mayfield Publishing Co., 1980.

Salmon, A. W. Motor skill learning. In *Human Skills* (2nd ed.). Edited by D. H. Holding. NY: John Wiley and Sons, 1989.

Schmidt, R. A. *Motor control and learning human* (2nd ed.). Champaign, Ill.: Human Kinetics Publishers., Inc., 1988.

Skinner, B. F. *Science and human behavior.* New York: Macmillan, 1953.

Skinner, B. F. Humanism and behaviors. In P. Kertz, *The humanist alternative.* Buffalo, N.Y.: Prometheus Books, 1973, pp. 98–105.

Smith, R. M. & Associates. *Learning to learn across the lifespan.* San Francisco, Ca.: Jossey-Bass Publishers, 1990.

Tibbetts, C. G. Adult learners: *Adult Learning,* May 1991, 9.

Utz, S. W. Motivating selfcare: A nursing approach. *Holistic Nursing Practice,* 1990, *4*(2), 13–21.

Utz, S. W., Hammer, J., Whitmire, V. M. et al. Perceptions of body image and health in persons with mitral valve prolapse. *Image,* 1990, *22*(1), 18–22.

Woods, N. Conceptualizations of self-care: Toward health oriented models. *Advances in Nursing Science,* 1989, *12*(1), 1–13.

Teaching and Learning Variables: A Holistic Perspective

Health teaching and nursing care in general are greatly influenced by variables in the practice environment. The practice environment is a broad arena that includes the physical, psychosocial, and other variables related to teaching and learning. When the practice environment is perceived in its broadest dimension, there is increased understanding of a client's health behavior, new strategies become available, and interventions may be more successful than if the focus of practice is exclusively client centered (Killien, 1985).

Unit II presents various dimensions of environmental awareness required in nursing practice.

5

The Environment

Barbara A. Graham

Most of us are relatively insensitive to our physical and social environments, and even less attuned to the personal spaces around us which vastly affect our health and well being.

(Ardell, 1977)

Environmental factors may facilitate or impede the teaching and learning process. Many nurses have witnessed a teaching activity marred by distractions in the environment. Even a well-conceived teaching plan designed by a skilled teacher can go awry if there is insufficient attention to the surroundings. In a teaching context, the environment encompasses physical, psychosocial, and related variables. These variables are an integral part of the teaching/learning plan.

VARIABLES IN THE PHYSICAL ENVIRONMENT

An important aspect of the teaching-learning environment is the adequacy of the physical surroundings. Health-teaching activities are often carried out under less than ideal conditions. A carefully developed lesson plan can be interrupted by distracting sights, noises, and odors. An otherwise well-planned teaching session can be marred by inadequate seating arrangements and crowded surroundings. In many instances, these distractions might have been avoided by a more thorough assessment prior to the teaching session. When possible, the physical surroundings are assessed in advance and an alternative setting is identified. An optimal learning environment includes the following: adequate space to accommodate the number of clients in the group and to allow for free movement about the room; safety features such as handrails and nonskid flooring for clients using wheelchairs, crutches, or walkers; an adequate number of comfortable chairs that are appropriate to the particular age group. Chairs must be checked ahead of time for comfort and proper functioning. If the learners are expected to take notes or need working space, desks or tables must be accessible. Another consideration is whether the room is appropriate for the activities planned. If an objective of the teaching session is group participation and discussion, chairs can be arranged in a circle or semicircle so that eye contact is easily made and communication facilitated. Arranging chairs in rows facing the teacher suggests a lecture format and perhaps the expectation of little input from group members. The room must have adequate lighting without glare or bright spots produced by the sun or an outside light source. The use of shades, blinds, and dimmer switches can control unwanted light (Van Hoozen, 1989). If activities require participants to read small print or to learn to operate a glucometer, for example, adequate lighting is essential. A magnifying glass and a pen light or flashlight are helpful for extra lighting and when reading small numbers and gauges. There must be a balance in brightness between the practice area and the area adjoining it with the task areas being twice as bright as the non-bright areas.

Audiovisual equipment must be checked prior to use, with replacement light bulbs and batteries readily available. The quality of films, slides, and other audiovisual media declines with use and can interfere with learning. Education materials must be updated and replaced when appropriate.

In planning a teaching session in an outpatient clinic, noise levels and room temperature is assessed in advance. In warm and humid weather, teaching can be scheduled for more comfortable times of the day, such as mornings and evenings. Nurses are aware that children and adults may be more alert in cool rather than warm room temperatures but that older adults may be less comfortable in a cool environment. In the event that building temperatures are too warm, the teaching session may be moved to an alternative site. It is important to orient clients to the physical facilities. Being made aware of entrances, exits, and the location of restrooms and other key areas will help clients be comfortable in the surroundings.

A room that is a designated teaching area can be made attractive and appealing. Hanging colorful pictures and wall posters will create a cheerful atmosphere. Ensuring that the teaching area is clean, waste baskets emptied, furniture arranged neatly without litter and clutter will also enhance the physical environment.

VARIABLES IN THE PSYCHOSOCIAL ENVIRONMENT

Equally important in health teaching is the psychosocial environment. Nurses may not have the advantage of extended contact with those they teach. Realistically, there will be occasions when only one teaching session is possible. Given these circumstances and to maximize learning the environment must receive special attention. Four basic characteristics of an environment conducive to learning have been described by Knowles (1980). They are: (1) respect for personality, (2) freedom of expression and availability of information, (3) participation in decision making, and (4) mutuality of responsibility in planning, setting goals, and evaluating activities. To accomplish the first, the atmosphere must be open and accepting. Clients are introduced and called by name. Personal recognition fosters a sense of self-worth and helps to create a feeling of mutual support and respect. The second characteristic is freedom to ask questions and share information. This is important in any teaching and learning interaction. An exchange of ideas between clients and the nurse-teacher can correct misinformation, provide feedback, and facilitate problem solving. Client participation in all phases of teaching and learning is encouraged. Nurses are alert to the clients' level of anxiety and the extent to which this may inhibit learning. An anxious client, or one who is in pain, may show a lack of interest and inattention, which is a cue to postpone the session. The nurse sets the emotional tone for the teaching session. Feelings about a client or the client's health condition can color the interpersonal environment and affect the ability of the nurse to connect emotionally with the client. Unrecognized feelings can create a barrier to the interpersonal environment that is essential for professional relationships (Arnold & Boggs, 1989).

RELATED VARIABLES IN THE ENVIRONMENT

Despite the large number of nurses in clinical practice and their high degree of patient-client contact, one cannot assume that health-teaching activities receive high priority status. First, nurses' involvement in health teaching will be limited unless they perceive it to be an integral part of their role. Nurses' perceptions are greatly influenced by the emphasis placed on health teaching during their educational preparation, *and* the extent to which they feel qualified to perform as a health teacher. Pohl's classic study revealed that many nurses do not feel they are educationally prepared to teach (1969). Although Pohl conducted her study in the late 1960s, there still are nursing education programs that may require students to teach but offer little theoretical content in teaching and learning. Gleit and Graham's (1984) national survey of health education content in baccalaureate nursing programs revealed that a student's exposure to teaching and learning concepts is often limited to general nursing textbooks such as medical-surgical and community health nursing textbooks. It is doubtful that the authors of these textbooks intended them to be major sources of health-teaching content. It would seem more educationally sound for students to be exposed to a number of different reading sources and specifically to those that emphasize the process as well as the content of teaching. Consistently planned experiences promote health teaching as a role expectation.

Another environmental consideration is the extent to which health-teaching activities are supported and rewarded. Although health teaching is cited in the American Nurses' Association Standards of Practice and the Patient's Bill of Rights, teaching efforts may not be as highly valued as other nursing functions. The quantity and quality of health teaching may be affected by staffing patterns, job descriptions, promotion criteria, and administrative support. If there is a staffing shortage, patient education may be compromised more than other services. When there is limited staffing, there may not be an alternative plan for carrying out health-teaching responsibilities. In a hospital setting, there are usually fewer staff during the evenings, weekends, and holidays. This may mean that health teaching must be accomplished at other times. An important consideration is for health-teaching responsibilities to be covered regardless of staffing inconsistencies.

Teaching activities must be clearly delineated in promotion criteria. Job descriptions and evaluations must make clear who is responsible for health teaching. For example, does the presence of a patient educator strengthen the overall health-teaching component *or* is there a tendency for staff to abdicate their teaching responsibilities? The establishment of policies and procedures related to patient education help to underscore the necessity of administrative support for patient teaching. Policies must clearly state the personnel responsible for this role.

Another consideration in the health-teaching environment is the extent to which the economy and the existing political climate support preventive health measures. Economic down turns can result in funded programs being totally eliminated or sharply curtailed. Unfortunately, when funding is reduced, health education may be one of the first activities to be curtailed. But gains have been made. Interest in health promotion and health education remains at a high level. The impetus for this movement was generated by Public Health Policy initiatives such as Healthy People and the 1990 Objectives for the Nation. These objectives and the more recently formulated Objectives for the Year 2000 clearly delineate the health gains to be made in different age groups across the life span from infancy to older adults. Achieving these national goals depends to a large degree on a knowledgeable and concerned public.

Many excellent health education materials are available. Nurses must be knowledgeable about health resources on the national, state, and local levels. Keeping abreast of new developments in the field and attending health education conferences and workshops will also add to the repertoire of a nurse teacher. Developing a network of nurses to serve as resources and as a support group is also beneficial.

SUMMARY

Environmental factors may facilitate or impede learning. Teaching efforts are more likely to be successful if attention is given to the learning environment. Adequate physical surroundings as well as a comfortable and nonthreatening atmosphere will allow learners to direct their energies to the activities at hand. Other variables in the environment such as administrative support and the nurse's perceptions of the teaching role greatly influence the quality and quantity of health teaching.

REFERENCES AND READINGS

Anderson, C. *Patient teaching and communicating in an information age.* Albany, N.Y.: Delmar Publishers, 1990.
Ardell, D. G. *High level wellness.* Emmaus, Pa.: Rodale Press, 1977.

Arnold, E., & Boggs, K. *Interpersonal relationships: Professional communication skills for nurses.* Philadelphia: W. B. Saunders, 1989.

Darkenwald, G. G. Enhancing the adult classroom environment. In E. R. Hayes (Ed.)., *Effective teaching styles.* San Francisco: Jossey-Bass, Inc., Publishers, 1989.

Dittmar, S. Rehabilitation. *Nursing process and application.* St. Louis: C. V. Mosby Company, 1989.

Gleit, C. J., & Graham, B. A. Preparation of nurses for the teaching role. *Journal of Patient Education and Counseling,* 1984, *6*(1), 25–28.

Killien, M. G. An environmental approach to nursing practice. In J. E. Hall & B. R. Weaver (Eds.), *Distributive nursing practice: A systems approach to community health* (2nd ed.). Philadelphia: Lippincott, 1985, p. 259.

Knowles, M. *The modern practice of adult education.* Chicago: Association Press, Follett Publishing Company, 1980.

Pohl, M. L. Teaching activities of the nurse practitioner. *Nursing Research,* Winter 1969, *4*(1), 4–11.

Posthuma, B. W. *Small groups in therapy sessions: Process and leadership.* Boston: Little Brown, and Company, 1989.

Rankin, S. H., & Stallings, K. L. *Patient education: Issues, principles and guidelines.* Philadelphia: Lippincott, 1990.

Sampson, E. E., & Marthas, M. *Group processes for the health professionals* (3rd ed.). New York: Wiley, 1990.

Van Hoozen, H. L., Bratton, B. D., Ostmoe, P. M., et al. *The teaching process theory and practice in nursing.* Norwalk, Ct.: Appleton-Century-Crofts, 1987.

Unit III

Learner Readiness: Factors Affecting the Client as a Learner

The old adage "You can lead a horse to water, but you cannot make him drink" has direct application in the teaching–learning process. A teacher may provide a variety of learning experiences, but only the learner can learn. Many factors influence an individual's readiness to learn about health. These must be understood by the nurse so that a thorough assessment can be performed and accurate nursing diagnoses related to learning can be made. This unit addresses the assessment of the learner.

Assessment of the learner focuses on assessing readiness to learn and the content area of learning need. Factors which influence an individual's readiness for learning can be understood and assessed by exploring three major categories. In this unit there is a chapter devoted to each of these.

Chapter 6 discusses the health state of the learner. Whether the learner is well, acutely ill, or chronically ill influences both willingness and ability to learn. Knowing how these factors affect the learner helps the nurse determine teaching strategies and the timing for these.

The influence of health values is discussed in Chapter 7. Nurses need to understand health as a value and how an individual's value systems affect readiness to learn. This facilitates identifying value-oriented factors to be assessed.

Chapter 8 identifies developmental characteristics. The physical maturation, cognitive development, and psychosocial development of an individual learner have an impact on the ability to learn and the motivation to learn certain things. Understanding aspects of development for various age groups will assist the nurse to focus on factors to assess.

The last chapter in this unit, Chapter 9, provides an in-depth discussion of the assessment process. Guidelines are provided to assist the nurse in learner assessment and to identify content areas for learning.

6

Health Status

Nancy I. Whitman

An individual's health status affects both experiential and motivational readiness to learn. Experiential readiness factors are those related to an individual's ability and energy to learn. Factors that determine willingness to put forth the effort to learn are labeled motivational or emotional readiness factors (Redman, 1984). To better understand how particular health states affect the learner, it is useful to consider health status in relation to three general categories. These categories are wellness, acute illness, and chronic illness. Individuals may also have characteristics of more than one state; for example, they may have a chronic condition and concurrently experience an acute illness. All individuals vary and learning readiness must be assessed on an individual level; however, there are characteristics common to each health state that allow examination of how learner readiness may be affected by that particular state.

WELLNESS

Readiness to Learn
The idea of "wellness" has evolved over the last several decades. Dunn (1977) proposed that high-level wellness was a pattern of behavior an individual developed to maximize his or her potential. The National History of Disease Model first proposed in 1970 (Robbins & Hall) indicates that individuals who are "well" are in one of three stages. They may be at no risk; they may be at risk from a variety of factors such as the effects of aging, environmental conditions, or the presence of a physical or psychosocial situation which causes stress; or they may have a precursor to disease present which causes no signs and symptoms of disease. Individuals in any of these three stages have no known health deficit, hence they are physiologically without energy-reducing demands that are caused by a bodily response to

TABLE 6–1. RELATIONSHIP OF HEALTH STATUS AND READINESS TO LEARN

Characteristics	Wellness	Chronic Illness	Acute Illness
Signs and Symptoms	None	Permanent physiological changes	Signs and symptoms present temporarily
Individual Stability	Stable	Variable	Unstable
Dependency	Low	Variable	High
Goal of Health Care	Prevention of illness Promotion of health	Long-term adjustment Management and monitoring of chronic condition	Survival Treatment
Potential Learner Readiness			
Experiential:	High	Variable	Low
Motivational:	Variable	Variable	Low

Adapted from Birchfield, M. E. Stages of illness: Guidelines for nursing care, Bowie, MD: Brady Communications, 1985.

illness. Energy is therefore available for learning. Well individuals can be independent in self-care including health promotion and disease prevention activities. The physiological status of the well individual can contribute positively to readiness to learn. Psychological factors in wellness are more variable.

Psychological factors related to readiness for learning include an individual's perception of self-responsibility for health and personal values and knowledge of risk factors. Health values are discussed in detail in the next chapter, but several important points will be emphasized here. For a well person, motivation to learn about any aspect of health care is based upon the acceptance of self-responsibility for health. In other words, the individual must recognize that he or she, not a physician, nurse, or other health care provider, is ultimately responsible for both his or her own well-being and the choices made that affect health. Some well individuals may not be inclined to learn health-generating or health-protection behaviors because they are not presently ill, do not perceive any vulnerability, and, consequently, see no reason to learn. On the other hand, there may be well individuals who participate in such health-generating behaviors as sound nutritional habits, regular exercise, and stress management activities. These individuals may be motivated to do this because they are aware of disease precursors or a risk of cardiovascular disease and they seek to control the precursors and reduce the risk of disease. Or they may be at no risk but may be consciously striving toward high-level wellness. Table 6–1 provides a summary of experiential and motivational learning readiness of the well individual.

Learning Content for Well Individuals
There are a number of health knowledge deficits commonly seen among healthy individuals. These deficits may be related to nutrition and weight control, stress

TABLE 6–2. HEALTH LEARNING NEEDS FOR INDIVIDUALS OF DIFFERENT HEALTH STATUS

Category of Health Content	Health Status		
	Wellness	Acute Illness	Chronic Illness
Nutrition	Balancing nutrients Weight control Normal elimination Understanding nutrition labels	Adjustment for disease Changes in elimination Equipment to aid nutrition and elimination	Balancing nutrients Weight control Adjustment for disease Changes in elimination Equipment to aid nutrition and elimination
Exercise and rest	Regularity Amounts Methods to promote rest or exercise Incorporation into life style	Hazards of immobility Adjustment for disease	Hazards of immobility Adjustment for disease Incorporation into life style Energy conservation
Stress management	Self-responsibility Diversions Relaxation techniques Use of support systems	Self-responsibility Pain management Rest and sleep Personal space Use of support systems	Self-responsibility Pain management Diversions Relaxation techniques Use of support systems Financial management Handling social systems
Illness care	Identification and treatment of minor illness When to call a professional How to enter the health-care system Over-the-counter medications	Illness related information: symptoms, treatment, tests, equipment, pain control, potential outcomes	Home care regimen Signs and symptoms of crisis When to call a professional How to enter the health-care system Adaptation of treating minor illness due to chronic disease Over-the-counter medications/implications with chronic disease Prescription medications

(continued)

TABLE 6–2. (*Continued*)

Category of Health Content	Health Status		
	Wellness	*Acute Illness*	*Chronic Illness*
Health monitoring	Life style appraisal Seven signs of cancer Breast self-exam/testicular exam BP monitoring Eye exams Dental exams Physical exams	Symptom monitoring Follow-up health care When to call a professional	Symptom monitoring Follow-up health care When to call a professional
Anticipatory guidance	Risk factors Environmental sensitivity Immunization Parenting Developmental crises Normal body functions Building self-esteem	Discharge needs: resumption of normal ADLs—diet, activity, work/school Prescription medications Potential complications	Financial management Developmental crises Disease trajectories Environmental sensitivity Body changes from illness Building self-esteem
Safety	Home, work, auto Hygiene Avoiding carcinogens Environmental sensitivity Smoking Alcohol and other drug use/abuse Safe sex	Ambulation Locomotion Hygiene Environmental sensitivity Dangers of equipment Smoking	Locomotion Adaptative devices Hygiene Home, work, auto Avoiding carcinogens Smoking Alcohol and other drug use/abuse

management activities such as meditation or yoga, management of common minor illnesses, and anticipatory guidance related to normal developmental crises such as childbearing and retirement. Table 6–2 provides a list of some common content for the health education of well individuals. Too often assumptions are made that individuals already know this content. The nurse needs to assess both interest and knowledge level before assuming these are not areas of learning needs.

ACUTE ILLNESS

There are a variety of interpretations for the term *acute*. It is often used to describe the duration of illness and specifically to differentiate from chronic illness, which carries the connotation of long-term duration. Acute illness also refers to diseases with sudden onset and severe effects. In this context, acute illness refers to illness or disease that is relatively time limited (as opposed to chronic illness) and either ends in death or resumption of the premorbid life style. Examples of acute illnesses include traumas such as burns and fractures, surgeries such as appendectomies and coronary artery bypass surgeries, and bacteriologic or viral diseases such as pneumonia and influenza. It is also important to recall that individuals with chronic conditions may experience acute illness episodes either as an exacerbation of a chronic condition or as a separate event. For example, the individual with asthma may experience pneumonia.

The threat of illness to the individual varies as a result of both the severity of the illness experience and the alterations in the self-concept arising from physical changes in body functions, structure, or appearance. Although the degree of threat will vary in individual situations, the stage of the illness experience determines how an individual may react. When examining acute illness and readiness to learn, it is helpful to consider the three stages of acute illness proposed by Birchfield (1985). These include the preacute stage, the acute stage, and the postacute or resolution stage.

Readiness to Learn

The preacute stage of acute illness is characterized by the presence of signs and symptoms. The decision to take action is based upon the level of concern generated by the threat of illness. This decision is based on physical, cognitive, and emotional components. Physical aspects include the presence of signs or symptoms such as pain, fever, or vomiting. The meaning that these signs and symptoms has for an individual is a function of the cognitive component. Emotional responses to the presence of the signs and symptoms and their meaning is the third component. When signs and symptoms are severe, or when they are perceived as threatening, individuals usually take action to determine what is wrong. If none of the three components at this stage are perceived to be significant, individuals may not take action at this time.

Once the decision is made that one is ill, the ill individual often seeks validation from friends and relatives and may ask for advice about illness care. At this point, individuals may be ready to learn about symptom control or how to enter into the health-care system. Sources of information tend to be friends and relatives rather than health-care professionals, however. Lay literature may also be used to learn about symptom control.

When the individual seeks health care, it is usually with a focus on determining a diagnosis or cause for the illness and seeking treatment. Thus, most individuals are cooperative in helping the health professional and are interested in learning about the health problem. While still in the preacute stage, individuals are able to continue self-care activities, at least to some extent, and have some available energy for learning.

During the acute stage of illness, individuals become dependent either on health-care professionals or other supportive individuals. Dependency may be a realistic and necessary condition because of the physical or psychological disequilibrium caused by the illness. The stress of the illness itself, the complexity of the treatment modalities, and, if hospitalized, the unfamiliar environment, can lead to a sense of powerlessness for the ill individual. Available energy is invested in coping with the physiological and psychological demands of the illness and the individual's focus is on survival. Readiness to learn, therefore, is extremely limited. Not only is energy itself diminished, but other distractors such as pain and fatigue are usually present. An ill individual's perceptions are limited and the immediate situation becomes paramount. The learning possible at this time usually relates to tests or treatments being done and is considered short-term learning. In other words, the material being learned relates to the situation at hand and once the situation is over, it is usually no longer necessary to retain it. As the physiological and psychological demands of the illness decrease and independence increases, the individual progresses to the postacute or resolution stage of illness. For most individuals, an improving physical condition and the necessity of returning to normalcy acts as an incentive to learning about avoiding complications and follow-up management. Individuals may also be ready for educational content related to preventive practices.

Individuals are usually at home during the final phase of illness. Even individuals hospitalized for treatment spend the majority of their postacute illness stage at home. This factor itself has serious implications for health-care teaching. During the time individuals are most ready to learn, they do not always have access to health-care teachers. In addition, individuals in the postacute illness stage are often fatigued as a result of the struggle for stability associated with the acute stage. Hence, teaching at this time necessitates consideration of the energy levels of the learner. For hospitalized individuals, appropriate discharge planning and referral is essential because of shorter hospital stays and the increasing complexity of care being given by families in the home. Practice caring for ill family members on hospital units and on field trips home help families make smoother transitions to home care (Baker, Kuhlmann, & Magliaro, 1989).

Learning Content Associated with Acute Illness

Content for the health education of individuals with acute illness falls into the same categories as those of well individuals. The focus of the content, however, is specific to the illness and its management. Important content in the categories of nutrition, exercise, and rest are related to adjustments necessitated by the illness.

In the preacute stage, individuals are eager to learn about the meaning of signs and symptoms being experienced or about tests that will be used for diagnostic purposes. Individuals for whom the acute event will be a surgical experience can be involved in preoperative teaching. Because of the organization of health-care systems today, this often takes place in an outpatient setting such as an ambulatory clinic.

Educational needs that are especially important for the acutely ill individual include information related to the illness and to safety. Illness-related material includes information about symptoms, diagnostic tests, treatment modalities, therapeutic equipment, and the usual outcomes of the illness. Individuals need to know what medications they are taking and what these medications can be expected to do. Other educational needs include the effects of the illness or treatment on ambulation and safety, special hygiene needs, and dangers related to any equipment being used. Most of the learning needs mentioned thus far are at the lower levels of the cognitive or affective domain. This is because patients who are acutely ill are not expected to act independently as a result of learning but only to participate with less anxiety in medical management.

Important content in the postacute stage includes learning behaviors that will promote reintegration into previous life style patterns. For hospitalized individuals this is part of discharge planning. Discharge teaching content includes material about resuming usual diet, activity, and job or school patterns. Information about medication names, uses, expected actions, and side effects is important as well. Before discharge, individuals also must learn what medical follow-up will be necessary, how to carry out any treatment to be continued at home, how to monitor progress, and what signs or symptoms indicate that the health-care practitioner should be consulted again.

Learning content associated with acute illness relates both to the illness itself and its effects on activities of daily living. In the dependent phase of illness, the focus is on the immediate situation and is primarily on an informational level. As independence increases, the level of education also increases. Behaviors for resuming self-care following the illness must be mastered. Table 6–2 summarizes learning needs associated with acute illness.

CHRONIC ILLNESS

Chronic illness is a significant health problem today. Chronic conditions occur in all ages of the population and have variable courses. Some chronic illnesses, such as many cancers and skin conditions, have periods of remission and exacerbation. During the exacerbations, these illnesses take on similarities to acute illnesses. Other chronic conditions, like cerebral palsy and spina bifida, are fixed conditions with long periods of stability; still others, like arthritis, may be controlled but continue to progress over time. Some individuals with chronic illnesses may function as well persons, but require special treatment or rehabilitation. Others must control their state of health through a therapeutic regimen of diet, exercise, drugs, and special treatments. The physical demands of chronic conditions vary, thus experiential readiness also varies. Individuals may be at different stages in adjusting to their chronic conditions as well. Understanding what stage of adjustment an individual is experiencing will assist the nurse in determining readiness for learning.

Readiness to Learn

Though adjustment varies among individuals, there are stages of adapting to chronic illness that have been identified. A variety of models, developed to trace the adjustment of individuals to loss, may be applied to individuals experiencing chronic illness (Engel, 1964; Kubler-Ross, 1969; Martocchio, 1985). While theorists label stages of adjustment differently, they all have in common three identifiable phases: initial avoidance, beginning approach, and then repetitious approach/avoidance cycles.

Avoidance behaviors mark the initial stage. These usually occur at the time of diagnosis. There is great anxiety, and defenses gathered to protect the self from the impact of the situation are ineffective in assisting the person to cope with the stress. Denial is a commonly used defense mechanism during this stage. Psychological energy is spent in maintaining the powerful defense mechanisms that protect the self from overwhelming stress. In addition to the strain upon psychological energy in this period, expenditure of physical energy to meet body requirements may also be great. Learning effectiveness during this time period is minimal. Nursing care is directed mainly toward reducing anxiety. Simple explanations are beneficial since only limited amounts of information can be processed. It is important for the nurse to focus on giving information and not require the client to make a lot of decisions during this time.

The next stage is characterized by behaviors to approach and begin to handle the chronic illness. The individual becomes gradually more and more aware of the realities of the situation. This stage typically begins when the physical condition stabilizes or when symptoms become too obvious to avoid (Birchfield, 1985). Initial defense reactions decrease as awareness of the situation increases. During this time the acute phase of the illness is usually brought under control. Once symptoms are controlled with a therapeutic regimen and there is beginning adjustment to the idea of chronic illness, energy levels become more stable. Readiness to learn is heralded by questions from the client about the illness and treatment. Teaching related to the client's current experiences is pertinent, but the client may have difficulty dealing with future-oriented educational content.

The last stage is characterized by repetitions of approach/avoidance behaviors. These continue to occur throughout the remainder of the individual's life. Education related to life style alterations necessitated by chronic illness, strategies for reintegration into the family and social system, problem-solving skills for coping with adjustments in living, as well as management of illness care regimens facilitate an individual's adaptation to chronic illness.

Some individuals adapt and attempt to integrate their chronic condition into their life style, attempting to reach normalcy as nearly as possible. They face reality and exhibit information-seeking behavior related to self-care management and implications of the long-term consequences. During this phase, these individuals focus on more positive factors and may express great interest in learning about their illness and management. Other individuals never fully adjust to the changes necessitated by chronic illness and may continue to predominantly use avoidance behaviors such as anger and resentment. Even those who do adapt to chronic illness have periods of depression or anger when losses are remembered. During these periods, motivation for learning is typically lower. Experiential readiness to learn may also vary during this stage. For some individuals, the chronic condition may be well controlled and the physical demands of illness stable. They have more energy for learning. Individuals who experience physical instability associated with their chronic condition will have variable levels of energy for learning.

Learning Content Associated with Chronic Illness

The same categories of learning content exist for chronic illness as for wellness and acute illness. In chronic illness, the content relates to adapting an individual's life style to facilitate management of the chronic condition and yet maximize wellness. All aspects of daily living affected by the disease provide topics of educational content. Under chronic illness in Table 6–2, specific content areas are listed. Topics such as balancing nutrients and adjusting the diet as necessitated by the disease, conserving energy, managing pain, home-care regimens, symptom monitoring, and using support systems are appropriate educational content for the individual who has faced the realities of the chronic condition. Content for those individuals who are in the acute stages of their illness is the content which is listed under acute illness and has been previously discussed.

SUMMARY

In summary, a particular health state affects readiness to learn by influencing energy levels and motivation, and hence the level of dependency of an individual as a learner. Figure 6–1 depicts the relationship between health status and learning dependency. During illness, physiological demands reduce an individual's energy for learning and invoke dependency in the teaching–learning situation as well as in the physical realm. Health state also influences the individual's perceptions of the situation. During an acute illness experience, an individual's perceptions are limited. Hence, learning readiness is focused on immediate needs recognized by the nurse–teacher. Teacher-directed learning is appropriate. With improvement in the acute illness condition, and in situations where chronically ill individuals have stabilized and accepted their illness, desire for independence increases. More expanded and future-oriented teaching is then possible. Individuals at this stage are ready to increase participation in determining educational needs. The readiness to learn of well individuals is primarily based on motivational factors. Perceptions of vulnerability, importance of health or other values related to health, and acceptance of self-responsibility for health are keys to their readiness to learn. Energy for

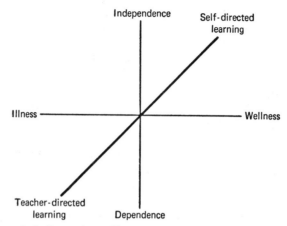

Figure 6–1. Comparison of health status and level of dependency.

education related to health is available. Whether individuals are motivated to expend the energy in this direction varies. Self-directed learning is possible for well individuals.

REFERENCES AND READINGS

Alexy, B. Goal setting and health risk reduction. *Nursing Research,* 1985, *34*(5), 283–288.

Balog, J. E. The concepts of health and disease: A relativistic perspective. *Health Values: Achieving High Level Wellness,* 1982, *6*(5), 7–13.

Baker, K., Kuhlmann, R. S., & Magliaro, B. L. Homeward bound. *Nursing Clinics of North America,* 1989, *24*(3), 655–664.

Barr, W. J. Teaching patients with life-threatening illnesses. *Nursing Clinics of North America,* 1989, *24*(3), 639–643.

Birchfield, M. E. *Stages of illness: Guidelines for nursing care.* Bowie, MD: Brady Communications, 1985.

Brillhart, B., & Stewart, A. Education as the key to rehabilitation. *Nursing Clinics of North America,* 1989, *24*(3), 675–680.

Craft, M. Education for the critically ill adolescent. *Dimensions of Critical Care Nursing,* 1983, *2*(2), 116–119.

Demuth, J. S. Patient teaching in the ambulatory setting. *Nursing Clinics of North America,* 1989, *24*(3), 645–654.

Dunn, H. L. What high-level wellness means. *Health Values,* 1977, *1,* 9.

Engel, G. L. Grief and grieving. *American Journal of Nursing,* 1964, *64,* 93–96.

Foster, S. D. Teaching patients to manage complex, long-term care. *MCN,* 1987, *12*(1), 57.

Harrison, L. L. A health promotion model for wellness education. *MCN,* 1990, *15*(3), 191.

Johnson, E. A., & Jackson, J. E. Teaching the home care client. *Nursing Clinics of North America,* 1989, *24*(3), 687–693.

Kubler-Ross, E. *On death and dying.* NY: Macmillan Publ. Co, 1969.

Lewis, K. Grief in chronic illness and disability. *Journal of Rehabilitation,* 1983, *49,* 8–12.

Martocchio, B. C. Grief and bereavement: Healing through hurt. *Nursing Clinics of North America*, 1985, *20*(3), 327–330.

McHatton, M. A theory for timely teaching. *American Journal of Nursing*, 1985, *85*(7), 798–800.

Milsum, J. H. Health, risk factor reduction and life-style change. *Family and Community Health*, 1980, *3*(1), 1–13.

Redman, B. K. *The process of patient education*. St. Louis: C. V. Mosby, 1984.

Robbins, L. C., & Hall, J. *How to practice prospective medicine*. Indianapolis: Methodist Hospital of Indiana, 1970.

Steele, J. M., & Ruzicki, D. An evaluation of the effectiveness of cardiac teaching during hospitalization. *Heart & Lung*, 1987, *16*(3), 306–311.

Ruzicki, D. A. Realistically meeting the educational needs of hospitalized acute and short stay patients. *Nursing Clinics of North America*, 1989, *24*(3), 629–637.

Woods, N. Conceptualizations of self-care: Toward health-oriented models. *Advances in Nursing Science*, 1989, *12*(1), 1–13.

7

Health Values

Carol J. Gleit

Lessening the gap between health information and health practice is a major challenge in health teaching today. The standardized role function of the patient or client educator has been perceived as telling patients or clients what to do, how to do it, how frequently, and why. The underlying assumption is that if people know what is beneficial to their health they will do it. We know that values are important in learning when we find that a topic is not learned, a learning objective is not achieved, or when someone decides not to follow prescriptions of health professionals, although there is accurate and adequate information about such a need. There is no doubt that "eagerness to cooperate" with the health professional's instructions facilitates the behavioral change, but frequently change does not occur or it is not complete.

Those not following health professionals' instructions traditionally have been labeled noncompliant. Noncompliance has been treated as a motivational or attitudinal problem on the part of the patient. It is only within the last several years that this problem has been systematically investigated. Noncompliance is in and of itself a value-laden term. The authoritative connotation is that the practitioner expects obedience as a legitimate right with the patient following rules that are for the patient's own good. The implication is that the practitioner knows what is best. If the patient ignores or rebels against instructions he or she is demonstrating irresponsibility. Another way of looking at noncompliance is that the patient is asserting the right to self-responsibility. Some authors, as Ardell (1988), Ryan (1988), and Haddon (1989), believe that a strong sense of personal accountability for one's own health is absolutely essential. Teaching clients to make their own decisions is seen as tremendously more important in this view than merely telling them to follow the instructions of health professionals. Basic conditions underlying this approach include: (1) creation of learner needs for understanding, (2) development of an atmosphere conductive to exploring the personal meaning of the health issue, and

(3) encouragement in actively exploring personal implications confronting the individual. Thus, values surrounding the term *noncompliance* may be quite disparate.

HEALTH AS A VALUE

In order to understand the effect of values, it is important to define the word *value* in the teaching–learning context. Definitions of values incorporate both cognitive and affective elements representing reasoning along with feelings, values, and attitudes. Although Raths et al. (1966), Krathwohl et al. (1964), and Carl Rogers (1969) view values from different perspectives, they are consistent in their belief that a value is learned, arises out of personal experience, forms a basis for behavior, has an internal locus of control, is held over time, and is evident in a consistent pattern of behavior. Raths et al. (1966) define a value as a belief which one chooses for oneself, cherishes, and consistently uses as a determinant of one's behavior. A value can be defined as a personal belief about the worth, desirability, goodness, truth, and beauty of a particular idea, object, derived from the individual's experience. Shaver and Strong (1976) define values as standards and principles for judging worth, criteria for judging people, objects, ideas, actions, and situations as good, worthwhile, desirable or bad, worthless, or in between these extremes. The Shaver and Strong definition differs from Raths' in that Shaver and Strong acknowledge that some values are the unconscious result of experience and that public affirmation and action is not always done. More recently, Ryan (1988) and Egan (1990) have incorporated valuing in their approaches to health teaching. The placement of values varies from individual to individual and for the same individual at different times. Good nutrition may not be important to someone at age 22 but may take on greater importance 10 years later. Values may be expected to change over time as new information is added that changes the cognitive or affective quality of those values. Values can be seen as action oriented and may give direction and meaning to one's life. Values can be considered the basis for decision making. What is important and relevant to a person is determined by that person's values. If a client is not aware of the values upon which decisions are based, there is unawareness of an essential component of decision making, and uninformed decisions result. Once the central role of values in decision making is recognized, values can be used deliberately and with awareness. When identified, values can be explored, clarified, and ranked. The result can be more deliberate and effective decisions. Assisting with generating and screening options may help the client improve decisions or decision making. For generating solutions, as many options as possible can be considered. Later these can be looked at one by one as to their feasibility or practicability. It is important to differentiate values from value judgments. Value judgments are assertions based on values. For example, a nurse saying, "Don't smoke cigarettes," to a patient is making a value judgment based on the nurse's own values. The value may involve self-responsibility or wellness life style. Because the value judgment typically does not state the value represented, it is important for a teacher to become sensitive to and aware of the use of value judgments, what the underlying values are, and whether there is consistency between the value judgment and a value. Once there is a conscious awareness of one's values, the values can become an internal control for behavior.

Health in itself is a value. Even the definition of health is difficult because it is multidimensional and difficult to measure and is open to individual interpretation. One's concept of health is tied into one's belief systems, how one defines health, and whether the value of health is low or high in one's hierarchical arrangement of values. A definition of illness also involves values. Some clients may seek advice from a health professional for a slight problem, while others seek advice only when there is grave illness. Some perceive illness as part of living, while others consider illness to infringe on well-being. Values, then, influence the motivation expressed by clients in seeking and using health services as well as the way they perceive health and illness. Response to treatment for illness is influenced by an individual's belief about the effectiveness of the treatment and the confidence placed in the health professional.

There is a relationship between information and values in decision making. Values may be powerful influences on whether an individual complies with recommended courses of health actions. Decision-making capabilities of learners may need assistance in order to change to a more health-generating behavior. Many of the more recent approaches to patient compliance have incorporated a reciprocal process between health teachers and learners (Speers, 1989; Egan, 1990). The term *information* can be used broadly to include, for example, reassurance, instant solutions, and long-term therapy. The nurse can assist the patient to build a behavioral commitment on the basis of the patient's beliefs and attitudes before the actual intervention begins. Using this line of reasoning, special diets, fitness programs, or a convenient medication regimen are not as likely to succeed if no behavioral commitment for the change has been made. No individual will follow instructions that the individual does not believe will work or will work toward a goal not valued. If client beliefs are taken into consideration, and if a treatment regimen is consistent with patient attitudes and values, the commitment to the behavior change is likely to be more lasting. Negotiation and mutual participation of the teacher and learner are most likely to bring about the behavioral change. This process takes into account the health practitioner's expertise in health and illness, and the patient's expertise on matters pertaining to the patient's own beliefs, values, and attitudes toward the situation. This method alleviates the notion of the patient's being delivered into the hands of the health professional and adapting a passive recipient stance or submission to health professional authority. The recent emphasis on self-responsibility in overcoming illness and maintaining health can lead an individual to adapt an active orientation toward health. This orientation fosters collaboration or partnership with the practitioner.

When there is a negotiated mutual contract (described in Chapter 13), both the health-care provider and the receiver have given their informed consent. In this case there can be a no-fault attitude toward noncompliant behavior, and the responsibility for the outcome of treatment is mutual. The contract encourages the compliant behavior, mutual understanding, and mutual responsibility. A mutual participative approach to changing health-damaging behaviors is more acceptable to patients and practitioners today than ever before. Many people no longer seem willing to grant health-care providers more knowledge and skill than they actually possess. In addition, practitioners are less likely to want the burden of taking responsibility for decisions that rightly belong in the patient's realm.

Readiness to Learn

Before instruction takes place, it is helpful for the nurse to determine whether the learner is likely to change health-damaging behaviors to those that are health generating. The client must also feel reasonably capable of carrying out the health-care plan. The term *readiness to learn* implies that the learner is likely to engage in positive action to change behavior. Determining readiness to learn is a crucial and separate step that occurs before the objectives and teaching plans are formulated. Girdano and Dusek (1988) define readiness as the possession of behaviors, attitudes, and skills and concomitant resources that make it possible for individuals to incorporate a new behavior into a permanent life style. Miller (1987) views readiness in a similar way. Many value-oriented factors influence an individual's readiness to learn. These include: awareness of diagnosis, previous knowledge and experience, motivational level, health locus of control, meaning of physical condition, psychological state, self-concept, and perceived need to learn. Individually determined beliefs and attitudes, feelings and values set the stage as to whether the behavior change will occur, be effective, be lasting or short-term. The health values involved usually are more than simple extremes of right or wrong, good or bad, true or false. The conditions under which behavioral change occurs typically involve conflicting demands and weighing of costs and benefits.

Readiness to learn is often difficult to assess because of a lack of definite guidelines. It is hoped that, with the format described in Chapter 10, progress can be made in this area. Many elements are involved in assessing readiness to learn, and they include factors from the various learning domains. An assessment of learner readiness is important before every teaching session. We used to think that nurses might need to spend a lot of time and effort in assisting the learner to see value in the learning outcome. With the implementation of Diagnostic Related Groups (DRGs), hospitalizations are more intense and shorter. This means that while the patient is hospitalized, less time may be available for teaching and other psychologically supportive nursing interventions, or more effective use of time available for teaching may be considered.

Affective Domain

Affect refers to the feelings and emotions that proceed from, lead to, accompany, underlie, or give color to a client's experiences and behavior (Egan, 1990). "I've been feeling sorry for myself ever since I've believed I have multiple sclerosis." The affective domain involves the feeling part of the individual. Learning to use a walker after a stroke involves motor skills, and also the affective domain as he accepts the reality of his situation. The concepts of feeling comfortable with breast feeding her baby, or giving oneself an insulin injection every day are part of affective learning. Changing values, attitudes, and feelings usually takes longer than increasing knowledge in the cognitive domain and may result from extensive one-to-one teacher–learner instruction or supportive small group sessions. Teaching in complex situations may begin with the affective domain. Someone in the midst of strong emotional upheaval is unlikely to attend to anything other than dealing with that emotional response. Nurses can assist the person to recognize and overcome obstacles to the desired behavior change. It is obvious that to be effective, learning must be individualized for each learner. The affective side of learning needs more attention. It is consistent with the humanistic philosophical approach to learning discussed in Chapter 4.

A change in attitude takes place slowly. The client must want to change the given behavior that the attitude influences. Structuring situations that elicit behaviors that would be manifest if the individual had the desired attitude can lead to more success in changing attitude. For example, a health-generating behavior (not smoking) will be followed by a changed attitude (seeing oneself as a nonsmoker). Some consider it easier to act the new way of behaving than to first think a different way and then act.

It is important to validate with the client the assessment of the client's readiness to learn. In addition, reassessment of the situation and the patient from time to time is important. The learner must ultimately decide whether or not to enter into the teaching situation. We can therefore say that the learner is taking responsibility for the learning.

SELF-CARE MODELS

The endpoint of teaching usually is that the client will manage on his/her own the behaviors that were learned. Self-care means "care performed by oneself when one has reached a state of maturity that enables him/her to take responsibility for consistent, controlled action" (Orem, 1980). Self-care and self-efficacy are related terms, as described in Chapter four. Bandura (1977) used the term self-efficacy to indicate that the more confident and capable an individual feels about performing health-related activities, the more likely the individual will try to change his behavior. High degrees of self-efficacy depend on the client's ability to clearly envision what needs to be done, to believe his participation makes a difference, and that he has the personal resources at hand to learn the skills and, subsequently, to maintain the changed behavior (Redman, 1985). By helping the client with more basic skills at the outset, he will gain a sense of accomplishment. For example, a client who begins by changing his breakfast to oatmeal and fruit from eggs, sausage, and gravied biscuits will be more likely to move on with changing other eating patterns.

Self-efficacy theory has been used in programs promoting life style changes (Creer, 1987; Indinnimeo et al. 1987; and Kirschenbaum, Sherman, and Penrod, 1987). Kirschenbaum et al. (1987) tested a complex program leading to self-directed hemodialysis patients. Their elderly program participants rapidly increased their self-directedness. Creer and Indinnimeo et al. in separate studies used self-efficacy theory with asthma patients. Larsson (1987), using a sample of adolescents with chronic headaches, found that self-help relaxation measures worked to lessen pain. Redman (1985), among others, states that self-efficacy theory can offer a more coherent framework for patient teaching than previously available.

Another model of self-care is the Health Belief Model, which focuses on the prevention of disease. Rosenstock's Health Belief Model, developed in the early 1950s, has been used extensively for predicting an individual's likelihood of positively engaging in health behavior. Taking action depends on one's perception of (1) one's level of susceptibility to the condition, (2) the degree of severity of the consequences that might result from contracting the condition, (3) the potential benefits of the health action in preventing or reducing susceptibility, and (4) barriers or costs related to starting or continuing the proposed behavior (Becker, 1974). Since its development, this model has proved a framework for a number of studies related to preventive health behavior and illness behavior, including chronic illness. Health beliefs are the concepts about health that the individual believes are true. They have both affective and cognitive components and may or may not be founded on fact. Health practices, or health-generating or health-damaging behaviors are activities that individuals carry out as a result of their health beliefs and definitions of health. These practices may or may not be recommended by health professionals and may or may not have been well thought out by the individual. Janz and Becker (1984) reviewed the literature testing the Health Belief Model, and found that costs and barriers are the most important reasons for engaging in health-generating behaviors. Susceptibility and severity of illness were not strong predictors of behaviors, unless the individual had a chronic illness.

Locus of Control

An important element in the Health Belief Model involves the learner's belief in the effectiveness of health-oriented actions as one part of perceived benefits. A significant influence on whether the person will follow a health-generating behavior is the belief that the state of health is within the realm of control, either that of the health teacher or the learner. The correlation between behavior and its outcomes is the basis of the concept locus of control, first published by Rotter (1954). Wallston et al. (1976, 1978) and Wallston and Wallston (1981) further developed the locus of control notion for health behaviors. The idea is that potential for enacting a behavior (for example, the likelihood that someone will engage in a regular jogging program) is affected by the person's expectation that the behavior will lead to better health or less disease and illness. The value of the outcome is likely to be at least partially dependent on that person's belief in the severity of the disease and his or her susceptibility to it. The value is also dependent on the person's concern for health, as well as for the benefits of the health behavior.

Wallston et al. (1976) and Wallston et al. (1978) have developed a Multidimensional Health Locus of Control Scale, similar to the original general Locus of Control Scale first developed by Rotter. Wallston and Wallston's scale specifically relates to health locus of control. Out of initial research on the instrument a revision was developed, reflecting three dimensions of health beliefs: (1) internal health locus of control, the belief that one can control many aspects of health with one's own behavior; (2) external health locus of control, in which others are powerful in personal health locus of control; and (3) the belief that chance happening is responsible for health or disease. Wallston et al. (1978) suggest that the use of this scale may be valuable in examining an individual's delay in seeking help with cancer's danger signals, reactions to side effects of drugs, and trust in health professionals.

There has been a fair amount of research on locus of control. Shillinger (1983) has reviewed much of the literature. Wallston et al. (1978) also reviewed research using Rotter's scale of locus of control and various health behavior forms. Findings are suggestive that locus of control is important as part of a comprehensive model of health behavior. The Rotter scale is a generalized view of control and thus is not limited just to perceptions of control in health actions. Several studies have reported that those with internal locus of control make better use of prevention strategies. Schroeder and Miller (1983) found that patients with an external locus of control were more responsive to having some decisions made for them, in a study of patients with peripheral vascular disease. Externals may also need help in setting realistic goals. Gotch (1983) in her study of locus of control with insulin-dependent diabetic adults did not find a systematic tendency for more external locus of control to be associated with lower diabetic regimen implementation.

More research in this field is needed to establish the base for locus of control. It may be that educational interventions can be tailored partly on the basis of an individual's locus of control, because beliefs in determinants of health may vary. It might be useful to choose teaching strategies for "internals" such as self-paced programmed learning, and other strategies for "externals," such as closely monitoring their progress.

"Internals" are seen to be more active seekers and users of information than "externals." Those with an internal locus of control would look for health programs in which active participation is stressed, and those who are more internally motivated would be better in programs that are nondirective, while those externally motivated would need a more directive strategy. Externally oriented individuals in some studies have been shown to feel less responsible for outcomes. From this, it would seem that those with an internal locus of control would have a more positive wellness life style.

Some suggest that belief in an internal health locus of control may require education involving self-direction, while education based on decision making by health professionals may be best for those with an external health locus of control. Those with a belief that health is due to chance may not benefit from either approach. Shillinger (1983) summarized differing directions for patient education in those with internal and external patterns. She advocates (1) choice of treatment, (2) involvement of the client in making choices, and (3) emphasis on individual responsibility and self-directedness for internally oriented persons. For those with an external locus of control one can (1) help individuals who believe in chance change to a belief that their health events can be controlled, (2) stress reliance on social support systems, and (3) improve decision-making skills. There is a definite need for more research that will specify the relationship of generalized and specific health-related locus of control as part of a comprehensive view of predicting health actions and developing educational interventions to change health-damaging behaviors.

La Montagne (1984) examined children's ways of coping preoperatively relative to locus of control, and found that "active" children were more internal than children who showed avoidant behavior. Marks et al. (1986) looked at the relationship between health locus of control and patient beliefs in the effectiveness of cancer treatment. Those with an internal locus of control showed a weak relation between depression and perceptions of disease severity. Those who perceived their illness as very severe showed strong negative correlations between expectations of self-control and treatment and depression. Huckstodt (1987) studied locus of control among alcoholics, recovering alcoholics, and nonalcoholics. The nonalcoholic group had the highest level of internal locus of control, those recovering ranked second, and the alcoholic group was the least internal.

SELF-CONCEPT

Self-concept is an important affective consideration in learning. Goals may be set to develop a more positive self-image in learners. Considerable research points to the relationship between positive self-worth and positive emotional and physical well-being. The idea is that if one feels good about oneself, there will be more active concern with feelings toward learning. Perceptions relating to aspects of self such as esteem, body image, needs, roles, and abilities may need revision on the learner's part. When an individual perceives a threat to these views of self, anxiety often occurs. It may be important for the nurse to assist the client in reducing anxiety before beginning a program of instruction.

The individual may need to redefine health. For example, a 68-year-old woman who can no longer play tennis may need to examine and redefine her concept of health in view of her age and abilities. There tends to be a circular effect of the self-concept, that is, we zero in on what we already believe about ourselves, whether positive or negative. If one's self-concept is positive, behavior is likely to lead to success; if negative, the self may be seen as undeserving, thereby making it difficult to learn. This may be a self-fulfilling prophecy; the self-corroborating nature of self-concept makes it stable and difficult to change once it is firmly established. Hallal (1982) showed a definite correlation between a positive self-concept and regular practice of breast self-examination. Girdano and Dusek (1988) speak of enhancing self-concepts of individuals in weight management programs.

The redefinition and examination of the self-concept may be crucial before an individual's values, attitudes, and basic beliefs can be changed. Educators need to become sensitive to the self-concepts of clients and skillful in helping them make changes in their self-concepts. Frequently this is not an easy task. Many individuals are not willing or able to reveal themselves to others, even significant others. Their self-reports may or may not be an accurate description of their self-concept. The healthiest of people do not always feel safe in revealing their deepest feelings to others (wives, lovers, therapists, and educators), even under the friendliest of conditions. Even if these constraints do not exist, sometimes people have difficulty in expressing their feelings accurately. A request for information, which seems an invasion of privacy, will be unlikely to produce accurate self-descriptions. In this case, health professionals tend to make inferences from observing clients' behavior, including their nonverbal behavior.

Self-concept is considered very important in teaching adult learners. There is an assumption that as a person grows and matures his self-concept moves from one of total dependency (as is the reality of the infant) to one of increasing self-direction. Andragogy (adult learning) assumes that the point at which an individual achieves a self-concept of essential self-direction is the point at which psychologically the individual becomes an adult. When this occurs, the person develops a deep psychological need to be perceived by others as self-directing. So, if an adult is not allowed to be self-directing, there is tension between the situation and the person's self-concept.

SUMMARY

Patient teaching undergirded by self-care models provides an excellent way for developing client self-responsibility. Self-responsibility can be seen as a core value in the teaching process, with the central idea that self-care is a learned behavior.

The helper–client relation in itself contributes to the learning needs of clients. If this process is effective, clients will be empowered to care more about themselves, trust themselves more, and begin to change old ideas (Egan, 1990). The relationship enables clients to tap into their own inner resources. This is essential for developing self-care skills and coping abilities.

Egan (1990) points out that if clients are not urged to explore and assume self-responsibility, they may not do the things needed to manage their lives better, or they may do something to aggravate problems they already have.

REFERENCES AND READINGS

Ardell, D. L. *Achieving high level wellness.* Emmaus, Pa: Rodale Press, 1977.

Bandura, A. Toward a unifying theory of behavior change. *Psychology Review,* 1977, *84,* 191–215.

Becker, M. (Ed.). *The health belief model and personal health behavior.* Thorofare, N.J.: Charles B. Slack, 1974.

Creer, T. L. Living with asthma: Replications and extensions. *Health Education Quarterly,* 1987, *14,* 319–331.

Egan, G. *The skilled helper: A systematic approach to effective helping.* Pacific Grove, Calif: Brooks/Cole Publishing Company, 1990.

Girdano, D. A., & Dusek, D. E. *Changing Health Behavior.* Scottsdale, Arizona: Gorsach Scarisbrick Publishers, 1988.

Gortner, S. R., et al. Improving recovery following cardiac surgery: A randomized clinical trial. *Journal of Advanced Nursing,* 1988, *13,* 649–661.

Gotch, P. M. Locus of control and implementation of health regimens in adults with insulin dependent diabetes. In Miller, J. F. *Coping with chronic illness: Overcoming powerlessness.* Philadelphia: F. A. Davis Co, 1983, 163–176.

Haddon, R. Tri-care: A new concept in health care. *Nursing and Health Care*, 1989, *10*, 4, 197–201.

Hallal, J. C. The relationship of health beliefs, health locus of control and self-concept to the practice of breast self-examination in adult women. *Nursing Research*, May/June 1982, 137–142.

Huckstodt, A. Locus of control among alcoholics, and non-alcoholics. *Research in Nursing and Health*, 1987, *10*, 23–28.

Hussar, D. A. Your role in patient compliance. *Nursing*, November 1979, 48–53.

Indinnimeo, L., Midulla, F., Hindi-Alexander, M., et al. Controlled studies of childhood asthma. Self-management in Italy using the "open airways" and "living with asthma programs: A preliminary report." *Health Education Quarterly*, 1987, *14*, 291–308.

Janz, N. K., & Becker, M. H. The health belief model: A decade later. *Health Educational Quarterly*, 1984, *11*(13), 1–47.

Krathwohl, D. R., Bloom, B. S., & Masia, B. B. Taxonomy of educational objectives: Handbook II: Affective domain. New York: D. McKay, 1964.

Kirschembaum, D. S., Sheriman, J., & Penrod, J. D. Promoting self-directed hemodialysis. *Health Psychology*, 1987, *6*, 373–385.

La Montagne, L. L. Children's locus of control beliefs as predictors of preoperative coping behavior. *Nursing Research*, 1984, *33*, 2, 76–85.

Larsson, B., Daleflod, B., Hakansson, L. et al. Therapist assisted versus self-help relaxation treatment of chronic headaches in adolescents: A school board intervention. *Journal of Child Psychology Psychiatry*, 1987, *28*, 127–136.

Lowrey, B. J., & Ducette, J. P. Disease related learning and disease control as a function of locus of control. *Nursing Research*, 1976, *25*, 358–362.

Marks, G., Richardson, J. L., Graham, S. W., et al. Role of health locus of control beliefs and expectations of treatment efficacy in adjustment to cancer. *Journal of Personality and Social Psychology*, 1986, *51*, 2, 443–450.

Marston, M. Compliance with medical regimens: A review of the literature. *Nursing Research*, 1970, *19*, 12–22.

Miller, H. When is the time ripe for teaching? *American Journal of Nursing*, July 1985, *85*, 7, 801–804.

Orem, D. *Nursing: Concepts of practice.* (2nd ed.) New York: McGraw Hill, 1980.

Rankin, S. H., & K. D. Stallings. *Patient education: Issues, principles, practices* (2nd ed.). Philadelphia: J. B. Lippincott Co., 1990.

Raths, L. E., Harmin, M., & Simon, S. B. *Values and teaching.* Columbus, Ohio: Chas. E. Merrill, 1966.

Redman, B. K. New areas of theory development and practice in patient education. *Journal of Advanced Nursing*, 1985, *10*, 425–428.

Rogers, C. *Freedom to learn.* Columbus, Ohio: Chas. E. Merrill, 1969.

Rotter, J. B. *Social learning theory and clinical psychology.* Englewood Cliffs, N.J.: Prentice-Hall, 1954.

Ryan, E. R. Viewing health education within the framework of the consumer's personal value system. *Nursing Forum*, 1987/88, *XXIII*, 2, 60–61.

Schroeder, P., & Miller, J. F. Qualitative study of locus of control in patients with peripheral vascular disease. In Miller, J. F. *Coping with chronic illness: Overcoming powerlessness.* Philadelphia: F. A. Davis Co., 1983, 149–163.

Shaver, J. P., & Strong, W. *Facing value decisions: Rationale building for teachers.* Belmont, Calif: Wadsworth Publishing Co., 1976.

Shillinger, F. L. Locus of control: Implications for clinical nursing practice. *Image,* Spring 1983, *15,* (2), 58–63.

Speers, A. T. Patient education: Theory and practice. *Journal of Nursing Staff Development,* 1989 (May–June), 121–126.

Taylor, C. B., Bandura, A., Ewart, C., et al. Exercise testing to enhance wives confidence in their husbands cardiac capability soon after uncomplicated acute myocardial infarction. *American Journal of Cardiology,* 1985, *55,* 635–638.

Wallston, B. S., & Wallston, K. A. Toward a unified social psychological model of health behavior. In G. Sanders, & J. Suls (Eds). *Social psychology and illness.* Hillsdale, NJ: Lawrence Erlbaum, 1981.

————, ————, Kaplan, G. D., & Maides, S. A. Development and validation of the health locus of control scales. *Journal of Consulting and Clinical Psychology,* 1976, *44,* 580–585.

Wallston, K. A., Wallston, B. S., & DeVellis, R. Development of the multidimensional health locus of control (MHLC) scales. *Health Education Monographs,* Spring 1978, 160–170.

Wiley, L. Nursing grand rounds: How can you improve patient compliance? *Nursing,* May, 1978, *9,* 40–45.

8

Developmental Characteristics

Nancy I. Whitman

Learner readiness, as previously discussed, includes both willingness (motivational readiness) and ability (experiential readiness) to make use of instruction. An individual's developmental stage greatly influences the ability to learn, and life stage influences willingness to learn about certain subjects at certain times. This chapter provides an overview of developmental factors that influence learner readiness during distinct life stages. The first portion explores the stages of childhood; the second part explores developmental factors influential for the adult learner.

CHILDHOOD DEVELOPMENTAL CHARACTERISTICS

Developmental theorists typically define various patterns of behavior seen in children according to stages or phases identified by an age range. In using age stages, one must keep in mind that the actual chronological age for transition may vary from child to child. Though no one-to-one correspondence of stage to age exists, age-related trends have been established. In the discussion which follows the typically recognized childhood stages are used to show the progression of three developmental learner-readiness factors—physical maturation, cognitive development, and psychosocial development.

Infant and Toddler

The two youngest age groups, infant and toddler, comprise children through about 3 years of age. Because of the dependency of this age group, in most health-care activities it is the parents rather than the children who are considered the learners. There are situations, however, in which older toddlers should be made a part of health-care teaching. Since the basis for later health habits is established in childhood, incorporation of these behaviors—washing hands and brushing teeth, for example—should begin in early encounters with the well child and the parents. In illness settings, the toddler who is to cooperate and cope emotionally with a procedure such as an injection or diagnostic test must be prepared. Understanding the very young child's psychomotor, cognitive, and social capacities allows the nurse to identify appropriate health content as well as developmental characteristics that will enhance or hinder learning. Because infants do not participate in health-learning situations, the discussion below focuses mainly on the toddler.

Physical Maturation. Great strides are made by toddlers in their overall growth, mobility, and erectness. This age child has a higher level of activity than at any other time (Eaton, 1983). Gross motor coordination allows the toddler to run, climb, and negotiate stairs. High-activity levels and constant practice developing motor skills coupled with limited judgment accounts for the high accident rate of this age group. Fine motor control and hand–eye coordination progress rapidly as well. Between the ages of 2 and 3, children learn to use a drinking glass with one hand, turn single pages of a book, and help dress and undress themselves.

Cognitive Development. Cognitive developmental progress has been analyzed and described by Piaget (Piaget, 1976; Piaget & Inhelder, 1969). He labels the period roughly corresponding to infancy and toddlerhood as sensorimotor. Learning occurs through visual, auditory, tactile, taste, olfactory, and motor experiences. The combination of developing fine and gross motor skills allows the young child to use movement to enhance learning. Manipulation of the child's own body and objects in the environment promotes explanation and understanding of the world. Grasping and dropping, pushing and pulling, chasing, and falling are among the important motor activities that promote learning. Children in this age group become increasingly aware of themselves through the result of their own actions and from others' reactions to their activities. They have a very short attention span, however, and are easily distractible. In addition, young children have a limited capacity to think about their own actions, to recall the past or anticipate the future. They experience time only in association with immediate events and have a difficult time delaying gratification of their needs. They can respond only to simple, one-step-at-a-time commands.

Although by age 3, the child has a vocabulary of 500 to 1000 words, action rather than words is still the major mode of expression. Movements are used to convey excitement, release tension, and to express love, aggression, self-assertion, and fear. Children of this age cannot distinguish fact from fiction. Their impression of the world is dependent on what they can see and touch. Fantasizing is also common, therefore, information inappropriately relayed may be the cause of fear-provoking misconceptions. The egocentricity of this age combined with limited cognitive capacity for understanding cause and effect often result in the child's feeling that an unpleasant event, or illness, is a punishment for something the child has done.

Psychosocial Development. Erikson (1963) identifies the psychosocial stage of infancy as trust versus mistrust and of toddlerhood as autonomy versus shame and doubt. Children in these age groups are working sequentially on developing basic trust in their world and then increasing independence and self-assertion. Consistent and loving parents, or other caretakers, are essential for accomplishing these tasks. Very young children need the security of having love and approval. A parent's expression of unhappiness is often as distressing to the toddler as a spanking. Routines are also valuable in fostering the toddler's security. Sometimes very elaborate ceremonies surround everyday activities of living and are essential to the accomplishment of a task.

Separation anxiety occurs when the infant or toddler is apart from the parents. This occurs in a variety of situations. When a young child is hospitalized, this has special implications for the nurse–teacher, since anxiety can adversely affect learning readiness. In addition to the insecurity created by separation from parents, an unfamiliar environment, physical examinations, and mobility restraints often compound the child's anxiety about the health-care setting.

Preschool

The preschool years are usually identified as encompassing ages 4 to 6. During this period, the family remains of primary importance, but the experiential environment of the child expands. Newly acquired skills allow the child to assert independence from parents and to perform some bodily care.

Because learning in early childhood occurs largely as a result of reinforcement during social interaction and through modeling, it is important in most situations to assess both the child and the parents.

Physical Maturation. During the preschool years, physical maturation of already developed basic skills continues. Gross motor skills become somewhat refined and fine motor skills become increasingly manipulative. The preschooler can manage self-feeding, going to the bathroom, washing and dressing. Some skills are still not totally coordinated, however. Fine motor skills necessitate large or grossly maneuverable equipment, for example, big buttons for dressing or large crayons and pencils for coloring. Even these still result in some imprecise efforts. The child has the psychomotor skills needed to do grossly coordinated activities, but does not have the judgment to do most skills without some supervision.

Cognitive Development. Piaget (1976) labels the preschooler stage of cognitive development as the preoperational period. Children at this developmental level still deal with experiences in a perceptual and egocentric way. It is their own feelings, sensations, and views that determine the reality of any situation. They are increasingly able to use symbols to represent their experiences, though. Pictures are mainly used, but words become useful symbols as the child progresses. Preschoolers are learning to classify objects according to groups and categories, but understanding is still incomplete. They conclude that objects fall into the same category if they have one or two similar characteristics. For example, a furry animal with a tail is a "kitty," therefore, all furry animals with tails become kitties to them. Preschoolers also have a beginning ability to count and can usually count to ten accurately.

The curiosity of this group is represented in numerous and seemingly unending questions. They ask about reasons or purpose (why?) but are not yet concerned about process (how?). Objects are instilled with a life of their own and perceived to have a meaning and purpose. A child may believe the sun rises so it will be light for the child to play. Reality is still not well differentiated from fantasy in the mind of the preschool child. For the 4-year-old, "bad" thoughts about killing people or setting fires may become so real that equally terrible punishments are imagined and feared. Evil is personified by monsters and bogeymen. Creative play, imaginary playmates, and vivid nightmares result from the preschoolers' active fantasy life.

Although the attention span of the preschooler is somewhat longer than that of the toddler, it is still brief. It is usually long enough for a story to be read or a record to be played. The preschooler still has a very limited sense of time. The 20-minute ride to grandmother's seems like forever. Timing of events is recognized in relation to activities that are part of the daily pattern. For example, it can be understood that bike riding can be done after lunch. The preschooler can follow simple directions of a step or two at a time.

Children's concepts of their bodies and of health and illness change with cognitive development. The first ideas about the body focus on global and observable activities, without differentiation of structure or function. As cognitive development proceeds, internal parts are recognized and differentiated at increasingly more complex levels of structure and function.

Preschoolers usually have highly subjective and egocentric views of their bodies. They display well-defined ideas of external body parts and spatial relations. They are able to name many external parts of the body; however, they have primitive concepts of internal organs (Vessey, 1988). They often include nonorgans such as food and blood, and confuse external and internal body parts in their descriptions (Crider, 1981). Organs cited are often misrepresented in shape and size as well. Though preschoolers can give rudimentary descriptions of functions of internal body parts, descriptions tend to include a single function and this varies among different children. For example, the heart may be described as a part for keeping you well, for love, or for pumping blood. By age 6, children can name some organs and talk about functions, though these are still perceived in terms of activities and states. For example, children can describe "taking in the good air and blowing out the bad air" and often accompany their explanation with exaggerated breathing actions. Some children identify skin as a wrapping and fear if it is cut or punctured, important parts will come out. This fear of mutilation, including castration, is a strong one and is derived from the child's limited understanding of the body coupled with a vivid imagination.

Ideas about illness in this young age group are also limited. As with explanations of the body, explanations of illness are global and include no articulation of cause and effect. Prelogical explanations of illness include accounts of illness attributed to external phenomena or caused by objects or people that are near, but not touching the child (Bibace & Walsh, 1981). For example, colds might be from cold weather or from when someone else gets near you. Preschoolers perceive illness in relation to their own world view, and may believe illness is a punishment for some wrong doing. Medical procedures are also described from the preschooler's egocentric view, according to perceptual cues such as smell or touch and for purposes such as "to steal blood" or "because I'm bad" (Steward & Steward, 1981).

In the preschooler's thinking, health and illness are separate. Health is usually identified by something the child can do, such as play with others or go outside. Preschoolers may identify health as arising from practices such as eating right, exercising, and keeping clean.

Psychosocial Development. During this period, labeled initiative versus guilt by Erikson (1963), the child initiates exploration of and struggles with mastery of his physical and social environment. This is done largely through play. Play now involves other children, and exposes the preschooler to new experiences, sensations, and attitudes. Social behavior is fostered as the child learns to wait for others, to control impulses, and to recognize the needs of other children. During play, children share their different viewpoints and ideas. They also imitate parents of the same sex role. Little girls model their mothers washing dishes and boys imitate daddy carrying the garbage. Play helps children understand the roles of people in their family and society. Young children also reenact their experiences through play. In this way, they are able to act out feelings to again experience joy and happiness, to master fears, and to move from passive to active roles. For example, the 4-year-old who has just had an immunization can master that fear and enforced passivity by playing "doctor" and giving a doll or another willing victim a shot.

School Age

The abilities of the school-age child vary greatly from beginning of this age group at 7 years until the end of the period at 11 years. The overall development of the school-age child at last brings together sufficient physical, cognitive, and psychosocial skills so that learning is not only possible but enthusiastically approached.

Physical Maturation. Gross motor skills are increasingly coordinated so that by age 8 to 9 there is good hand–eye coordination incorporating skilled control and timing of motor movements. Playing marbles, handling tools, and hitting moving targets such as a baseball are all popular ways school-age children use their increasing dexterity. Children of age 8 to 9 and older are also able to learn the psychomotor skills necessary for some self-care management in illness. For example, a child at this age can learn to give insulin injections or manage an inhalator.

Cognitive Development. In the period of concrete operations, the beginning of logical thought processes and reasoning develops. Piaget (1976) describes this cognitive developmental period as one in which the child is able to see the cause and effect of concrete processes.

There is increased mastery of symbols including language, ability to classify, and awareness of conservation of matter and reversibility. School-age children are able to understand that medicine may come in the form of a liquid or a pill and still have the same effect on the body. They know and can express ideas about relationships between people and objects. The school-age child still interprets the world quite literally, and ideas about the abstract are still vague. Often the ability to use language is more advanced than the understanding of the terminology being used.

By age 7 to 8, beginning decision-making skills are developed. This allows children to take action based on the interpretation of events. For example, when a headache occurs, if at home, the child may lie down; at school, action may be initiated to see the school nurse. The school-age child can assume self-responsibility for activities of daily living. Because ideas are based on personal experiences and observations, prior to age 12 to 13 most children are not well equipped to make independent judgments related to novel or uncommon experiences. This accounts for some children's experimentation with alcohol or smoking at a young age.

Although during the school-age years thought processes become more logical and reasonable, the child is still limited in conceptualizing the abstract. Time orientation includes the past and present and some vague ideas about the future. School-age children are increasingly able to take action in the present, which will have an effect in the future, but they are readily discouraged if the effect does not occur within the predicted amount of time.

During this developmental period, children learn strategies for concentration and remembering (Berger, 1988), and the attention span increases sufficiently to facilitate longer periods of study. One or 2 hours can often be devoted to a subject of interest. Thought processes are developed sufficiently to allow children to follow directions involving several specific tasks and to appreciate views other than their own.

Though descriptions are primarily at the concrete level, children between the ages of 7 and 11 display definite ideas about their bodies and how the body functions. Younger children in this group can usually identify the brain, bones, heart, blood, and blood vessels; children about age 10 to 11 add the stomach; later kidneys, nerves, muscles, intestines, lungs, and other specific internal organs are included (Crider, 1981). Although children are increasingly able to differentiate between internal and external body parts, some descriptions are still vague and nonspecific, and functions and relationships of internal organs may be confused (Pidgeon, 1986).

Accounts of illness are less egocentric and more in keeping with medical and cultural explanations. Children are increasingly able to link cause and effect in relation to illness. Initially, they identify causes of illness as objects or people external to themselves; as they continue to mature in their thinking, they grasp the idea that illness is located inside the body even though the cause may be external (Bibace & Wallace, 1981). They also recognize the effect of germs in causing illness; however, they often do not understand germs fully and identify the presence of any germ as meaning immediate illness (Wood, 1983). Young school-agers often describe illness in terms of social consequences or role alterations; for example, they miss school or people feel sorry for them (Banks, 1990). Prior to age 8 or 9, they have difficulty determining health or illness states according to body cues (Kalnins & Love, 1982). As children mature in their thinking, illness concepts change from more global descriptions to specific features or symptoms. Multiple-step medical routines can be understood and children can follow these as long as there are no deviations. Medical procedures are correctly described, but functions may be interpreted literally; for example, a child may worry that a CAT scan of the brain may find bad thoughts (Steward & Steward, 1981).

Older school-age children are beginning to understand health as a state that involves interaction of body, mind, and environment. They are more likely to define it as positive concept rather than the mere absence of illness. They can list specific acts or rules for staying healthy or getting sick (Kalnins & Love, 1982).

Psychosocial Development. Erikson (1983) places the school-age child in the stage of industry versus inferiority. Mastery of academics, peer relationships, and physical skills are tasks the child strives to accomplish and school is the major locus of accomplishments. Self-esteem is influenced by experiences of accomplishment and attitudes of peers, family, and other significant adults. Children often become self-critical as they become increasingly aware of their own abilities and perceptions of inability. They are also more aware of society at large and susceptible to influences outside of the family.

Because accomplishments are so essential to this age group, factors that cause disruption of this process are of concern to the child. Fears about disability, loss of status, and loss of control are common in times of stress. Fear of disability often occurs when children are observed with crutches, bandages, wheelchairs, or braces. Since school activities are such an important focus, disruption by illness or hospitalization interferes with academic work and social contacts, and children often fear they will fall behind and be left out of the group. Illness also may cause loss of control of body functions, and hospitalization certainly causes loss of control of many activities that the school-age child is otherwise able to independently undertake.

Adolescence

The adolescent, ages 12 to 18, is approaching adult abilities. During this period of life, maturation occurs both physically and psychologically as the adolescent prepares for the self-sufficiency and self-responsibility of adulthood.

Physical Maturation. Gross motor mobility and fine motor manipulations reach adult capacity during adolescence. Skills, already present and well coordinated, become increasingly refined and may become highly developed with special practice. During this developmental period, many athletes are discovered and begin preparing for competitive events. There are periods during adolescence in which rapid physical growth temporarily results in some clumsiness and poorly coordinated muscle movements. Secondary sexual characteristics also appear and develop during this period.

Cognitive Development. By this stage, the individual has reached what Piaget (1976) labels the period of formal operations. This means that the ability to abstract, conceptualize, and internalize develops. Because of the capacity to mentally organize and visualize the processes involved, complex scientific theory related to cause and effect and process can be understood. The adolescent can handle multiple verbal directions and rules.

The ability to interpret and use language, to understand the complexity of nuance and satire, develops in the adolescent. Vocabulary is extensive. Adolescents can understand implications of future outcomes as well as evaluate past events and present implications.

Older children are able to understand more abstract concepts of health and illness and express these more specifically in terms representing scientific and prevailing cultural beliefs (Banks, 1990; Bibace & Walsh, 1981; Pidgeon & Olson, 1986). Body functions are explained in physiological terms. However, some ideas about the body may remain unclear because the adolescent may be embarrassed to discuss the topic.

Illness is identified as a nonfunctioning or malfunctioning body part, or process, which is the outcome of a specific sequence of events. Symptoms are understood as manifestations of the physiological malfunctions. Multiple causes of illness, including psychophysiological causes are recognized. For example, an explanation of a heart attack might include the physiological cause, the heart not pumping right, as well as recognition of the effects of psychological events such as worry and stress. Medical procedures are readily explained and the probable impact to the procedure can be understood (Steward & Steward, 1981).

Adolescents are able to understand health as a concept difficult to describe. They are also able to understand ideas about health promotion and maintenance, thus identify healthy behaviors. Nonetheless, feelings of invincibility may cause the adolescent to use unhealthy behaviors and to take unadvisable risks. In addition, despite the ability to provide more complex explanations of the process of illness and treatments, the adolescent's understanding is not always rational, and may blend fact, fantasy, and emotion (Pidgeon & Olson, 1986).

Psychosocial Development. The adolescent encounters the task labeled by Erikson (1963) as identity versus identity diffusion. This is a time of struggle to assert independence, establish one's own values, and determine "self." The individual is dependent on group belongingness and increasingly aware of his or her own appearance and functions compared to an ideal image. The need to be and look like peers and idealized heroes governs most of the adolescent's actions. Personal values are shaped by what is important to others and what type of behavior is rewarded.

In developing independence, the adolescent is concerned about personal space, privacy, and confidentiality. Relationships with parents may alternate between ignoring, alienation, and tolerance. Other authority figures are sometimes approached with similar conflicting attitudes.

Stresses experienced by the adolescent during times of illness or hospitalization include fears of death and disability as well as loss of identity, loss of privacy, and loss of control. The adolescent, so often uncertain about identity and abilities, is threatened by illness, the possible changes in body function or appearance that it may bring, and others' reactions to those changes. The ability to conceptualize allows the adolescent to understand the implications of illness and the permanence of death. Illness usually brings about enforced dependency upon others for bodily care as well as other activities of living. This causes conflicts in the adolescent's striving for independence as well as embarrassment about the body.

Summary

Children of all ages can be health learners. An understanding of the developmental characteristics that govern the learning abilities of a child at any given age is essential for identifying appropriate assessment areas, health activities, and strategies to optimize learning.

DEVELOPMENTAL CHARACTERISTICS OF ADULTS

The period of life referred to as adulthood is divided into different developmental stages, just as is childhood. Although theorists characterize each stage somewhat differently, there is commonality in the timing of the stages. Adulthood comprises the years from adolescence until death. Young adulthood includes the ages of about 20 to 40 years, middle adulthood ages 40 to 65 years, and late adulthood over 65 years. By young adulthood, the growth of physical and cognitive structures is complete. Although changes continue throughout life, in the adult these changes are slower in developing and less dramatic than in the child. Certain characteristics describe the adult learner irrespective of age, but there are also age-related implications. The following discussion relates to the adult learner. Then, age-related factors are explored.

The adult learner is quite different from the younger learner. As has been seen in the previous discussion, the readiness to learn for the child varies with the level of physical, cognitive, and related psychosocial development. Since adult physical and cognitive capacities are fully developed, these have less of a differentiating effect. Instead, readiness is determined by life tasks and recognized problems. Readiness to learn evolves mainly from developmental tasks related to social roles and aspects of work, family, and leisure. Motivation is sparked by the existence of a problem that needs solving. Where children's learning is subject centered, adult learning is problem centered. For adults, the application of learning is present oriented. Because they are problem centered learners, they are also able to identify their own readiness to learn. New behaviors must be clearly relevant to an adult's situation in order for a learning need to be perceived.

Another difference between the child and adult learner is the level of dependency of the learner. The child is dependent in many ways and this carries over to learning as well. Children usually respond to a teacher as an authority figure. With growth, there is a move toward less other-directed learning and increasing self-directedness. Adults often prefer, therefore, to direct their own learning. When this is not allowed, the result of this loss of control may cause resentment in the adult. An individual may withdraw from the learning situation or learn less effectively.

Experiences provide rich resources for adult learners. For children, experiences happen to them and are viewed as external events. For adults, experiences help define who they are and provide valuable foundations for further learning. Experiences allow adults to more quickly grasp relationships. Adults have more stored information on a topic and hence can cross-reference new ideas to existing ones readily. Past experiences, as part of an already established system of ideas, also make the adult learner more resistant to change.

The rate of learning also varies between child and adult learners. Most children learn fairly quickly and are tolerant of learning isolated facts and concepts. Adults, however, as previously stated, are problem centered and are therefore resistant to learning material not applicable to practical problems. During the process of aging, changes also occur that may increase the time necessary for completing learning tasks. These changes are discussed in more detail in the section on late adulthood.

Barriers toward learning are different for children and adults. Although the child may be distracted from learning by outside events, there are few other responsibilities competing for learning time. The child of 5 and older is also accustomed to a formal learning environment. Barriers to learning in childhood are usually those related to developmental capacities. In adults, barriers may be situational or emotional. Additional responsibilities, or concerns about those responsibilities, like child care, work, and community activities, may interfere with time and energy for learning. Adults also may have anxieties for being learners. They may feel too old to learn, that they have been away from learning too long, or that past experiences have not prepared them for the learning situation. Unpleasantness from the school-room years ago may generate fear or anxiety. The adult may be fearful of the risk of failure as a learner.

As is evident from the discussion above, there are a number of differences between the child and the adult learner. Table 8–1 lists the learner characteristics and the basic differences. The remainder of this chapter provides a discussion of differences in the developmental characteristics of the three stages of adulthood. This will provide further basis for assessing the adult learner.

Young Adult

During young adulthood, ages 20 to 40, individuals become independent in all facets of life. Decisions regarding education, occupational choice, and life style are completed and acted upon.

Physical Maturation. Although physical abilities are very individual, persons in their twenties are at their peak. All body systems are functioning optimally. Muscle tone and coordination are at the maximum, so athletic endeavors are at their best during this period. There are few psychomotor skills that an individual of this age group could not master if so inclined.

Cognitive Development. Young adults have reached full cognitive capacity but may continue to learn either formally or informally. They are concerned about

TABLE 8–1. COMPARISON OF LEARNER CHARACTERISTICS BETWEEN CHILDREN AND ADULTS

Characteristics	Children	Adults
Readiness to learn	Based primarily on biological development	Determined by life tasks, roles and immediate problems
Application of learning	Postponed application; subject centered	Immediate application related to relevant problems
Orientation to learning	Dependent; other-directed learning	Independent; self-directed
Value of experiences	Experiences seen as external events	Experiences are internalized: they provide a foundation for further learning and may contribute resistance to change
Rate of learning	Quickly masters isolated facts and concepts	Resistant to learning nonrelevant material; the aging process increases the time needed to complete some learning tasks
Barriers to learning	Few competing responsibilities for learning time; accustomed to formal learning through school experiences	Family, work, or community responsibilities may compete for learning time and energy; anxieties about self-image as a learner may threaten

society's values, the world in which they live, and life style choices. Perceptual and cognitive capacities allow critical analysis and problem solving. Application of these abilities may be for personal decision making or in social or occupational roles.

The young adult has both the cognitive capacity and physical strength and skill to learn things of various levels of difficulty. Past experiences provide a foundation for further learning. Because the adult is problem oriented, interest will be in areas that are both relevant and have immediate application. Developmental tasks discussed in the following section refer to some areas of interest for the young adult. The young adult experienced in being independent and self-directing can be involved in planning both the content to be learned and the methods of learning.

Psychosocial Development. The young adult in American society is expected to be independent. This expectation necessitates the establishment of living arrangements and financial self-sufficiency. In order to do this, the young adult faces many new experiences and choices. Decisions about education, career, marriage, and beginning a family are ones that will influence life style in the future as well as in the immediate time period. Often young adults seek to learn more about the implications of various life style choices. In the area of health, they may wish to learn about sexuality, family planning, child-rearing practices, home and occupational safety, and stress management. Current emphasis on physical fitness has made exercise, nutrition, and preventive health practices relevant areas of interest as well.

Erikson (1963) labels the conflict of the young adult as intimacy versus isolation. Working to establish a commitment to others, to develop trust and satisfy relationships in love and work are important tasks for the young adult. Health learning needs identified to help meet these tasks are some of the same as those listed above.

Middle Adult

The years of middle adulthood, ages 40 to 65, are often looked at as years of stability. Families are grown and parents have more time to pursue other interests. Careers are well developed, permitting optimum professional and occupational contribution.

Physical Maturation. Although at age 40 most adults function as well as they did during their twenties and thirties, a number of physiological changes take place. Many of these do not affect learning directly, but may affect self-image, and this in turn can affect learning. Changes may also precipitate a desire to learn more about the body, developmental changes, and health monitoring. Different body parts age at different rates. During middle age, hair grays or some is lost, decreased skin turgor causes wrinkles, fatty tissue is redistributed toward the middle of the body, decreased basal metabolism often results in weight gain, and loss of muscle tone leads to varicose veins and some decreased strength. In addition, hormonal changes may cause a variety of symptoms. These culminate in menopause in women. Men may or may not experience physical symptoms as androgen levels decrease. Hearing and visual acuity both diminish slightly. Energy is also expended more rapidly and recovered more slowly during middle adulthood.

Cognitive Development. Learning capacity remains unimpaired during middle age. In fact, past experiences, flexibility, and confidence achieved from other experiences often facilitate learning. Motivation to learn knowledge that can be applied remains high. Changes in strength, vision, and hearing that may affect learning should be assessed on an individual basis.

Psychosocial Development. This stage is one of self-assessment. Transition to middle age, as described by VanHoose and Worth (1982) occurs when an individual realizes that he or she has reached the halfway mark of life and that life is finite. Individuals reexamine their lives, reevaluate their goals and achievements, and look at remaining options. Often career or personal life changes are made at this time of life.

Adults in middle age also view their bodies differently. Physical changes are visible so individuals look older, and change in energy levels also make them feel older. "Change of life" experiences also affect self-concept. Erikson (1963) labels the conflict of middle adulthood as generativity versus self-absorption and stagnation. Individuals move from the self and family orientation of young adulthood to a concern about the larger community and future generations. Service projects and cultural endeavors are undertaken. Individuals, freed from previous family responsibilities or more secure in occupational roles, develop new interests and leisure-time activities. Other life events that affect the individual in middle adulthood include the joy-without-responsibility of grandparenthood and the care of and loss of elderly parents. Both financial and recreational planning for retirement also occur. Health education desired may be in the area of environmental protection, relaxation and diversion, or enhancement of self-concept.

Late Adult

The population of late adulthood comprises those over the age of 65. Often this group is referred to as "the elderly" and stereotyped as feeble, slow moving, irritable, and not interested in learning anything new. Although there are physical, cognitive, and psychosocial developments during late adulthood, most elderly adults are active and healthy; only a minority, the frail elderly, are too ill to care for themselves. Knowing the changes that occur during older adulthood will help nurse–teachers focus on areas to assess so that teaching strategies can be modified and learning maximized for each individual older adult.

Physical Maturation. After the age of 65, there are physiological changes in all body systems. Before discussing these changes, it is important to emphasize that the age of onset and degree of involvement vary among individuals. Those changes affecting the neurologic, cardiovascular, respiratory, and musculoskeletal systems have the most effect on health learning.

The neurologic changes involve both sensory and cerebral systems. Both vision and hearing diminish. Nine out of 10 elders need glasses, and usually obtain these; one of three could benefit from a hearing aide but these are not as readily obtained (Berger, 1988). Visual acuity is impaired as the lens of the eye becomes rigid and opaque, decreased pupil size causes less light to reach the retina, and sensitivity to glare increases. Accommodation takes longer and depth perception is decreased (Weinrich, Boyd, & Nussbaum, 1989). Poorer discrimination among blue, green, and violet hues and decreased ability to discriminate detail also occur. High-pitched sounds are less well heard due to degeneration of central and peripheral auditory mechanisms. Individuals may have difficulty discriminating the sound of high-frequency consonants like s, f, and k. Older people also tend to hear male voices better than female voices (Kick, 1989). In addition to visual and auditory changes, there are changes in tactile perceptions. Older adults have less sensitivity to touch, pressure, and temperature (Weinrich, Boyd, & Nussbaum, 1989).

Cerebral systems are also affected by neurologic changes. Investigations suggest that there is a decrease in the integrative function of the nervous system. This often results in a diminished sense of balance and fine movement.

Gradual declines affect other body systems as well. Cardiovascular and respiratory changes affect the circulation of oxygen and other nutrients and the amount of available oxygen. Cardiovascular changes cause the heart to work harder to accomplish circulatory tasks. Respiratory efficiency also declines. Together, these can result in easier fatigue and decreased attention span, especially under stress. As muscle mass deteriorates, muscle tone and strength decline. However, exercise and physical activity play an important role in maintaining physical strength and endurance. The level of motor strength can affect the mastery of psychomotor skills. Degenerative changes in the joints can make movement stiffer and more restricted. Inactivity also aggravates this stiffness so it may be difficult for some older adults to maintain a prolonged sitting position. The loss of kidney function along with the use of diuretics shortens the time some elderly can sit (Picariello, 1986).

Cognitive Development. The organization of knowledge remains stable during adult life, and older adults do not seem to differ from young adults in rate or breadth of comprehension, but they do differ in memory and integration of ideas when large amounts of material, especially irrelevant material, is involved (Light, 1990). Lack of memory can affect the older adult when trying to learn material that would build upon that previous information. More difficulty is seen when elders attempt to process new classifications of material as opposed to material that is familiar or logically related to other known information. Older adults are also not able to divide their attention well and may have difficulty concentrating. They also require more time to respond. Monotony, boredom, and isolation may also contribute to a decrease in cognitive function (Kick, 1989).

Psychosocial Development. The developmental task of late adulthood, labeled ego integrity versus despair by Erikson (1963), involves acceptance of one's own life as it has been lived. Most elderly individuals still value independence and may struggle to look after themselves and maintain their own households. It is important for the elderly individual to maintain a sense of self-worth in coping with physiological changes sometimes aggravated by illness, environmental changes, and the adjustment to a retirement life style.

The older adult can learn skills that will help maintain as much independent function as possible and that will permit functioning as fully as possible within limitations. Often acute illness and accidents can be prevented. Aging is not the same as disease, but symptoms are often overlooked and labelled as "signs of growing older." Many pathophysiological conditions also affect the older person's ability to learn. Chronic obstructive pulmonary disease, cardiovascular disorders, and depression are common.

SUMMARY

From the foregoing discussion, it is possible to see that there are a variety of developmental factors that must be assessed in order to plan an individualized approach to health teaching. When working with children, it is especially important that the nurse determine cognitive and psychosocial development. These will influence the level of the teaching strategies chosen and help identify whether parental or peer involvement would facilitate learning. If psychomotor skills are part of a health-learning need, it is imperative to assess physical maturation to determine if the abilities foundational to the new skills are present.

When assessing the adult, emphasis upon the developmental areas is different than when assessing a child. The average adult possess cognitive capacities to learn, so assessing the precise level of cognition becomes less important. It is still important to determine the existing knowledge about the content area to be studied. This is especially important when dealing with illness-related topics that are not as well understood by the general public as by health professionals. Misconceptions or lack of knowledge of terminology must be identified. Since physical skills are developed fully in the average adult, the assessment of this area should focus on past experience with skills and the adult's feelings about manipulative competencies. This can help the nurse determine the amount and type of practice that will be needed to master psychomotor skills. Assessment of older adults needs to focus on the physical changes experienced by a given individual. Assessment of the psychosocial development of the adult will provide information that can help the nurse work with the adult learner to identify areas of relevant health learning.

Assessment of the developmental level of the learner is an important step for determining appropriate teaching strategies. Knowing developmental stages and sequence can assist the nurse to focus on key assessment data. The next chapter provides guidelines for incorporating the developmental factors discussed in this chapter into learner assessment. Chapter 12 discusses in detail how to use developmental assessment data in planning appropriate teaching strategies for learners of various developmental levels.

REFERENCES AND READINGS

Ager, C. L. Teaching strategies for the elderly. *Physical and Occupational Therapy in Geriatrics*, 1986, *4*(4), 3–14.

Alywahby, N. F. Principles of teaching for individual learning of older adults. *Rehabilitation Nursing*, 1989, *14*(6), 330–333.

Banks, E. Concepts of health and sickness of preschool- and school-aged children. *Children's Health Care*, 1990, *19*(1), 43–48.

Berger, K. S. *The developing person through the life span* (2nd ed.) NY: Worth Publishers, 1988.

Bibace, R. & Walsh, M. E. Children's conceptions of illness. In Bibace, R. & Walsh, M. E. (Eds.). *New directions for child development: Children's conceptions of health, illness and bodily functions.* San Francisco: Jossey-Bass, 1981, pp. 31–48.

Crider, C. Children's conceptions of the body interior. In Bibace, R. & Walsh, M. E. (Eds.). *New directions for child development: Children's conceptions of health, illness, and bodily functions.* San Francisco: Jossey-Bass, 1981, pp. 49–66.

Eaton, W. O. *Motor activity from fetus to adult.* 1983. Paper.

Erikson, E. H. *Childhood and society.* NY: W. E. Norton & Co., Inc., 1963.

Fielo, S. B. & Rizzolo, M. A. Handle with caring: Meeting elderly clients' special learning needs. *Nursing and Health Care*, 1988, *9*(4), 192–195.

Fox, V. Patient teaching: Understanding the needs of the adult learner. *AORN*, 1986, *44*(2), 234–238.

Fozard, J. L. Vision and hearing in aging. In Birren, J. E. & Schaie, K. W. (Eds). *Handbook of the psychology of aging* (3d ed.). San Diego, CA: Academic Press, Inc., 1990, 150–170.

Gratz, R. R. & Piliavin, J. A. What makes kids sick: Children's beliefs about the causative factors of illness. *Children's Health Care*, 1984, *12*(4), 156–162.

Gessner, B. A. Adult education: The cornerstone of patient teaching. *Nursing Clinics of North America*, 1989, *24*(3), 589–595.

Kalnins, I. & Love, E. Children's concepts of health and illness and implications for health education: An overview. *Health Education Quarterly*, 1982, *9*(2&3), 104–115.

Kick, E. Patient teaching for elders. *Nursing Clinics of North America*, 1989, *24*(3), 687–693.

Kim, K. K. Response time and health care learning of elderly patients. *Research in Nursing and Health*, 1986, *9*(3), 233–239.

Knowles, M. *The adult learner: A neglected species* (3d ed.) Houston, TX: Gulf Publishing, 1984.

Light, L. L. Interactions between memory and language. In Birren, J. E. & Schaie, K. W. (Eds). *Handbook of the psychology of aging* (3d ed.). San Diego, CA: Academic Press, Inc., 1990, 275–309.

McDowd, J. M. & Birren, J. E. Aging and attentional processes. In Birren, J. E. & Schaie, K. W. (Eds). *Handbook of the psychology of aging* (3d ed.). San Diego, CA: Academic Press, Inc., 1990, 222–274.

Padberg, R. M. & Padberg, L. F. Strengthening the effectiveness of patient education: Applying principles of adult education. *Oncology Nursing Forum*, 1990, *17*(1), 65–69.

Piaget, J. *The grasp of consciousness: Action and concept in the young child*. Susan Wedgwood (Trans.). Cambridge, MA: Harvard University Press, 1976.

Piaget, J. & Inhelder, B. *The psychology of the child*. Helen Weaver (Trans.). NY: Routledge and Kegan Paul, 1969.

Picariello, G. A guide for teaching elders. *Geriatric Nursing*, 1986, *7*(1), 38–39.

Pidgeon, V. Children's concepts of illness: Implications for health teaching. *Maternal-Child Nursing Journal*, 1986, *15*(3), 23–35.

Pidgeon, V. & Olson, S. A comparison of illness concepts of school age children and adolescents. *Issues in Comprehensive Pediatric Nursing*, 1986, *9*, 209–221.

Porterfield, L. & Harris, B. Information needs of the pregnant adolescent. *Home Healthcare Nurse*, 1985, *3*(6), 41–43.

Pridham, K. F., Adelson, F., & Hansen, M. F. Helping children deal with procedures in a clinic setting: A developmental approach . . . competence and self-esteem. *Journal of Pediatric Nursing*, 1987, *2*(1), 13–22.

Reichenback, M. B. A framework for the nature and development of health beliefs in children. *Maternal Child Nursing Journal*, 1986, *15*(3), 119–127.

Spirduso, W. W. & MacRae, P. G. Motor Performance and aging. In Birren, J. E. & Schaie, K. W. (Eds). *Handbook of the psychology of aging* (3d ed.). San Diego, CA: Academic Press, Inc., 1990, 183–200.

Steward, M. S. & Steward, D. S. Children's conceptions of medical procedures. In Bibace, R. & Walsh, M. E. (Eds.). *New directions for child development: Children's conceptions of health, illness and bodily functions*. San Francisco: Jossey-Bass. 1981, pp. 67–83.

Tumminia, P. A. & Weinfield, A. M. Teaching the learning-disabled nursing student. *Nursing Educator*, Winter 1983, 12–20.

VanHoose, W. H. & Worth, M. R. *Adulthood in the life cycle.* Dubuque, Iowa: Wm. C. Brown Co., 1982.

Vessey, J. A. Care of the hospitalized child with a cognitive developmental delay. *Holistic Nursing Practice,* 1988, 2(2), 48–54.

Vessey, J. A. Comparison of two teaching methods on children's knowledge of their internal bodies. *Nursing Research,* 1988, *37*(5), 262–267.

Waidley, E. K. Show and tell: Preparing children for invasive procedures . . . a picture book. *AJN,* 1989, *85*(7), 811–812.

Weinrich, S. P., Boyd, M., & Nussbaum, J. Continuing education: Adapting strategies to teach the elderly. *Journal of Gerontological Nursing,* 1989, *15*(11), 17–20.

Wood, S. P. School-aged children's perceptions of the causes of illness. *Pediatric Nursing,* 1983, *9,* 101–104.

9

Assessment
of the Learner

Nancy I. Whitman

A "sense of appropriate timing is essential in teaching" (Murray & Zentner, 1985, p. 170). Assessment of readiness factors can help nurses more accurately choose the appropriate time for teaching and learning. In addition, assessment of readiness factors provides the nurse with data for predicting the efficacy of learning and helps identify situations where specific strategies must be used to facilitate learner readiness and learning.

THE ASSESSMENT PROCESS

Assessment is an integral part of the teaching–learning process and is essential in determining an individual's readiness for learning. Just as in the nursing process, it is the first step in the teaching process and is followed by diagnosis, planning, implementation, and evaluation. Assessment begins with the systematic collection of data relevant to the teaching–learning situation. Data are then organized and categorized so that analysis is facilitated. Through analysis, educational needs are identified.

Data collection includes obtaining information relevant to learning readiness factors previously identified and obtaining information about health content areas for learning. Each of these is discussed separately here.

Assessment of the Learner
The three categories previously identified as the main categories for determining readiness for learning—health status, health values, and developmental characteristics—provide the framework for assessment of the learner. In addition to these, it is important to assess prior learning experiences upon which the learner can build. Table 9–1 provides a list of each main category and subcategories to be assessed.

TABLE 9-1. LEARNER READINESS: FACTORS AFFECTING THE CLIENT

Factor Categories	Experiential Readiness Factors	Motivational Readiness Factors
Health status	Physiological state: Energy level Sensory status Comfort status	Psychological state: Anxiety/fear level Adjustment to health status
Health values		Perception of control over health Expectations of outcomes: Beliefs of susceptibility to illness Perceived benefits and barrier of health action
Developmental characteristics	Psychomotor skills Cognitive abilities Learning disabilities	Life stage Psychosocial development
Prior learning experiences	Existing knowledge base Learning style	Attitudes toward learning: From past experiences From within social/cultural groups

Health Status

An assessment of this area encompasses the assessment of both physical and emotional status. During a physical assessment, a nurse should evaluate the client's energy level, comfort status, and sensory status. Energy level is an important determinant of the physical strength available for learning. If energy level is drastically reduced, learning may not take place, or it may take more time. For example, a newly diagnosed diabetic recovering from ketoacidosis or a first-day postoperative patient must invest all available energy into physiological needs. In these situations, it is unlikely that much energy will be available for learning. As the body state stabilizes, however, the level of energy usually increases, and readiness to learn improves. Assessment of a client's comfort status will assist in identifying possible barriers to learning. It is possible for the nurse to help minimize many discomforts and therefore maximize learning. In addition, sensory impairments such as visual deficits or hearing losses can limit learning ability. Psychological health status is influenced by anxiety, fear, or adjustment to the health state. An individual may be physiologically stable after a laryngectomy necessitated by recently diagnosed cancer. He may not be ready to learn, however, because psychological energy is being invested in coping with the diagnosis of cancer. Another client, still struggling with a change in body image associated with a colostomy, will not be emotionally ready to learn to care for the appliance. Identification of physiological and psychological strengths and stressors also helps determine the structure, organization, and timing of the teaching–learning interaction.

Energy Level. The client's energy level can be ascertained by observing the client's level of activity. Is he or she able to move easily without frequent rests or easy fatigue? How much sleep or rest does he or she require each day? If the client is recovering from surgery, the answers to these questions will be very different from those of the client who is visiting the clinic for hypertension screening or the client with severe chronic obstructive pulmonary disease. Most individuals also have a certain time of day when their energy is at its peak and they are most productive. Discussing this with the client or observing what is accomplished each day will also help determine energy level.

Comfort Status. Assessment of the client's comfort status involves assessing factors that have both physical and psychological effects on comfort. Usually first identified are physical factors affecting comfort, the primary one being pain. The nurse can determine if the client is experiencing pain by observing body posture, movement, and facial expression, and by discussing the pain experience with the client. Sometimes it is possible to postpone teaching until pain diminishes. When that is not possible, such as in the case of chronic pain, plans can be made to minimize the pain and to time the teaching–learning interaction to occur when pain is reduced as much as possible. Other common physical discomforts include nausea, itching, fatigue, hunger or thirst, and the need to eliminate urine or feces. Each of these must be assessed and managed before beginning the teaching–learning interaction. When it is not possible to eliminate the discomfort and the teaching–learning interaction needs to proceed, the discomfort should be recognized and the teaching plan structured to keep the discomfort at a minimum. Shorter, spaced teaching sessions help accomplish this.

Psychological discomforts can also hinder the learning process. The fear of dying or anxiety about scars can interfere with learning about surgery. Guilt related to the cause of hospitalization or anger about the timing of required medical care may hinder learning about preventive health behaviors. Fear, anxiety, guilt, anger, and grief are commonly occurring emotions that interfere with attention to learning (Potter & Perry, 1991). These emotions must be recognized by the nurse and managed before the teaching–learning interaction can be productive.

Sensory Status. Sensory status is the third part of the physical assessment. Basic to all communication are the channels of conveying a message. Visual, auditory, and perceptual abilities provide channels for communication and are therefore important determinants for the effectiveness of teaching–learning interactions. These abilities also help determine the type of teaching–learning experience that might be effective.

Visual acuity influences the learning aids that can be used. Posters or pamphlets with large, easily legible print would be appropriate for those learners with some visual deficits. If the learner wears corrective lenses, the nurse should know this and ensure that they are worn for teaching–learning sessions. Eye contact is often an indicator of interest; lack of eye contact may be a cultural phenomenon or an indication of discomfort about the topic being addressed (Anderson, 1990). Visual perception that interferes with eye contact can affect the teaching–learning interaction.

Since our primary channel of communication is oral, assessment of the auditory channel is imperative. As the nurse observes the client's reaction to oral communication, the question should be, "Can the client hear normal voice tones?" and "At what distance are they heard?" It is also important to determine if the client wears an auditory aid. Knowing if the client finds certain sounds distracting will also help the nurse plan for the teaching–learning interaction.

Assessing perceptual abilities involves determining the client's awareness of stimuli and ability to interpret what was experienced. Determining the client's level of consciousness is the first step in assessing perceptual abilities. A nurse–teacher needs to determine the individual's awareness of and responsiveness to environmental stimuli. This may be impaired by a disease state or by psychological events such as fear or anger. Evaluating an individual's responses to questions about life experiences and health state allows the nurse–teacher to assess both the quality and rate of response. The thoughts expressed by the client will provide data for evaluating comprehension, coherence, and reality orientation. Continuing discussion over a short period of time will help determine the client's ability to concentrate and the attention span.

Adjustment to Health State. The emotional state of the client is equally important to assess when considering health state. Since emotions can interfere with the ability to learn, an assessment of the client's emotional status is essential. As discussed in Chapter 6, adjustment to illness includes both approach and avoidance behaviors as temporary or permanent losses are dealt with. Assessment of the level of adjustment can help determine readiness for learning. In the avoidance stages, the individual will not be ready to concentrate on learning. As an individual begins to adapt to the realities of the new situation, however, teaching is likely to be effective and the teaching plan can be introduced. Questions that will facilitate assessment of the client's level of adjustment include, "How would you describe your health?" "How do you feel right now?" "Do you have concerns about your health/illness?" and, if yes, "What concerns you most?" "How do you think you can best stay healthy?" and "What do you think you need to do to best take care of yourself during this illness?"

An assessment of the client's current health status can provide indications about his or her readiness to learn. In addition, it can provide clues for the nurse about some content areas for learning. To validate an anticipated area for learning, the nurse can ask the client if there is anything he or she would like to know or learn that would improve the client's health. If several areas of learning need are identified, ranking these as to what is most important to the client helps determine priorities.

Health Values

Individuals first learn about health from their families. Families are influenced by the larger sociocultural group to which they belong. Cultural orientation affects health beliefs and health practices. Chapter 14 provides specific information on cultures commonly encountered in our health-care systems. The nurse–teacher needs to understand that attitudes toward health and about health behavior will influence participation in the teaching–learning interaction. An individual's perceptions and expectations related to the health situation will provide clues to health values. Perceptions of control and expectations related to the outcome of health behavior need to be assessed.

Perceptions of Control Over Health. One's perception of control provides clues about feelings of power or powerlessness (locus of control) and one's ability to influence a situation. Some individuals strongly believe that their own actions, for example, taking vitamin pills and eating nutritionally balanced meals, help maintain their good health state. Others feel that nothing they do will affect the outcome of a situation and that their lives are controlled by luck or fate (Hussey & Gilliland, 1989). Self-control and luck or fate are two perceptions of types of influence upon health. A third is the perception that someone else has control. Many individuals invest their feelings of control over health to health professionals, that is, nurse, doctor, or other therapist. The determination of where this control is invested is important for planning effective teaching strategies. An approach for clients who have a strong belief in self-control or internal locus of control may be that of self-care, while for those believing in control outside of themselves, or external locus of control, a more directive approach may work better (Shillinger, 1983). Asking questions about how individuals would behave in an illness situation and from whom they would seek help can provide information about perceptions of control.

Expectations of Outcomes. In addition to feelings of control, expectations of outcomes are influenced by health values. These include beliefs related to the likelihood of becoming severely ill and the benefits or barriers perceived in taking health actions. A perceived threat of illness, perception of positive outcomes from taking health action, and minimal impediments for taking the health action may motivate health behavior in some situations. Chapter 7 provides a more thorough discussion of health values and their implications. The assessment of health values may begin by asking the following questions: "What would you do first if you (or some member of your family) became ill?" "Whom would you call for assistance if you became ill?" "When you are ill, what can you do to help get better?" "What do you expect to happen when you (specifying health behavior as appropriate)?" "How likely is it that you will become ill?" "Is there anything you could do to help you become more healthy/better?" (If positive) "What would make it easier for you to do _____? What makes it difficult for you to do _____"? Observations of congruence between statements and behaviors also provide useful data.

Developmental Characteristics

Learner readiness is influenced by developmental characteristics that determine the level at which the learner is able to function. These characteristics can be divided into three main categories for the purpose of assessment—physical maturation, cognitive development, and psychosocial development. Physical maturation includes psychomotor skills and coordination. Cognitive development refers to the intellectual skills the learner possesses and capacity for self-responsibility. Life-stage tasks are important components of psychosocial development.

The developmental characteristics of a certain age group help predict the cognitive abilities and motor skills that can be expected and subsequently incorporated into a learning program. For example, it is not possible to teach a 5-year-old with diabetes how to give his or her own insulin because the child does not possess the necessary psychomotor abilities for manipulating a syringe nor the cognitive capacity to understand the mechanics or rationale for the injection. An older child or adult, however, does typically possess the developmental skills needed for learning the injection technique. Psychosocial development also follows characteristic patterns. Knowing these patterns can be helpful in determining important tasks for individuals at certain phases of life. This, in turn, promotes more accurate identification of readiness for learning about certain health-related topics. A 26-year-old mother, for example, may be interested in learning about her child's growth and development, but a 16-year-old mother may be more concerned with her own self-image and developing independence.

Determining the age of the client is a good way to begin the developmental assessment. Age will provide clues to the client's developmental tasks and the usual rate of learning. Once the age is known, the nurse has a frame of reference for what to assess within the other categories of developmental characteristics.

Physical Maturation. Physical maturation is likely to be more variable among children of different ages than it is among a population of normal adults. A child aged 4 is just learning to master the fine motor control necessary to handle a large crayon, the child aged 6 is learning to control a pencil to print, and the child aged 8 is learning to write. Most adults, however, possess the fine motor capacity for controlling a pen or pencil with which to write. (Do not assume that all adults can write, though. This is an important factor to assess.) The task to be learned will determine what psychomotor skills, if any, the learner must possess to be able to master the task. Most health-care tasks involve fine motor skills. For example, changing a colostomy bag, manipulating an insulin syringe, or applying a dressing all require a degree of fine motor coordination. Even taking a pill requires the ability to open a medication bottle and obtain a single small capsule or tablet. Through observation of activities of daily living, the nurse can determine the learner's physical maturation. Observing dressing and eating skills can provide good evidence of fine motor skills and coordination. Asking the client to rate his or her own manual dexterity and the amount of practice needed to learn a physical skill can also be helpful. Finding out if the client can write will help the nurse–teacher determine the appropriateness of learning experiences that include making lists or keeping records.

Cognitive Development. The nurse must also be aware of the client's cognitive level. Assessing an individual's formal educational experience is helpful, but it is insufficient as the only factor upon which to base a cognitive assessment. The nurse also needs to assess the client's verbal skills, reading abilities, cognitive level, and memory. Knowing an individual's grade level gives some idea of reading skills, of the ability to use mathematical skills, and of the ability to deal with abstract concepts. Educational level can also provide an indication of vocabulary level. But educational attainments can give only a gross idea of an individual's abilities. Everyone is aware of people who have graduated from high school and cannot read!

Assessing verbal language skills and reading abilities is important. Asking learners what grade they completed gives an indication of their reading ability, but even when clients have adequate reading skills, understanding and interpretation may be limited. Asking them to read a pamphlet or brochure and discuss its contents will provide some information about both reading ability and level of comprehension. The learner's vocabulary dictates what terms and phrases are best used in teaching; however, the extent of the learner's vocabulary does not indicate what can be learned, rather how nurses should teach.

Determining whether the client can relate to the world from an experiential or a symbolic standpoint is basic to assessing cognitive level. Does the client relate experiences in a concrete or symbolic manner? What symbols—visual or verbal—does the client understand? Are cause-and-effect relationships understood? Can the client think in the abstract? Ability to abstract is frequently tested by having a client explain a proverb, for example, "A bird in the hand is worth two in the bush." An individual who has the ability to abstract will describe the meaning of the proverb in general terms, that is, something of lesser value which you have access to is more valuable than something of greater value to which there is no access. The concrete thinker will focus on or ask questions about the birds and bush rather than ascribe meaning to the statement. The client's time frame of reference also helps determine cognitive capacity. Can the client relate to past experience and anticipate future events, or is the present the only frame of reference?

The ability to learn is dependent upon memory. Immediate memory is remembering information immediately after it is presented. Recent or short-term memory involves recall after several minutes to an hour. Remote or long-term memory includes remembrances after longer periods of time—hours, days, or years. In short-term learning, for example, learning how to cooperate during an x-ray, recent memory needs to be intact. For long-term learning like that required for giving self-injections over a lifetime, remote memory is important. To test for memory, the nurse can give information and ask the client to recall it at appropriate times after it is presented. The nurse–teacher can structure the assessment for short-term memory. "I'd like to test your memory skills. Repeat this series of numbers after me." Other questions that are less structured but provide the same data may be based on any recent events that the client has experienced that the nurse can validate (Malasanos, et al., 1990). Questions about the client's past (birthplace, date of admission to the hospital, highest grade of education completed) that can be validated by written records or other individuals can be used to assess long-term memory abilities. Other questions that are helpful when assessing memory include: "Do you find remembering things easy or difficult?" "What helps you to remember?" "Does taking notes or seeing pictures help you in learning?"

The presence of a learning disability can interfere with an individual's learning. Though these may be identified at school-age when the child has difficulty with a skill easily mastered by others of the same age, learning disabilities in some individuals are not diagnosed. Characteristics often seen in learning-disabled persons include:

1. Difficulty with reading, comprehending, spelling, writing, math computations, or problem solving.
2. Difficulty in organizing and presenting ideas.
3. Difficulty in following oral directions.
4. A discrepancy between the ability to write ideas and to express them orally (Tumminia & Weinfield, 1983).

Persons with learning disabilities have normal intelligence but their ability to learn is impeded by sensory and motor dysperceptions (Tumminia & Weinfield, 1983). Learning disabilities can be of various origins: genetic (Turner syndrome), congenital (prematurity, drugs), and constitutional (injuries). Specific learning problems include dyslexia, disability in reading; dyscalcula, difficulty with mathematical processes; and dysgraphia, difficulty printing or writing (Berger, 1988).

Obviously, nurses are not trained to help remedy a client's learning disability. However, they do need to note learning problems and avoid labeling the individuals as "slow," "retarded," or "uninterested." In some instances, nurses only offer one method of learning. When the learner cannot learn, or does not learn, the person is labeled "dumb" or "uninterested." Assessing how the individual learns best is essential. For example, if an individual has difficulty reading because of dyslexia, oral and audiovisual instructions can be used. Specialists in learning disorders at local colleges and universities and those within the local school systems can help tailor teaching efforts to meet the special needs of the individual with a learning disability.

Related to cognitive development is the client's ability to assume responsibility for the client's own decisions and actions. Until about age 8, cognitive functioning is not adequate to support safe, independent decision making, because there is limited capacity to understand cause and effect. The self-responsibility level in some older, cognitively impaired individuals also differs from the normal and is important for the nurse to assess. Assessing self-responsibility can be done by observing or discussing with the client self-care behaviors and preventive health actions.

Psychosocial Development. Assessing psychosocial development gives the nurse insight into what may be happening in a client's life during a specific time. Although there are predictable developmental patterns that provide a helpful frame of reference, each client must be individually assessed. At each stage of life, there are certain normative tasks to be accomplished. Since life-stage tasks are dynamic, reassessment is needed at periodic intervals for each individual. In young adulthood, for example, involvement may be centered around raising a family, managing a home, or launching a career (Berger, 1988). The orientation toward these tasks can determine readiness to learn about related health care. A young parent may be interested in child health and safety, while the career-minded person may prefer more self-oriented health education. To assess life-stage tasks, the nurse–teacher can discuss current goals with the client. If a client has several goals, it may be helpful to rank them. Knowing the patterns of life-stage task progression (see Chapter 8) will also help the nurse–teacher focus on specific areas in the discussion with the client. This can facilitate assisting the client to identify specific health-related areas of interest.

Previous Learning Experiences. All individuals can learn; in addition to physical, cognitive, and psychosocial developmental factors, the level at which learning can begin is affected by factors arising from previous learning experiences. These include attitudes towards learning, existing knowledge base, and learning style.

Attitudes toward learning arise from other educational experiences and from within the social group. Cultural or socioeconomic factors influence social group attitudes about health and about learning, and therefore contribute to learning potential. Previous learning experiences also contribute to an individual's interest in learning. A child who has had a bad experience with a nurse in the past may unconsciously not trust nurses nor want to learn from them. An adult may not follow health recommendations because of a past experience ("I didn't take the medicine because when I took it before I got sick"). If past learning experiences have been positive, the individual may be more willing to learn; if they were negative, the individual may avoid learning. Helping individuals interpret past learning experiences in relation to their new learning can be helpful.

Although general data about the client's overall knowledge of health and medical terminology may be helpful, it is usually better to assess one area related to an identified learning need in a step-by-step manner. Identifying a content area provides a framework for the assessment and allows a depth to the assessment that the general approach does not. Once the specific content area has been identified, knowledge of anatomy and physiology, bodily functions, illness recognition and management and monitoring, preventive health practices, and correlation of life-style patterns to the health state can be assessed appropriately.

Wright (1985) demonstrated that learners learn better when the style of learning offered—kinesthetic, visual, or auditory—matched the individual's strong cognitive style. Another dimension widely known to influence learning style is field dependence. Determining whether an individual has the characteristics of a field-independent or field-dependent learner can help indicate the types of learning that will be most productive. Field-dependent individuals prefer a passive role in the learning process, are more affected by criticism, and motivated by social approval. These individuals typically like to learn best when material is organized and they are given cues about what to learn. Field-independent individuals, on the other hand, like active participation in learning, are goal directed, less influenced by outside factors, and motivated by challenge. They learn better when they organize their own material for study and test out new ideas (Garrity, 1985). While it is not necessary to "classify" learners into these categories, certain questions can help elicit information helpful to planning learning activities that take learning style into consideration.

Determining a client's preference for learning style can be done by asking the client about his or her preferred access to new information and past positive learning experiences. If the client prefers to watch the news on television rather than read the newspaper or listen to the radio, enhancing learning by visual representations such as pictures, slides, or film strips may be more acceptable than reading materials, audiotape, or live lectures. Asking the client how he or she would prefer to learn about a health topic of interest can also provide valuable information. If the client indicates a preference for asking a health professional, then one-to-one instruction might be the most appropriate. If reading is preferred, providing useful, accurate, up-to-date reading materials would be a useful approach. If the client states a preference for a health class, providing information about local classes on the topic of interest would be appropriate. The client can also be asked to describe a past experience in learning that was beneficial. These data can also give the nurse cues about learning preferences.

The client's description of his or her own interpersonal interactions can help the nurse determine if a lecture or discussion would be a better way to approach the subject matter. The client whose self-description is as a quiet or shy individual might do better in a lecture, while a more talkative, outgoing client might prefer a discussion style of learning. Nurses do most of their teaching on a one-to-one basis. For some individuals, this may be the preferred style of learning, for others a group setting facilitates more active interchange and enhances learning. Although nurses do not always have control over whether teaching–learning sessions will be on an individual or group basis, the client's preference should be considered when possible.

The client can provide valuable information about his or her individual learning style that can help the nurse plan effective learning strategies. Even though individuals may have a preference, combining the preferred method of learning with others is a strategy often recommended to optimally facilitate learning.

A complete assessment of the learner is important to provide data for planning teaching–learning strategies. Learner assessment is a continuing process, however, and does not stop after the initial interaction with the client. It is not usually possible to gather all data on an initial visit or even during subsequent interactions. Table 9–2 provides a guide for assessing the learner.

Content Areas for Health Learning

Although it is impossible within the scope of this text to identify assessment criteria for all health-content areas, there are eight categories of behaviors about which nurses are exceptionally knowledgeable and in which health-care consumers commonly have learning needs. These include:

- Nutrition
- Exercise/physical fitness
- Sleep and rest
- Stress management
- Safety
- Health monitoring
- Anticipatory guidance
- Illness care

TABLE 9-2. GUIDE FOR LEARNER ASSESSMENT

Health Status

Energy Level
Is activity nonlabored, without rest or easy fatigue?
How much sleep/rest is needed each day? (Is this different from the usual pattern?)
What is the client able to accomplish in a day at this given time?
Is energy level higher at one time of day than another?

Comfort
Physical:
   Pain? (What can be done to minimize? When is it at minimum?)
   Nausea? Itching? Fatigue?
   Is the client hungry or thirsty?
   Does the client need to go to the bathroom?
Psychological:
   Fear? Anxiety? Guilt? Anger? Worry? Grief?

Sensory Status
Vision:
   Can the client see at normal distances? Need corrective lenses?
Hearing:
   Can normal voice tones be heard?
   From what distance are normal voices heard?
   Does the client wear a hearing aid?
Perceptions:
   Level of consciousness?
   Ability to concentrate? Attention span?
   Thought processes?

Adjustment to Health State
Does client describe health state accurately? Realistically?
How does the client feel now?
Does the client express concerns about health (illness)?
   If yes, what concerns are rated as most important?
What does the client identify as measures for staying healthy (or improving health?)
What does the client think is necessary during this illness? Who should do it?
What would the client like to know about the health (illness) state?

Health Values

Perception of Control:
What would the client do first on hearing that a family member became ill?
Who would be called for assistance?
When the client is ill, what is done to help the client get better? Who does it?

Expectations of Outcomes:
Does the client feel that illness is likely to occur?
What does the client expect to happen when experiencing . . . (fill in specific illness health
   behavior as appropriate)?
What would make it easier to do . . . (answer from above)?
What would make it easier to manage?
What makes it difficult to manage?
What does the client expect to happen when participating in . . . (specify health action or
   behavior)?
What would make it easier to participate in this?
What makes it difficult to participate?

(continued)

TABLE 9–2. (*Continued*)

Developmental Characteristics

Physical Maturation
How well developed are the client's fine motor skills?
Does the client have good hand–eye coordination?
How does the client rate his or her own manual dexterity?
How much practice does the client usually need to learn a new psychomotor skill?
Can the client write?

Cognitive Development
Formal educational experience?
How does the client use verbal language?
What is the level of reading ability?
Level of cognition:
  Does the client use experiences and perceptions or symbols when explaining the
    surrounding world?
  What is the client's understanding of past, present, future relationships?
Memory:
  How good is immediate recall? Recall after 15 minutes to an hour? Recall after longer
    periods of time?
  What improves the client's ability to remember?
  How responsible is the client for self-care?

Psychosocial Development
Life-stage tasks:
  What are the client's goals?
  What are the health-related aspects?

Prior Learning Experiences

Attitudes towards learning
  Were past experiences positive or negative?
Health knowledge:
  What is the client's knowledge about an identified content area?
  What is the understanding of medical terminology?
  Does the client have a preferred way of learning?
    Visual input—television or pictures? Reading?
    Auditory input—listening to speakers, audiotapes?
    Interactive input—health classes, one-to-one with a health professional?

There are basic questions for the nurse to ask when gathering data from the client in preparation for teaching about one of these content areas. The questions which appear in Table 9–3 are not inclusive but provide a baseline for content assessment. Clients' answers will indicate further directions to pursue. In addition, the nurse–teacher can gather data by observing client behaviors related to each of the areas listed. The next section of this chapter reviews the process of data collection appropriate for the teaching–learning situation.

Data Collection Methods

There are a variety of methods that can be used to collect data. Written records, if they are available, are often the best first source of information. These provide

TABLE 9–3. QUESTIONS FOR ASSESSING CONTENT AREAS

Nutrition
Describe your usual eating times each day.
What do you usually eat at those times?
Are you satisfied with your eating habits?
If not, what would you like to change?

Exercise
Describe the exercise you get each day.
Are you satisfied with that amount?
If not, what would you like to change?

Sleep and Rest
How many hours of sleep do you get each night?
Do you have difficulty getting to sleep or staying asleep? If yes, describe.
Do you feel rested when you awaken?
Do you have the energy you need to accomplish your day's activities?
Do you wish to change your sleep/rest pattern?

Stress Management
How do you react when you are under stress (tense)?
How do you unwind?
Is there anything in your home, work, or personal life now causing you to be more tense than usual?
Do you feel you are successful in coping with tension?
If not, what other things do you feel would assist you?
Do you smoke? Drink coffee?
Do you drink alcoholic beverages? If yes, what kind and how much?
Do you take any recreational drugs or prescription drugs to help you relax? If yes, what do you take? How often?

Safety
What kinds of things do you do to protect yourself from accidents or injury at home? at work? driving?
Are you satisfied with those practices?
If not, what would you like to change?

Health Monitoring
How often do you (your family members) see a health-care provider? Who?
Are there any specific conditions that you have monitored regularly? What? How often?
Are you interested in other information about health screening?

Anticipatory Guidance
Are you expecting any life changes? Are you doing anything to prepare for them?
(If a parent) What growth and development progress do you see in each of your children?
Do you have questions about what is occurring now or will occur in the next developmental stage?

Illness Care
What do you do to prevent (manage) illness?
Who do you call when an illness occurs which you don't know how to handle?
Do you know how to get a physician when you need one?
Are there any specific illnesses you would like more information about? What are they? What would you like to know?

background data related to age, sex, occupation, location of home, family members, and health state. This information can be used in preliminary planning for further data collection. For example, if you discover that your client is a homebound senior citizen recovering from a broken hip, your focus might initially be related more to health status variables than if your client were a healthy adolescent. Written records may provide other information relevant to the teaching–learning situation that can be validated by interview or observation.

An interview provides the nurse–teacher with the opportunity to explore what the client wants to learn, provides the foundation for establishing a relationship, and aids identification of preexisting factors that can facilitate or impede learning. The structure of the interview may be formal or informal. Some new teachers feel security in establishing a time frame for the interview and proceeding through this in a preplanned manner. Others prefer to conduct an informal interview while giving a bath, making the bed, or performing other technical tasks. An excellent opportunity for an informal interview about a specific topic is during a procedure being done by the nurse which will eventually need to be performed by the client. The client and nurse can focus their discussion on what the client knows and would like to know about the procedure. At times, clients may not have had enough experience to predict learning needs, or for other reasons they may not be ready or able to identify their needs. During the interview, nurses may use the strategy Bille (1981, p. 55) labels as "therapeutic seeding." This strategy involves "planting" the idea of a learning need. For example, a formerly sedentary patient recovering from a myocardial infarction may not identify the need to learn an exercise regimen. A nurse can suggest that "many patients who have had heart attacks are interested in learning an exercise plan to incorporate into their lives." Or, to the mother who has just delivered her second child and does not recognize sibling rivalry as a factor to consider, the nurse may verbalize that idea. Sometimes therapeutic seeding engenders an immediate recognition of the need for education. At other times, clients need time to think through ideas. Nurses can "fertilize" ideas through occasional references to them and their potential outcomes.

The interview provides the opportunity to elicit information about what the client already knows about health promotion, illness prevention, and body functions, as well as the practice of specific health behaviors. Misinformation may also be identified during the interview. With some clients, self-administered assessment tools may be used as a preliminary step in the assessment process. Questions listed in Table 9–3 could be put into a format that would allow clients to answer them independently. Following the administration of a self-assessment tool, the nurse needs to provide time to discuss responses with the client.

Observations can also provide assessment data. Skill inventories may be used to assess psychomotor abilities. For example, a checklist for observing all the steps involved in insulin injection or in self-catheterization may be used to determine learning needs related to these skills. Table 9–4 provides an example of a skill inventory. The nurse observes the client perform the task and notes which steps are and are not done. This provides the basis for reviewing the skill. Observations of the environment may also provide clues to learning needs. The elderly client with

TABLE 9-4. SKILL INVENTORY FOR INSULIN INJECTION

Steps	Done	Not Done
1. Chooses appropriate injection site (based on rotation pattern).		
2. Cleans skin with alcohol and places swab nearby.		
3. Removes needle cover aseptically.		
4. Grasps skin between thumb and first finger.		
5. Thrusts needle into skin at 45° or 90° angle.		
6. Pulls back on plunger to see if blood appears.		
7. If blood appears, withdraws needle, reprepares insulin and begins again with step 1. If no blood appears, injects insulin steadily within 5–10 seconds.		
8. Removes needle quickly.		
9. Compresses site with alcohol swab for 5 seconds.		
10. Breaks needle off syringe.		
11. Disposes syringe and needle in special container.		

scatter rugs and cluttered furniture or the young mother with unlocked cupboards full of hazardous substances may need to learn about safety in the environment.

In addition to using written records, interviews, and observations for data collection, other individuals can be sources of information. Surveys may be conducted among a target group. Committees of people familiar with a certain population may be approached and asked to identify health-learning needs of that select group of people. Family members and friends can be valuable sources of information.

Through the use of combinations of the methods described above, nurses collect data relevant to the teaching–learning process. There are several factors that can affect the success of any assessment. Since a nursing diagnosis made without adequate supporting data will lead to incorrect assumptions, it is important to briefly summarize those factors that affect the data collection process.

Interviewing. The success of the interview depends upon the degree of rapport with the client, the timing of the interview, the amount of time available, the client's health condition, and the environment, as well as the skills of the interviewer. To initially establish rapport, the nurse should inform the client of the reasons for the questions to be asked. All of us tend to guard what we say to another individual. Helping a client understand that the answers to your questions will help "better determine the learning needs and preferred ways to learn" provides the rationale for the questions to be asked. Showing a genuine concern for the client also helps develop rapport. The interview should be conducted at a time when the client is most comfortable and the nurse is not rushed. Pain, fatigue, and anxiety interfere with data collection. When these are present the interview should be deferred until they are minimal. The environment should be relatively free of disrupting factors— noises and visits by other medical personnel—and privacy should be assured. The nurse should always sit down to provide eye contact and appear unhurried. It is usually best to place a time limit on an interview, but the nurse should not appear to have insufficient time to listen to the client. The time limit should be realistic for the interview as well as appropriate to both the client's condition and the nurse's other responsibilities. The rationale for a specific time allotment for the interview should be explained. When a client senses undue time constraints, information given is usually not complete. In addition, an effective nurse–teacher will identify the client's preferred style of communication, preference for address (first name or more formal address), and style of nonverbal communication (Tripp-Reimer & Afifi, 1989).

Successful interviewing takes practice. Usually the interview begins with broad, nondirective, open-ended questions that encourage the client to speak freely. Next, slightly more directive questions that are topic specific, but still put no limits on responses, are used. A third type of question is a limited choice, directive question. This puts specific limits on the topic and the expected responses. Since this type of question yields only one- or two-word answers, it adds little data. It should be used only when broad questions have provided data necessary to narrow the interview and open-ended questions are not yielding the specific information needed. A nurse learns from experience when to focus more specifically in one area. The skilled interviewer, if forced to use limited-choice questions, will follow these up with further open-ended responses ("Tell me about that."). Table 9–5 provides examples of each type of question.

During the interview, it is important to use language familiar to the client as well as to use words that are not value laden. The nurse also needs to minimize suggestions or bias when forming questions. For example, asking the client to describe meal times and foods usually eaten, rather than to describe breakfast, lunch, and dinner, allows the client to list the meals. It does not assume that the three traditional meals are eaten.

Well-formulated questions are important, but equally important is listening to the answers. The client should be given enough time to answer each question, and the nurse should listen carefully to the answer. Active listening facilitates a more appropriate response. Questions can be used to clarify or encourage expansion on the topic.

TABLE 9–5. EXAMPLES OF TYPES OF QUESTIONS FOR INTERVIEWING A POTENTIAL LEARNER

Type of Question	Examples
Nondirective open-ended	How are things? What brings you here? What questions do you have today?
Directive open-ended	What questions do you have about your surgery? What would you like to learn about hypertension? What kinds of things do you do to protect yourself from accident and injury?
Directive limited choice	Do you have difficulty getting to sleep or staying asleep? Have you experienced many accidents and injuries?

In addition to questioning, the interviewer may use techniques of silence, confrontation, and nonverbal responses when interviewing. Silence, when effectively used, can show interest and support. It may be augmented by nonverbal communication such as a nod of the head or leaning forward to encourage further verbalization. Confrontation is a method of pointing out to the client feelings and behaviors. It helps focus the individual's attention on the feeling or behavior and also lets the client know you understand what was said. "You look confused" is a confrontation that may be appropriate during a teaching–learning interaction. Multiple sources about communication are available for the novice interviewer.

Observation. Observation is a part of the interviewing process. The nurse observes the facial expression, body posture, and mannerisms of the client throughout the interview. Although body language cannot be interpreted in the same way for all individuals, patterns of behavior may provide clues to the nonverbal message the client is sending.

Other observations may provide data related to health education needs. Observations of the client's personal hygiene, health behaviors, and environment—when validated with the client or observed in several different time periods—can be helpful. It is important to emphasize that conclusions should not be drawn from a single observation. Patterns seen in multiple observations by the nurse or by other health-care providers, and behaviors validated with the client through discussion are those which are useful to the nurse when analyzing the data.

Analysis of Data

Once the data collection phase of assessment has been completed, the nurse organizes and then analyzes the data. Data are usually organized mentally by the nurse and compared against the nurse's knowledge of health knowledge, skills, and attitudes in similar situations. Most of these fall within the categories discussed previously—nutrition, exercise, sleep and rest, stress management, illness care, health monitoring, anticipatory guidance, and safety. Examples of specific content needs in each of these categories for clients with acute and chronic illnesses and for clients who are well appeared in Chapter 6. Once data have been thoroughly analyzed, specific nursing diagnoses may be identified. These are diagnoses about actual or potential health problems which exist owing to knowledge and skill levels or value orientations. Although the system of nursing diagnoses continues to develop, the nursing classification system developed by the North American Nursing Diagnosis Association provides a frame of reference for diagnostic statements related to the educational needs of clients. There are numerous diagnoses listed by this group which include lack of education, knowledge, or skills as a possible related factor. Examples of nursing diagnoses often related to a knowledge or skill deficit include (Carpenito, 1989):

Nutrition
    Nutrition, altered: Less than body requirements
    Nutrition, altered: More than body requirements

Exercise and rest
  Sleep pattern disturbance
  Fatigue

Stress management
  Coping: Comprised, ineffective family
  Coping: Ineffective individual

Illness care
  Noncompliance (specify)
  Skin integrity, impaired
  Decisional conflict

Health monitoring
  Noncompliance (specify)

Anticipatory guidance
  Parenting, altered
  Self-concept disturbance: Body image, self-esteem, personal identify
  Health maintenance, altered

Safety
  Injury: Potential for

Many nurses practice with clients who are healthy, and do not have deficits or health problems, yet have learning needs that nurses can meet; for example, new parents who need to learn infant care, or school children who need to learn healthy life style behaviors. Thus, during the assessment it is important to identify strengths that can be used to maximize learning. Some examples of strengths in the same general areas as previously discussed have been suggested by Carpenito (1989):

Nutrition
  Effective nutritional-metabolic pattern

Exercise and rest
  Effective activity-exercise pattern
  Effective sleep-rest pattern

Stress management
  Positive self-perception

Illness care
  Effective health management

Health monitoring
  Effective health management

Anticipatory guidance
  Positive role-relationship pattern

Safety
  Positive cognitive-perceptual pattern

Obviously, the type of teaching interventions and the level of these will be different depending upon whether diagnoses focus upon deficits or strengths. Once a nursing diagnosis related to a health-learning need has been established, the nurse moves to the planning stage of the teaching–learning process.

SUMMARY

Assessment is the first stage of the teaching–learning process. It forms the foundation for all succeeding steps. For this reason, it is important that assessment data be as complete as possible. In this chapter, the process of assessing the learner was discussed. Learner-readiness factors were identified and defined. Specific methods for collecting data for the teaching–learning situation were suggested. In addition, nursing diagnoses that relate to learning needs were suggested. The following unit focuses on the remainder of the teaching process. General strategies as well as those for specific populations are addressed.

REFERENCES AND READINGS

Anderson, C. *Patient teaching and communicating in an information age.* Albany, NY: Delmar Publishers Inc., 1990.

Antai-Otone, D. Concerns of the hospitalized community psychiatric client. *Nursing Clinics of North America,* 1989, *24*(3), 665–673.

Armstrong, M. L. Orchestrating the process of patient education: Methods and approaches. *Nursing Clinics of North America,* 1989, *24*(3), 597–604.

Baker, K., Kuhlmann, R. S., & Magliaro, B. L. Homeward bound. *Nursing Clinics of North America,* 1989, *24*(3), 655–664.

Berger, K. S. *The developing person through the life span* (2nd ed) NY: Worth Publishers, 1988.

Bille, D. A. (Ed.). *Practical approaches to patient teaching.* Boston: Little, Brown, 1981.

Carpenito, L. J. *Handbook of nursing diagnosis 1989–1990.* Philadelphia: J. B. Lippincott, 1989.

Carpenito, L. J. *Nursing diagnosis: Application to clinical practice* (3d ed.). Philadelphia: J. B. Lippincott, 1989.

Collett, C. Assessing the patient education needs of the elderly. *Medical Times,* 1988, *116*(11), 95–99.

Garrity, J. Learning styles: Basis for creative teaching and learning. *Nurse Educator,* March-April 1985, 12–15.

Gessner, B. A. Adult education: The cornerstone of patient teaching. *Nursing Clinics of North America,* 1989, *24*(3), 589–595.

Higgins, M. G. Learning style assessment: A new patient teaching tool? *Journal of Nursing Staff Development,* 1988, *4*(1), 14–18.

Holland, S. Teaching patients and clients: The benefits of communicating. *Nursing Times,* 1987, *83*(9), 56–58.

Hussey, L. C. & Gilliland, K. Compliance, low literacy, and locus of control. *Nursing Clinics of North America*, 1989, *24*(3), 605–611.

Leff, E. W. Ethics and patient teaching. *MCN*, 1986, *11*(6), 375–376.

Luker, K. & Caress, A. L. Rethinking patient education. *Journal of Advanced Nursing*, 1989, *14*(9), 711–718.

Malasanos, L., Barkauskau, V., Moss, M., & Staltenberg-Allen, K. *Health assessment* (4th ed.). St. Louis: C. V. Mosby, 1990.

Miller, A. When is the time ripe for teaching? *American Journal of Nursing*, 1985, *85*(7), 801–804.

Miller, J. F. *Coping with chronic illness*. Philadelphia: F. A. Davis, 1983.

Murray, R. B. & Zenter, J. P. *Nursing concepts for health promotion* (3d ed.). Englewood Cliffs, N.J.: Prentice-Hall, 1985.

Partridge, R. Learning styles: A review of selected methods. *Journal of Nursing Education*, 1983, *22*(6), 243–248.

Potter, P. A. & Perry, A. G. *Basic nursing: Theory and practice*. St. Louis: C. V. Mosby, 1991.

Sachs, B. Cognitive screening for adolescent health education. *Journal of Pediatric Nursing*, 1987, *2*(2), 113–119.

Shillinger, F. L. Locus of control: Implications for clinical nursing practice. *Image: The Journal of Nursing Scholarship*, Spring 1983, *15*(2), 58–63.

Smith, C. E. Overview of patient education: Opportunities and challenges for the twenty-first century. *Nursing Clinics of North America*, 1989, *24*(3), 583–587.

Streiff, L. D. Can clients understand our instructions? *Image: Journal of Nursing Scholarship*, 1986, *18*(2), 48–52.

Tripp-Reimer, T. & Afifi, L. A. Cross-cultural perspectives on patient teaching. *Nursing Clinics of North America*, 1989, *24*(3), 613–619.

Tumminia, P. A. & Weinfield, A. M. Teaching the learning-disabled nursing student. *Nurse Educator*, Winter 1983, 12–20.

Wright, J. E. Using cognitive channels in patient education. *Dimensions of Critical Care Nursing*, 1985, *4*(5), 308–313.

Strategies for Health Education

Content in this unit provides information relative to nursing practice strategies, which comprise the active component of nursing practice. Chapter 10 describes the teaching process, focusing specifically on planning, implementing, and evaluating teaching. Chapter 11 specifically addresses teaching strategies that nurses use in assisting clients to learn management of illness, and attaining or maintaining a maximum level of wellness.

The next four chapters in this unit provide information about strategies for teaching in specific situations. Chapter 12 describes strategies useful for various aged learners. The amount of learner participation, structure of the lesson, content considerations, and enhancement of learning are discussed according to age group. In addition, implications for short-term and long-term learning for each age group are addressed.

Chapter 13 provides information about teaching health values. Teaching and learning in the affective domain is discussed and a variety of models for facilitating this are presented.

Teaching populations with special needs is discussed in Chapter 14. Strategies for the educationally disadvantaged and learners with physical and mental handicaps are presented. In addition, health-care practices of common minority cultures and related implications for teaching are addressed.

Chapter 15 describes teaching strategies for groups. Discussion focuses on group characteristics, assessment, and specific approaches for teaching groups.

The final chapter identifies the variety of sources from which health education materials can be obtained. Specific organizations and their addresses are cited so that nurses are aware of where they may have access to teaching materials.

10

The Teaching Process

Marlyn Duncan Boyd

The teaching process is a planned and purposeful activity that nurses use to increase the likelihood that individuals will learn. The teaching process follows the same steps as those in the nursing process: assessment, planning, implementation, and evaluation (Figure 10–1). Each of these steps involves a series of tasks; each of these tasks contributes to the overall success of the process. The steps of the

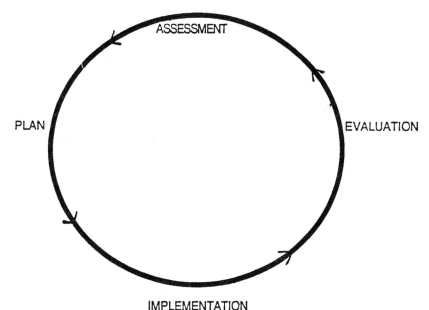

IMPLEMENTATION
Figure 10.–1. The Teaching Process.

teaching process are discussed in this chapter. Strategies to help the nurse facilitate an individual's learning and to promote the adoption of positive health behaviors are discussed in Chapter 11.

ASSESSMENT

The assessment stage of the teaching process is perhaps the most crucial element, because what the nurse accomplishes in this stage will influence all of the following stages. The systematic and thorough collection of data relevant to the teaching process is the basis from which learning needs are identified, objectives are developed, and a workable plan is formulated. Data collected during the assessment helps nurses identify what the learner knows and what he or she wants and needs to learn. Chapter 9 outlined appropriate data collection methods, areas that need to be assessed before developing a teaching plan, and strategies that can help the nurse collect appropriate data. This chapter discusses the tasks that follow data collection, beginning with how to prioritize learning needs.

PLANNING

Prioritizing Needs

The ways nurses prioritize needs, write goals and objectives, and organize teaching content are all based on learning theories. In the clinical setting, few nurses adhere to only one theoretical approach to teaching. Rather, they use a variety of approaches depending upon their assessment of the learner, the task to be learned, and the learning environment. Individuals' learning needs are prioritized to facilitate teaching and learning. Prioritizing needs can help the nurse use time more effectively. In many situations, nurses must carefully allocate their time, taking into consideration their many responsibilities. A lack of time for teaching can be the result of staffing patterns, work assignments, short hospital stays for patients, a client's desire to prematurely terminate a session, or an unexpected emergency. Insufficient time for teaching can also be the result of poor planning by nurses. To maximize their time, and to facilitate client learning, nurses must often prioritize the learning needs of individuals.

There are several methods that can be used to prioritize learning needs. These are based on various learning theories. A commonly used method is Maslow's Hierarchy of Needs. Maslow (1970) suggests that humans have five broad categories of needs (Table 10–1) and that before one can satisfactorily meet higher needs, lower needs must be at least partially met. This theory would suggest that a nurse's first priority would be to assess how well an individual is meeting physiological and survival needs. Then, if a deficit is found, the nurse would formulate a diagnosis and plan to help the person successfully meet the need. For example, if an individual who is without a job is admitted to the hospital with malnutrition, the nurse would, aside from helping to improve the person's physical well-being, assess why

TABLE 10-1. HEALTH-RELATED ASPECTS OF MASLOW'S HIERARCHY
OF HUMAN NEEDS

Level Five: Self-Actualization
Tasks to accomplish in this level might include helping promote healthier communities
   through political activism or becoming involved in the fight against world hunger.

Level Four: Self-Esteem
Tasks to accomplish in this level may include improving one's own health as well as
   promoting healthier life styles for your family.

Level Three: Love, Affection, and Belongingness
Tasks in this level may include caring for an ill family member or providing a healthier life
   style for your family (improving nutrition, etc.).

Level Two: Safety and Security
Tasks in this level may include ensuring a safe home environment, using seat belts, or
   obtaining immunizations.

Level One: Physiological and Survival Needs
Tasks in this level could include adequately meeting food, water, and air needs.

Adapted from Rankin S. H., & Duffy, K. L.: Patient education: Issues, principles and guidelines. *New York:
Lippincott, 1983, pp. 127–128.*

this person went without food. A diagnosis might be, "Nutrition, alteration in: less than body requirements related to the lack of information about how to obtain no-cost or low-cost food." The resulting plan might involve consulting social services and educating the patient about community resources.

Another method for prioritizing needs involves taking into account, on a daily basis, both the client's learning needs and the amount of time the nurse has available to teach. By assessing each person's learning needs, the nurse can better allocate time and ensure that primary learning needs are met for each individual. The three categories of needs are (George, 1982):

- *Immediate need* (urgent) versus a *long-range need* (can be met at a later time)
- *Specific need* (related specifically to the learner's condition or treatment plan) versus a *general need* (something done for all learners)
- *Survival need* (the learner's life may depend on it) versus a *well-being need* (helpful, but not essential)

Examples to illustrate these categories would include deciding whether to teach a patient who has been unexpectedly discharged and who will be leaving in an hour (immediate need) or spending the time teaching a patient who will be leaving in 3 days (long-range need); teaching a preoperative patient how to turn, cough, and deep-breathe (specific need) versus explaining that vital signs are routine to a patient admitted for a physical (general need). The nurse also needs to decide which should be done first—teaching a client with cardiovascular disease to report any changes in angina (survival need) or teaching a mother about infant developmental tasks (well-being need).

When prioritizing learning needs, the nurse must take into consideration the individual's needs and readiness to learn and the amount of time available for teaching. Nurses can meet immediate and specific needs and plan to meet more general needs in the future. It is important to remember, too, that teaching does not have to entail blocking out a half-hour of time. Teaching can be integrated into routine nursing activities such as giving baths and medications. Integrated teaching or "action dialogues" can help the nurse maximize the use of available time and help space teaching–learning sessions, giving the learner more time to process the information (Strauss & Glaser, 1975). In addition, well-planned teaching can be a shared responsibility among health-care professionals. What is essential is that clients' needs be prioritized and a plan designed to ensure that their learning needs are met.

Setting Goals

After nursing diagnoses related to learning have been made and prioritized, goals are set for teaching–learning sessions. Goals are broad, general statements about what is expected as the outcome of an individual's learning. Goal statements help us further define what needs to be accomplished to meet an educational need. These are end-product statements—what the nurse hopes the final outcome of teaching will be. Such statements do not provide the specifics about how the goal will be accomplished. Behavioral objectives are the "how to" statements. Table 10–2 gives examples of goal statements and behavioral objectives. Goals can be subdivided into short-term goals and long-term goals. Using the prioritizing system mentioned earlier, short-term goals would be those that help the individual meet immediate and specific needs. For example, a short-term goal statement might be "Mrs. Jones will properly self-inject insulin × 3 prior to discharge." A long-term goal statement would be "Mrs. Jones will be able to discuss the benefits of exercise for the diabetic." Goals must be realistic for the individual and must allow for the amount of time that is available for teaching.

Goal setting is usually a joint venture between the nurse and the client or patient. The outcomes of goal setting are usually more successful if the goal is the result of a client's expressed need or interest (Bille, 1977; Cahill, 1987; Van Hoozer, et al., 1987); the client, if at all possible, should set the goals for learning and behavioral change. He or she may set goals after the nurse has provided adequate information so that informed choices can be made. Sometimes a client may not be able to take part in goal setting. In such instances, the nurse can incorporate significant others or, if need be, set the goal. Under such circumstances, the goal may change after the individual is able to take a more active role in the teaching–learning process. Someone who has recently experienced a cerebral vascular accident and has expressive and receptive aphasia may not be able initially to be actively involved in setting goals. As the person improves, however, involvement will increase. Initial goals set by the nurse may need to be revised depending on the individual's expressed needs. Another benefit of mutual goal setting is that it encourages an individual to actively participate in health management—to share the responsibility for health outcomes. It can also help to maintain or increase an individual's sense of autonomy.

TABLE 10–2. MEDICATION TEACHING PLAN

Primary Goal: Patient will remain free from complication of TB chemotherapy.

Secondary Goal: Patient will understand major elements of the chemotherapy plan.

Prerequisites: Classes 1 and 2.

Patients are taught about the medicines one at a time. Patient must meet minimum objectives for each drug before proceeding to next drug.

Objectives:

In each of the classes that follow, the patient will:

1. State the name of the prescribed drug when shown the pill or tablet.
2. State the dosage of the prescribed drug.
3. Describe the action of each drug (cidal or static).
4. Recount the most *common* and *major* side effects of each drug.
5. List the names of drugs or foods that interfere with the action of TB drugs or are interfered with by TB drugs.
6. State when each medication should be taken.

Materials Needed: For each class the instructor should have a sample of the medicine in its most common dose(s). Also any posters of *individual* drugs. Do not use materials that show several medicines at one time. A blackboard can also be used to illustrate points.

Methods of Presentation: Parts of these classes are incorporated in daily medication administration. (Name, dosage, time taken.) These concepts and the remaining objectives should be covered in regular classes in quiet surroundings and *away* from the pressures of daily meds. Class size may be 1:1 or 1:small group. (Obviously, all members of the group would be receiving the medicine.)

Sources:

Stead, W., & Dutt, A. Chemotherapy for tuberculosis in the 1980s. *Clinics in Chest Medicine,* May, 1980, 243–253.

Addington, W. W. The treatment of tuberculosis. *Archives of Internal Medicine,* December 1979, 129.

Nursing 80 Staff. *Nurse's guide to drugs.* Intermed Communications, 1980.

Adapted from TB Teaching Plan, Blue Ridge Division, University of Virginia, Division of Nursing, 1982. Used with permission.

Behavioral Objectives

Behavioral objectives are the "how to" statements that express in specific, measurable terms *who* will do *what* as *measured by what and by when*. These statements are used by those who subscribe to the theory that learning has taken place when behavior changes can be observed. Since a great deal of health care necessitates the accomplishment of a specific task, behavioral objectives are commonly used by nurses. Behavioral objectives are designed to deal with only one behavior at a time and are yardsticks for measuring an individual's success as a learner. They also help nurses to acknowledge learner readiness, plan continuity of care, and appropriately sequence teaching, and prioritize learning needs (Redman, 1988).

When writing behavioral objectives, it is very important that nurses know exactly what must be accomplished by the learner in order to reach the learning goal. Too often, an individual needs to develop effective problem-solving skills and the nurse focuses only on the client's ability to memorize signs and symptoms.

TABLE 10-3. A CLASSIFICATION OF VERBS RELATED TO A COGNITIVE TAXONOMY

Knowledge: Emphasis on recall, specifics, or universals.

choose	answer question	complete a work, phrase,
define	label	or statement
identify	list	record
review	locate	confer (to gain information)
survey	match	review (to obtain facts)
read	select	
indicate	copy	

Comprehension: Emphasis on grasp of meaning, intent, relationships, in oral, written, graphic, nonverbal communication.

classify	interpret	convert
describe	measure	compare the importance of
estimate	recognize	put in order
expand	suggest	compute
explain	summarize	review to explain
express	trace	

Application: Emphasis on applying appropriate principles or generalizations.

arrange	discuss	perform activity
apply	implement	plan activity
calculate	coordinate (activities)	prepare
construct	use information, tools	present
make	collect information	solve
draw	keep records	compile data
demonstrate		schedule
differentiate		administer test

Analysis: Emphasis on breakdown into constituent parts and on the way they are organized.

analyze	review to analyze	make inferences
debate	form generalizations	organize
determine	deduce	interpret relationships
differentiate	draw conclusions	

Synthesis: Emphasis on putting together elements or parts to form a whole.

combine and organize	coordinate (program design)	write (original)
design	produce	plan program
develop		

Adapted from Bloom, B. S. (Ed.): Taxonomy of educational objectives; the classification of educational goals. Handbook I: Cognitive domain. *New York: Longmans, Green and Co. 1956.*

Someone with angina not only needs to know the signs and symptoms of ischemia but should also be able to decide what to do with an anginal onset. Table 10–3 list verbs that can be used to construct behavioral objectives. If the goal for the learner is to problem solve, the behavioral objective would include terms such as *analyze, discuss,* or *solve.* If the concern is that the learner only be able to identify or list signs and symptoms, then knowledge-level cognitive terms are used. These terms can help identify what level of learning is to take place.

In order to be part of a behavioral objective, *what* the client will be doing needs to be stated in objectively measurable terms. Any verb used must therefore be action oriented. A statement such as "Mrs. Jones will understand how to give a baby a bath" is not a behavioral objective. How can "understand" be objectively measured? What behavioral change would be evident? A better way to state this would be: "Mrs. Jones *will bathe* her new baby." The term *bathe* can be observed. In addition to an action verb, a behavioral objective must also include criteria for assessing how well a behavior is accomplished and any condition under which the behavior will be performed. In the example given, there are no specifics to indicate how well Mrs. Jones will bathe her baby, or the conditions under which she will do this.

Criteria can be specific measurements such as percentage or frequencies. For an example using a percentage, see example A in Table 10–4. Whenever a degree of accuracy is used as a criterion, there also must be some standard against which it is measured. If the standard is universal, it need not be stated, as in example A. When a specific standard is used, this must be identified (example B). This ensures that different nurses who evaluate learning outcomes are measuring the same thing. Frequency used as a criterion is exemplified in objective C. Example E is a behavioral objective for Mrs. Jones (cited earlier).

Conditions identify any special circumstances under which the behavior is

TABLE 10–4. EXAMPLES OF BEHAVIORAL OBJECTIVES

By When	Under What Conditions	Who	What	How Well
A. Sunday, 3/5		Mr. Harris	Will draw up his insulin	With 100% accuracy
B. Thursday evening		Mrs. Vavaldi	Will list	All of the steps for cast care outlined in "Home Cast Care Instructions"
C. Tomorrow (10/23)	From her menu	Susie Jacobs	Will choose	At least 3 foods that are high in protein
D. On my next visit	With his wife preparing the site	Mr. Campbell	Will apply his colostomy bag	So that it does not leak
E. Tomorrow evening	After the nurse has gathered the equipment	Mrs. Jones	Will bathe her baby	Incorporating principles of safety and hygiene outlined on Baby Bath Sheet

performed. If the learner is to use a specific tool or aid, this is considered a condition. In example C, "from her menu" is a tool to be used, therefore a condition. D provides an example of a condition of aid. Although criteria occur in all behavioral objectives, conditions do not. Examples A and B are complete behavioral objectives that do not include conditions.

The time component—the *when*—is an essential element for behavioral objectives. This element needs to be realistic. Too often nurses set both themselves and their clients up for failure by expecting too much too soon. For example, it is unrealistic for patients and nurses to have a preoperative teaching plan, for patients admitted the evening before surgery, that states that patients will learn the anatomy and physiology of their conditions, understand general anesthesia and reasons for postoperative pulmonary hygiene, provide a return demonstration of pulmonary and musculoskeletal exercises, discuss their fears and anxieties, take a tour of the operating room holding area, and understand routine postoperative procedures. Obviously, some teaching should have occurred before the patient's admission, but this is not always the case. The nurse must therefore assess the situation, prioritize teaching needs, and decide *what* is the most important, *when* it can realistically be accomplished, and *what* the patient or client can realistically learn in the time available.

The time element in behavioral objectives needs to be specific as well. "Before discharge" is not sufficient. A specific time or date should be used and changed if necessary, if the learning does not progress as anticipated. Also, specific times and dates help nurses avoid procrastination—today is today.

Perhaps, the most difficult behavioral objectives for nurses to write are those that describe learning or behavioral change in the affective domain (values, beliefs, attitudes, emotions). The key to writing affective behavioral objectives is to focus on measurable behaviors. A nurse cannot feel whether or not a mother of a child born with a birth defect loves her child, but, she can observe actions that typically indicate love and acceptance. For example, before the nurse talks to the mother about the importance of bonding to the mother and the child, she observes that the mother does not hold the child unless it requires feeding. When she does hold the child, she does not hold it close to her body, does not try to maintain eye contact, and refers to the child as "it." Behavioral objectives for the teaching session on the importance of bonding might include: Within 8 hours following a discussion of the importance of bonding, the mother will: (1) pick up her infant two or more times without it requiring care, (2) hold her infant against her body for a minute or more two or more times, (3) look into her baby's eyes at least once within 5 minutes of picking up the baby, (4) refer to the baby in a possessive manner, i.e., by name, "my precious baby," "Mommy's sweetheart."

Once nursing diagnoses related to learning are made, and goals and behavioral objectives set, the nurse needs to decide what teaching strategies will best facilitate learning and accomplish these goals and objectives.

Strategies for effective teaching that promote learning and behavioral change are discussed in the following chapter.

IMPLEMENTATION

Implementation involves putting the teaching plan into action. The process of implementation is a dynamic, didactic encounter between the nurse and the learner. The implementation of the teaching plan may not progress exactly as envisioned—patients may be tired, clients may want to pursue new health concerns, or other factors may interfere with the session. Throughout the implementation, the nurse must continue to assess, plan, and evaluate to keep abreast of the evolving needs, concerns, and abilities of the learner. The success of implementation of a teaching plan depends a great deal upon the nurse's knowledge and the skills required for teaching and the learner's readiness and motivation to learn. The information provided in this book, when used, will help increase the nurse's success as a teacher.

EVALUATION

Evaluation is an ongoing, crucial component of the teaching process. Evaluation involves judging to what extent the teaching has been successful (this is process evaluation) and to what degree individuals have learned (this is product or summative evaluation). Evaluation in health teaching should be a mutual process between the teacher and the learner. This mutual process insures that the learner is involved in all the phases of the teaching–learning process. Evaluation also produces the "evidence" to prove to what extent nursing interventions have been successful.

Evaluation is really an ongoing component of assessment, planning, and implementation. As nurses move through the phases of the teaching process, they must continually evaluate the data that are collected, the appropriateness and efficacy of the plan, and the impact of implementation strategies. For example, during the assessment phase nurses must ask themselves questions such as: "Have I covered all the necessary areas?" "Is there anything else that I need to know before I begin to synthesize the data and identify nursing diagnoses?" When beginning to develop the plan, they should ask: "Will this effectively meet the learner's needs?" "Are the goals and objectives obtainable?" "Can we accomplish this in the amount of time available?" During the implementation, it is important to continually be evaluating teaching performance, the impact of teaching aids, and the learner's response. For example, does a frown mean the learner does not understand? Am I talking too fast? Am I involving the learner sufficiently? What is the reason for a lack of understanding? Is the noise in the hall distracting?

Evaluation serves many functions as part of the teaching process. Evaluation outcome measures helps the nurse to plan her teaching and know what to look for as evidence of learning; ongoing evaluation helps the nurse to reinforce appropriate behaviors, detect misinformation, and correct improper technique. Evaluation helps the nurse avoid ongoing errors in her teaching technique and helps to increase patient's learning and behavioral change. Likewise, ongoing evaluation helps the nurse save time by identifying problems as they arise instead of waiting until teaching is finished to find out that the patient has been lost since the beginning. Evaluation also provides the necessary measurable criteria for documentation to show that the nurse's teaching efforts produced learning and behavioral change (Cahill, 1987).

PROCESS EVALUATION

Process or formative evaluation is aimed at monitoring the ongoing process of the nurse's teaching effectiveness, the teaching process, and the learner's response. Process or formative evaluation is a must if behavioral objectives are to be met. As the teaching is in progress, the nurse needs to constantly be evaluating how the teaching is going. Am I talking too fast? Am I on the same vocabulary level as the patient? Am I making my points clear to the patient? How well the nurse functions as a teacher in orchestrating the teaching process can make the difference between learning and confusion for the patient. In addition to self-evaluation, the nurse might try having patients complete a short satisfaction questionnaire about how well they perceive that she taught (Table 10–5). If time and materials permit, the nurse might try tape recording or videotaping her teaching. Likewise, a periodic peer evaluation may prove helpful in pinpointing strengths and weaknesses of teaching.

Process evaluation of the teaching process can include questions such as, "Why aren't all the patients getting to the two daily preop classes?" "How can we avoid running short on booklets on the evening shift?" "Why aren't all the cardiologists referring patients to the program?" "It's hard to get more than 15 minutes of the patients' time without being interrupted—Can I shorten the material or decrease interruptions?" "The patients seem bored during the film—Should I use it or try a different strategy to get the material across?" Process evaluation is just that—evaluating how the teaching process is going. Process evaluation encompasses evaluating patients, personnel, materials, and the environment and how they facilitate or impede the teaching process.

TABLE 10–5. PATIENT TEACHING SATISFACTION QUESTIONNAIRE: SAMPLE QUESTIONS

Direction: Please place a check mark beside the answer that best describes how you feel about your teacher and what she taught.

1. Did the teacher discuss with you what you wanted to learn about? _____ Yes _____ No
2. Was your teacher pleasant? _____ Yes _____ No
3. Was the information well organized? _____ Yes _____ No
4. Did she present the information too fast? _____ Yes _____ No
5. Did she encourage you to ask questions? _____ Yes _____ No
6. Did she answer your questions to your satisfaction? _____ Yes _____ No
7. Would you recommend this teacher to a friend that has the same problem? _____ Yes _____ No

Finally, process evaluation encompasses assessing the learner's response to the teaching process. Is he or she bored, confused, tired? Does the learner feel a part of the process? Is the learning environment a positive one? How does he or she respond to the teaching? Periodic evaluation of the learner, his response to the teaching, and his progress toward the successful mastery of the behavioral objectives saves time and helps insure that the learner will be successful. The guiding question behind process evaluation is, "What can be done to better facilitate learning?"

OUTCOME OR SUMMATIVE EVALUATION

Process evaluation helps to ensure that nurses do not wait until the end of their efforts and find that they were all wrong. An ongoing or process evaluation is used to make adjustments in midcourse. Summative or product/end evaluation, on the other hand, helps nurses measure the effects or outcomes of their teaching efforts. Outcome evaluation is often thought of as counting wedgets, a very quantitative affair. Behavioral objective outcomes are measurable and lend themselves easily to quantitative evaluation methods. Behavioral objectives let the nurse and the patient know to what extent learning has taken place (Table 10–6). Behavioral objectives can be used to evaluate the progress of an individual patient or they can be looked at for numerous patients to identify teaching process problems or successes. Although quantitative data tend to be the mainstay of outcome evaluation, another very helpful component of outcome evaluation should be the use of qualitative data.

Qualitative data include impressions formed through data collection a well as professional judgments. For example, when teaching a patient to change the stoma appliance, the nurse may note that the patient carried through with the technique flawlessly, therefore successfully meeting the behavioral objectives; it may, however, also be noted that the stoma is described as "revolting," and that the patient "hates doing the stoma care," and keeps questioning why it needs to be "done so often." Next to the behavioral objective, the nurse might write "has not accepted necessity for stoma care, also having difficulty accepting stoma." Analysis of these data might lead to an addendum to the original plan on whether to consider consulting a psychiatric liaison nurse or initiating a public health referral.

Outcome evaluation can be accomplished by using a variety of tools; however, the tools *must* measure objectively. Many evaluation tools incorporate behavioral objectives. These include written tests, checklists, interviews, observations, and health records.

Written tests can be useful as evaluation tools. They do not change over time. They can be self-administered and can provide before-and-after results, not only showing that learning took place but how much. Good written tests take time to construct and must be pretested. Too often, written tests cue appropriate responses, do not test essential information, or are difficult to read and understand. Another factor to consider when using written tests is that many individuals feel threatened by them, especially older adults and those with low literacy skills. Also, for individ-

TABLE 10–6. PATIENT TEACHING PLAN

Diagnosis: Knowledge deficit related to new medication.
Standardized Care Plan: Teaching the Patient and Family About Long-Term Digitalis Therapy.

Patient Problem	Patient Outcome	Start Date/Date Discussed Plan	Initials
Long-term digitalis therapy	1. Can recite the rationale for digitalis therapy.	Indicate to whom instructions specified in plans below were given: patient and/or _____ (relationship: _____) 1.1 Teach that digitalis is a cardiac drug which improves the strength of the contractions of heart while slowing down the pulse rate.	1.1.
		1.2 Have patient describe rationale for digitalis.	1.2
	2. Can count radial pulse and record accurately.	2.1 Teach how to count a radial pulse.	2.1
		2.2 Have begin recording radial pulse on a sheet of paper 4 to 5 days prior to discharge.	
		2.3 Have the nurse assigned to the patient check for accuracy of recorded pulse rate.	2.3
		2.4 Teach not to take the digitalis pill should the pulse rate fall below _____ (per M.D.). Instruct to call _____ if pulse falls below this rate.	2.4
	3. Can state dose schedule, and side effects of digitalis.	3.1 Teach to take pill at ordered time(s).	3.1
		3.2 Instruct in the importance of daily use of digitalis.	3.2

Initials	Signature/Status	Initials	Signature/Status	Initials	Signature/Status
____	____	____	____	____	____
____	____	____	____	____	____

Used with permission from University of Virginia Hospitals, Division of Nursing, 1979.

uals who have poor vision, arthritis, or learning disabilities such as dyslexia, responding to a questionnaire can be extremely frustrating and even painful. Written tests are therefore not appropriate for all learners as a means of evaluation.

Written tests can be true–false, multiple choice, matching, cloze, or essay. True–false tests primarily test for knowledge acquisition. Individuals can falsely elevate a score by guessing and words like "always," "never," and "all" can confuse readers.

Multiple choice questions are more difficult to develop although they can be used to test knowledge, comprehension, analysis, synthesis, and evaluation. Multiple choice tests should be relatively short—two pages—so as not to tire an individual. Only the most important aspects of the learning therefore should be tested. "Nice-to-know" information testing should be avoided.

Matching test items can test for knowledge, comprehension, and application. They are often ambiguous. Guessing and cueing can often artificially inflate scores. When developing a matching list, make sure to include more items on one side to decrease the reader's chance of guessing the right answers.

A cloze comprehension test is perhaps one of the best test methods to measure recall and comprehension. Using the cloze technique, every nth word, usually every fifth, is omitted from a paragraph and the reader fills in the blanks. The cloze method has several advantages over multiple choice tests. It can be easily constructed. If only exact answers are accepted, it can be unambiguously scored, and it is a more sensitive measure of comprehension (Felker, 1980).

Essay tests are particularly good for evaluating comprehension, analysis, synthesis, and evaluation. Essay questions must be explicit in detail and a list of points that should be included in an adequate response must be developed along with the questions. Essay questions may not be the best way to evaluate learning in health education. Essays require that the learner have a great deal of skill in organizing thoughts and in writing skills. In addition, essay responses usually take a great deal of time. The same essay question might be better used by presenting it orally. For example, "Tell me how you will make sure your house is safe for your toddler."

Checklists can be a quick and easy way of evaluating and documenting learning. They can also incorporate behavioral objectives and learning contracts. Checklists can be developed in a variety of ways. Table 10–7 gives one example of a checklist, another is found in Chapter 9 (Table 9–4).

Interviews or oral questioning are common methods of evaluation. Interviews can be guided by the nurse asking open-ended questions or the nurse can follow a form listing specific questions. Interviews are particularly useful when attitudinal information is needed. Interviews also allow the nurse to clarify misconceptions, provide reinforcement, and give feedback to the learner. Interviews can be time consuming and therefore the nurse should plan the interview strategy to maximize the information obtainable in the amount of time available.

Observations of an individual's health behaviors are essential if we want to document changes in health behaviors, acquisition of psychomotor skills, or changes in attitudes. During observations, the nurse can provide positive reinforcement, correct inappropriate techniques before they become bad habits, and provide

TABLE 10–7. TEACHING CHECKLIST

TB Teaching Plan	
Treatment Record	**Addressograph Plate**

Allergies (written in red ink)

Date Ordered Class (No.)	Treatments, Nursing Orders	Hr	Dates
1	Orientation to BRH	————	————
2	Orientation to 2 WW	————	————
3	Respiratory Isolation	————	————
4	TB—Anatomy, Infection	————	————
5	TB—The Disease Process	————	————
6	TB—Risk Factors	————	————
7	TB—Tests & Procedures	————	————
	A—Skin Test	————	————
	B—Sputum Collection	————	————
	C—X-rays	————	————
	D—Venipuncture	————	————
	E—Thoracentesis	————	————
	F—Bronchoscopy	————	————
	G—IV Fluids	————	————
	H—NG Feedings	————	————
	I—O_2 Therapy	————	————
	J—Postural Drainage	————	————
	K—Cupping and Clapping	————	————
	L—Suctioning	————	————
8	TB—The Goals of Tx	————	————
9	Orientation to Nursing Unit	————	————
	Part A—Physical Layout	————	————
	Part B—Info Pamphlet	————	————

Adapted from TB Teaching Plan, Blue Ridge Division, University of Virginia, Division of Nursing, 1982. Used with permission.

coaching and support for the learner. Checklists can be a helpful adjunct to observations. They can be shared with the learner and can be used in documentation.

Health records can be used to document learning and behavioral change. For example, blood pressure flow charts can give some indication of whether or not an individual is following the treatment regimen, weight charts can chronicle a dieter's progress, and nurse's notes and medical notes can outline a patient's behavior. References to specific parts of a health record can be used in documentation as well.

Overall Evaluation

A thorough evaluation of teaching and learner outcomes should enable nurses to answer these two questions: Was the teaching appropriate? Did the individual learn?

If the answer to either question is no, further evaluation is needed. Teaching methods used may have been flawless, but other factors may dictate whether or not they were effective. Common problems that inhibit the effectiveness of teaching include lack of adequate assessment, poor planning, choice of inappropriate teaching methods or teaching aids, lack of adequate time for teaching, lack of effective communication skills and teaching strategies, lack of rapport between the nurse and the learner, lack of learner involvement throughout the teaching process, and lack of documentation leading to chaotic and fragmented teaching.

Common problems that inhibit patient and client learning include pain, anxiety, psychological problems, health and cultural values, fatigue, literacy level, and learner readiness. These factors have been discussed elsewhere in this text.

If there is a problem with the teaching process or with an individual's learning, an assessment must be made as to why. The nurse can, of course, evaluate the process but the learner's input into the assessment is critical. The nurse's perception of problem areas may not be the same as those of the learner. Once problem areas have been identified the learner must be incorporated into planning revisions.

Not every teaching session will be successful nor will every individual learn as easily and as much as a nurse hopes. Too many factors contribute to the overall process; it is unlikely that nurses can control or manipulate all of them. By being aware of what needs to be assessed and of how to plan, implement, and evaluate, nurses can increase the likelihood that both they and the learner will be successful.

DOCUMENTATION

Adequate documentation of the teaching–learning process is crucial. It catalogues the nurse's involvement in teaching; it notes the systematic and planned approach to teaching; it is a communication medium between health professionals; it helps agencies meet mandates for federal programs such as Medicaid; and it serves as a legal statement about the nurse's interventions and the patient's or client's response.

Documentation of teaching and learning can be accomplished through the use of flow charts, checklists, care plans, or traditional anecdotal notes. Whatever the method that is used, it is essential that the information is a part of the individual's permanent health record. For example, flow charts or checklists are often used to chronicle teaching; they are, however, primarily used as a communication medium for staff and are thrown away once the patient is discharged. Unless other documentation has been made, there is no permanent record of teaching efforts or their outcomes. Legally, the nurse would have little recourse of proof in such a situation.

For documentation purposes, it is important that nurses detail *what* was done and *how* the effect was evaluated. Chapter 2 lists considerations from a legal perspective for charting. Common forms of documentation include those found in Table 11–2 (the behavioral contract), Table 10–6 (the behavioral objective), and Table 10–7 (a behavioral checklist).

SUMMARY

The teaching process involves many activities and considerations. This chapter has outlined how to move from the nursing diagnosis to evaluation. The importance of evaluation and documentation were emphasized. The teaching process requires that the nurse have knowledge and skills that can promote learning. As with other nursing activities, the application of the teaching process becomes more finely tuned and easier to perform with continued use. It is essential that health teaching follow a planned, systematic process to increase the likelihood of success.

REFERENCES AND READINGS

Armstrong, M. L. Orchestrating the process of patient education. Methods and approaches. *Nursing Clinics of North America,* 1989, *23*(4):597–604.

Bille, D. A. A study of patients' knowledge in relation to teaching format and compliance. *Supervisor Nurse,* 1977, *8*:55–62.

Cahill, M. (Ed.). *Nurse reference library: Patient teaching.* Springhouse, PA: Springhouse Corp, 1987.

Felker, D. (Ed.). *Document design: A review of the relevant research.* Washington, D.C.: Carnegie Mellon University and Siegal & Gale for the American Institutes of Research, 1980.

Fresette, S. L. A model for improving cancer patient education. *Cancer Nursing,* 1990, *13*(4):207–215.

George, G. If patient teaching tries your patience, try this plan. *Nursing '82,* May 1982, 50–55.

Harrison, L. L. A health promotion model for wellness education. *Maternal Childhealth Nursing,* 1990, *15*(2):113.

Hjelm-Karlsson, K. Comparison of oral, written and audiovisually based information as preparation for intravenous pyelography. *International Journal of Nursing Studies,* 1989, 26(1):53–68.

Lipetz, M. J. What is wrong with patient education programs? *Nursing Outlook,* 1990, *38*(4):184–189.

Maslow, A. *Motivation and personality.* New York: Harper & Row, 1970.

Peterson, S. K. Evaluation of a resource center for cancer patients. *Health Education Research,* 1989, 4(4):495–500.

Redman, B. *The process of patient teaching,* 6th ed. Chicago, IL: C. V. Mosby Co., 1988.

Strauss, A. L. & Glaser, B. *Chronic illness and the quality of life.* St. Louis: C. V. Mosby Co., 1975.

Van Hoozer, H. L., Bratton, B., Ostmoe, P., et al. *The teaching process: Theory and practice in nursing.* Norwalk, CT: Appleton-Century-Crofts, 1987.

11

Strategies for Effective Health Teaching

Marlyn Duncan Boyd

Teaching strategies should be chosen after the assessment has been made and must reflect what is to be learned and the learner's abilities and preferences for learning. It is certainly permissible to plan ahead in choosing teaching strategies, but, the planning must include a variety of ways for the learner to obtain the material and/or skill. Think of teaching strategies as a repertoire of potential tools to facilitate learning. The nurse will not use all of her potential tools with every patient—it would not be necessary nor wise. She does pick and choose the strategies based on her assessment, time available, patient preference, and guiding educational principles. Perhaps the two most common mistakes nurses make in using teaching strategies is that too few are used (oral teaching only) and inappropriate strategies (written material too complicated, films too technical, miss–match of strategy with expected learner outcome, for example). This chapter will help prepare the nurse to avoid these mistakes and better facilitate learning.

TEACHING STRATEGIES

The broad category of teaching strategies can be subdivided into instructional methods, educational strategies, behavioral strategies, and teaching aids. When deciding how to facilitate learning, the nurse must choose methods and materials appropriate for the task to be learned. Instructional methods refer to the way the nurse plans to conduct the teaching–learning session. Common methods include one-to-one, lecture, discussion, demonstrations, and role playing. Lecture, demonstration, field trips, case presentation, and role playing are presented in Chapter 15 as methods appropriate for groups. Here we will discuss strategies for one-to-one teaching and then provide information about educational and behavioral strategies and teaching aids.

One-to-One Teaching

One-to-one teaching is usually accomplished through oral communication—the exchange of words, ideas, and feelings—and through nonverbal body messages. This is perhaps the most common form of information exchange and learning. Oral communication serves several functions: it helps to establish rapport; it is a means of giving information and instruction; and it allows for immediate feedback. Too often, oral communication is ineffective on the part of the nurse and is not understood or retained by the client. Part of this problem is the result of ineffective communication skills or ineffective teaching methods. Studies have shown that, in general, people forget about one half of all oral instructions within 5 minutes of receiving them (Ley, 1973). In addition, laypersons often do not understand common medical terms (Cosper, 1977; Fitzpatrick et al., 1988).

Although one-to-one communication is often ineffective, it is frequently preferred by patients for learning (Boyd & Feldman, 1984), and it is especially important for those who are educationally disadvantaged. Such individuals often use oral communication as a primary source of information. More information about teaching the educationally disadvantaged is presented in Chapter 14.

Strategies for Effective Oral Communication in Teaching

Effective oral communication and patients' resulting satisfaction from the encounter are strong facilitators of learning and behavioral change (Roter, 1988). Effective teaching is a combination of the use of good communication skills and effective educational strategies. Before beginning a teaching session, the nurse must prepare an appropriate and conducive learning environment. Outside stimuli such as distracting sights, noxious odors, and noises should be minimized if possible. When in the hospital setting, draw the bedside curtain, close the door, or, if possible, take the patient to a quiet area. Help make the patient as comfortable as possible, both physically and emotionally. Providing comfort measure such as rolling up the head of the bed, elevating edematous feet, or drawing the curtains against brilliant sunlight will help minimize distractors. If the patient or client is worried about a parking meter that is running out, or getting home before the children return from school, or whether family members will be coming during visiting hours, these concerns will dilute the amount of attention given to the teaching session. The nurse can try to plan teaching to coincide with times when the patient is the most relaxed and receptive.

The beginning of the teaching session sets the stage for much of the success of the interaction. It is important that the learner know what to expect. Reviewing the goals and objectives for the session and emphasizing the potential benefits of learning with a positive attitude can be helpful.

Because patients and clients tend to forget much of the oral information presented to them, the nurse must carefully plan the teaching session. Advance organizers are especially important; these can help patients and clients remember more. Advance organizers help "clue" individuals about what is going to happen and what will be expected of them. Such statements would include: I am going to tell you about:

- How your heart works.
- What caused your heart attack.
- What you must do to help yourself now that you've had a heart attack.

Then continue the teaching session with, "Now, first let me tell you how your heart works . . ." (Boyd, 1983; Ley et al., 1973). It is very important to involve the individual in the teaching session; this increases recall of information and patient satisfaction (Roter et al., 1988; Bille, 1977). Open-ended questions such as "Tell me what worries you the most about . . ." and "How do you feel about . . .?" can help the nurse gather information about the individual's needs and actively involve the learner. Questions such as "Now, tell me how you'll know if your finger's infected," and "How will you know if your 'sugar' is getting low?" help the patient or client focus on important concepts and provide a means for ongoing evaluation of the teaching–learning process. Because people tend to remember best the information presented in the first one third of the interaction (Ley, 1972), plan to present the most important information first, especially in time-restricted teaching settings like clinics and emergency rooms.

Individuals who are educationally disadvantaged or those who are investing much of their energy to meet physiological demands often have short attention spans. Teaching sessions should not continue past the point where the person can no longer concentrate on the material being presented. Signs of lack of attention can include: loss of eye contact or eyes "wandering," frequent changes in posture, an inability to answer questions, and attempts to change the topic. The nurse should be aware of these signs and end the session by recapturing the most significant points. If possible, the teaching sessions should be spaced so as not to tire the patient or client. If this is not possible, provide frequent breaks within the teaching session. At the beginning of each session, review what has been covered in the past session(s); repetition strengthens recall. When providing instructions, remember to be specific. Specific information increases recall and has a more effective impact on behavior (Ley, 1973, 1976; Padberg & Padberg, 1990). It is more effective to say, "Lose 10 pounds by your next appointment," than it is to say, "Lose weight."

The choice of vocabulary used in teaching is dictated by the individual learner's vocabulary level. During assessment and teaching sessions, note the person's use, if any, of medical or technical words. Are they used in the proper context? If so, you may use these terms during the teaching session. If the terms are used inappropriately, you will need to clarify the misuse. Do not make the assumption that if individuals use a few medical terms appropriately they will understand other medical terms. For example, a patient with a long history of hypertension may use the words "hypertension," "systolic," "diastolic," and "diuretics" correctly, but when confronted with a new condition, such as diabetes mellitus, will need to be introduced to the new vocabulary. Assess slang terms for body parts and bodily functions used by the patient and use these to define frequently used medical terms. Give the patient a list of terms that will be used frequently and define these, using the level of vocabulary appropriate for the patient. This can be done orally or in writing. If the learner's condition can be referred to by using various terms, be sure to include all of these in the list. A patient in a coronary care unit, who had had a heart attack, anxiously asked the nurse if they (the doctors) had found anything else wrong. Puzzled, the nurse responded, "No, you've only had a heart attack." The patient replied by saying, "Well, the doctors have told me I've had an M.I., a heart attack, a myocardial infarction, a coronary occlusion, and an infarct. Do you think I'll make it?"

"Closure" is essential for teaching sessions, as well as a summary of essential information and an evaluation of what the individual has learned. Closure is a means of tying loose ends and alerting the learner that the session will be ending. Statements that can alert the individual that the session will be ending are, "This is the last thing we have to discuss today," "We will be finishing in a few minutes," or "I have finished going over. . . . Is there anything you want me to review before we finish?" A summary helps to reinforce essential information for the learner and helps to clarify any misconceptions. Learners can be asked to summarize the essential elements of the session; this actively involves them and can also serve as a method of evaluation. The nurse can also use this time of closure to encourage the learner and give positive reinforcement for the learning that has occurred. It is important that the client feel a sense of satisfaction and achievement.

Throughout the teaching session it is important to maintain a therapeutic relationship. Cline (1983) lists several frequently occurring barriers to effective communication:

1. Ignoring the presence of the person or ignoring attempts to communicate. Examples include giving silence when a reply is expected, leaving the client's presence when he or she is speaking, engaging in tasks unrelated to the conversation, or changing the topic abruptly.
2. Using communications that prohibit or discourage the participation of the other person. Such communications include interrupting, monopolizing the conversation, or using closed-ended questions.
3. Using behaviors that cause distance to increase between yourself and the client. Distance-increasing behaviors include avoiding eye contact, using impersonal language ("How are *we* doing?"), concealing personal feelings or denying the other person's feelings or meanings ("You don't really mean that.").
4. Using messages that are contradictory or ambiguous. Ambiguous messages include "Lose weight" rather than "Lose 10 pounds." Other problem messages include using verbal and nonverbal messages that contradict each other or responding only to parts of the client's message.

Effective oral communication skills are an essential component of the teaching–learning process. Nonverbal communication also contributes to a successful teaching session.

Nonverbal Communication

Individuals often express their feelings and thoughts through behavior. Motor activity is a normal way of discharging energy, of relieving tension, and of expressing inner feelings. Behavior is often purposeful, like closing your eyes during a scary movie, or it can be unconscious, such as a nervous patient clenching and unclenching the fists. Nonverbal behavior and its meanings vary somewhat from cultural influences, gender variations, socioeconomic status, social distance, power relationships, and affective states.

Common nonverbal communication variations across cultures include how much eye contact is given, how much touching occurs, and how pain, happiness, or sorrow are expressed. For example, people place themselves in varying degrees of closeness during communication. Across ethnic groups, it has been found that Mexicans place themselves closest, Anglos next, and blacks the farthest apart (Mehrabian, 1972).

Gender differences show, for example, that women are more competent than men in both expressing and perceiving emotions. Women make eye contact more often than men. Women, typically, have superior verbal skills and ask more questions (Wientraub, 1983; Weisman & Teitelbaum, 1989).

Socioeconomic status, social distance, and power relationships can affect nonverbal behavior. As individuals get to know each other better, they use more covert expressions. Within power relationships, the dependent member is more sensitive to nonverbal cues (Wientraub, 1983; Weisman & Teitelbaum, 1989).

Affective states influence our behavior. Anxiety, sadness, joy, and fear can affect our voice tone, speech pattern, posture, and walk. Most researchers believe that nonverbal behavior is a more accurate conveyer of emotion than spoken messages (Wientraub, 1983). Posture can convey liking, boredom, or interest. Eye contact can convey liking or anger. O'Brien (1978) lists several types of nonverbal behaviors and their possible meanings (see Chapter 9, Table 9–7).

Nonverbal communication can give the nurse clues to help make accurate learner assessments and plan teaching strategies. Nonverbal communication is often hard to assess and difficult to interpret. Many times, nonverbal messages do not match verbal ones. For example, patients may state that they are ready to learn, yet they frequently gaze out the window or get up to walk about the room. Nonverbal behavior can either reinforce or negate what is said orally.

Nonverbal behavior can be classified in three broad categories: (1) immediacy, (2) relaxation, and (3) responsiveness. Immediacy refers to the degree of "closeness" between individuals who are interacting. Relaxation is defined as the extent of postural relaxation or tension exhibited by individuals. Responsiveness is the extent of awareness of and reaction to another person. Mehrabian (1972) has further divided these categories as shown in Table 11–1. The nonverbal behavior of communicators can be assessed by assigning numbers to the categories. For example, body orientation would be scored +4—high immediacy (directly facing the other person) to −4—low immediacy (turning 180 degrees away from the other person).

Several studies have shown that nonverbal behavior is a very important component of a teaching–learning interaction. Researchers have found that immediacy is correlated with liking and patient satisfaction with interactions. Immediacy has also been shown to be associated with higher levels of patient comprehension of information. Eye contact has also been associated with liking. Those body postures of

TABLE 11–1. MEHRABIAN'S THREE MAJOR AREAS OF NONVERBAL COMMUNICATION

I. Immediacy
  A. Touching: bodily contact between communicator and client.
  B. Distance: physical distance between communicator and client.
  C. Forward lean: number of degrees that a plane from the communicator's shoulders to hips is away from the vertical.
  D. Observation: occurs when one individual looks directly at the face of another.
  E. Body orientation: measure of the torso's rotation.

II. Relaxation
  A. Arm position asymmetry: degree of asymmetry in arm position.
  B. Sideways lean: degrees of lean away from the vertical.
  C. Leg position asymmetry: degree of asymmetry in leg position.
  D. Hand relaxation: ranges from very tense to relaxed.
  E. Neck relaxation: measures degree of head support and level of gaze.
  F. Reclining angle (or backward lean): the negative of forward lean.

III. Responsiveness
  A. Facial activity
  B. Vocal activity
  C. Speech rate
  D. Speech volume

Adapted from Mehrabian, A. Nonverbal communication. New York: Aldine-Atherton, 1972, and Larsen, K. M., & Smith, C. K. Assessment of nonverbal communication in the patient-physician interview. Journal of Family Practice, 1981, 12(3), 481–488.

the therapist that most positively influenced patient understanding were forward body lean and body orientation (directly facing the client) (Larsen & Smith, 1981; Mehrabian, 1972; Weisman & Teitelbaum, 1989).

It is important, during the teaching session, that an on-going assessment be made of the learner's nonverbal messages. What are they saying? Is the learner anxious, tense, tired? Is he or she preoccupied with other concerns? Do the nonverbal messages match the learner's verbal ones? If not, point this out. For example, you might say, "Mr. Jones, you said you wanted me to come this morning to teach you about how to take your nitroglycerin at home, but you keep dozing off. Would later this afternoon be a better time for you?"

Nonverbal communication is an important component of the teaching–learning process. The teacher can use body language to convey interest, concern, and respect for the learner. In addition, by reading the nonverbal messages, the nurse can assess whether learners are ready to learn, whether verbal and nonverbal messages are congruent with each other, and how learners are responding emotionally to the session.

EDUCATIONAL STRATEGIES

Green (1979) identified several educational strategies that can be used to promote learning. Many of these were used in the preceding teaching session illustration. These and other strategies are discussed here.

Specificity

The more specific—to the point—a communication is, the more effective it is, especially in the areas of retention of information and behavior change (Ley, 1975, 1976). For example, it is much more effective to instruct a client to "walk one mile every other day" than to say, "Get some exercise." Simplicity is also important. Long, running narratives can lose the learner to boredom or frustration. They can also camouflage important content.

Repetition

Repetition strengthens learning. Whether the information is presented repeatedly in one form (oral) or whether it is presented using multiple methods, retention increases. In addition, when more than one of the body's senses is used, individuals learn better (Bille, 1977; Klausmeier & Ripple, 1975; Cahill, 1987). It would therefore be helpful to augment one-to-one interactions with written materials, audiovisual aids, and other means of reinforcing the learning.

Brevity

As mentioned earlier, individuals tend to forget approximately one half of what they hear within 5 minutes (Ley, 1973). This finding has been found to be accurate about 77 percent of the time. This should not discourage information giving but encourage us to find better ways to communicate and teach. Additionally, it appears that the passage of time does not adversely affect recall. Joyce et al. (1969) found that patients were able to recall 48 percent of what they were told immediately following a medical visit and 40 percent 4 months later. Nurses must also remember that their goal is not to make individuals experts in a particular aspect of health care, but to help them become knowledgeable and skilled enough to safeguard their health. Present, emphasize, and summarize key information, do not overload the learner with nice to know information.

Organization

The way health content is organized and presented can affect how well it is received, understood, and remembered. The use of advanced organizers can increase recall by as much as 50 percent (Ley et al., 1973). Learning can be disorganized, ineffective, and confusing for the learner if advanced organizers are not used (Ausubel, 1963). Advanced organizers help the learner to know what to expect and in what order. Advanced organizers also help cue the learner about what is important to remember. For example, "Today I will be going over the four signs and symptoms of infection. You will need to remember these. The first sign is . . ." Logical organization from simple to complex and from concrete to abstract provide learning building blocks.

Primacy

Ley (1972) found that regardless of the type of information delivery (oral, audiovisual, or written) patients remembered the first third and the last one fourth of the information best. This finding further supports the need for nurses to plan relatively short teaching sessions and use advanced organizers to point out the key elements of the teaching session and summarize essential points.

BEHAVIORAL STRATEGIES

Behavioral strategies refer to those techniques used to change specific behaviors (Dunbar et al., 1979). Common behavioral strategies include contracting, tailoring, graduated behavior change, and self-monitoring. Behavioral strategies are discussed in the following section.

Contracting

Contracting refers to the process in which the teacher and the learner mutually set rules regarding a specific behavior and formalize a commitment to change the behavior. Mahoney and Thoresen (1974) list five guidelines for a contract:

1. The contract should be fair.
2. The terms should be very clear.
3. The contract should be generally positive.
4. Procedures should be systematic and consistent.
5. At least one other person should participate.

Mahoney and Thoresen (1974) acknowledge that a contract may be made with oneself; the individual may be more successful, however, if the contract involves another person. See Table 11–2 for a sample contract which lists the specific components.

A learning contract can be negotiated anywhere—hospital, home, clinic, medical office—and is a joint venture between the teacher and learner. Behavioral contracts, because of their nature, work best when there is continuity of care. A learning contract, like a behavioral objective, deals with one behavior at a time. Often the behavior that needs to be changed is very complex and must be broken down into smaller behavioral tasks. For instance, losing weight may be the broad goal for a behavioral contract, but the specific behavior may be that the client will agree not to snack between meals for 4 days out of each week until the next clinic

TABLE 11–2. A SAMPLE CONTRACT

I *(Client's name)* will *(behavior)* by *(date)*. In return *(teacher or other participant)* will *(nurse responsibility)*. When successful, Jim Smith will *(reward)*.

(Client's signature/date)
(Nurse's signature/date)

I *Jim Smith* will *lose 5 lbs* by May 5, 1986. In return *Paula Jones, R.N.,* will spend 15 minutes at my next clinic visit to discuss stress reduction techniques. When successful, Jim Smith will purchase a new cassette tape.

Jim Smith/April 18, 1985
Paul Jones, R.N.

visit. In exchange, the client may ask that his wife take out the garbage on the days that he successfully avoids snacking. Once this contract has been fulfilled another contract can be negotiated. It is important that the patient choose the reward—what will motivate one person may not motivate another. Rewards must be individually specific.

Behavioral contracts serve several therapeutic functions. They encourage learner involvement in the health plan, they prompt a firm commitment by both parties involved, they allow for positive reinforcement for behaviors that are specific for each individual, and they provide incentives for behavioral change. Behavioral contracts have been used successfully to promote weight loss (Dinoff et al., 1972), improve hypertension control (Steckel & Swain, 1977), and abstain from alcohol (Bigelow et al., 1976) to mention a few of their successful uses. For a discussion of the use of contracting as a strategy in value education, see Chapter 13.

Graduated Behavioral Change
Graduated behavioral change indicates that behavioral change takes place in increments over a period of time. Graduated behavioral change may or may not be part of a formal contract. By promoting gradual behavioral change, the teacher acknowledges that behavioral change is often difficult and that gradual change may be a more feasible way of altering behavior. For example, a hypertensive individual may be advised to lose weight, decrease the use of salt, quit smoking, and relax. Obviously, to adhere to the recommendation the individual must make radical life style changes and such changes may seem overwhelming. The client also may be more prone to failure. Helping the client successfully change one behavior at a time increases the chances for long-term success. Again, it is most important that the patient choose what behavior he or she wants to try to change first. It is essential that they experience success. It may be the behavior easiest to change or the most essential to improve health.

Tailoring
Tailoring should be an integral part of each teaching plan. Tailoring refers to the process of making a teaching plan "fit" the particular needs and characteristics of an individual. Tailoring is frequently used to set medication schedules, plan wound care, and plan teaching sessions. By adapting teaching or treatment regimens to an individual's personal habits and routines, it is more likely that the person will be receptive to teaching and carry through with health-care recommendations (Hallburg, 1970; Haynes et al., 1976).

Self-Monitoring
Self-monitoring is a method used to help individuals become aware of their behavior. It often consists of an individual recording when a certain behavior occurs, where it occurs, what happened before the behavior, and how the individual felt before and during the behavior. A common use of self-monitoring has been diet diaries. There is increasing evidence that self-monitoring can be an effective method

for promoting behavioral change (Maletzky, 1974; Nelson et al., 1976). As with behavioral contracts, individuals who agree to monitor their behavior must be able to identify the behavior, know how to record it properly, and be consistent with recordings. Self-monitoring may best serve as a self-regulating mechanism. Once individuals are aware of their behavior they can then take appropriate steps to correct it.

The successful use of instructional methods and educational and behavioral strategies is contingent upon the nurse making a thorough assessment and developing a realistic plan. Once these tasks have been accomplished, the nurse chooses which methods and strategies will be the most likely to facilitate learning. Another important component of the teaching process is the use of appropriate instructional or teaching aids. The following section outlines commonly used teaching aids, how to assess their appropriateness, and how to develop written materials.

TEACHING AIDS

Often nurses either do not use media to enhance their teaching or they rely solely on media with the mistaken notion that information dissemination is teaching. Neither of these approaches is appropriate.

One-to-one teaching can be augmented and reinforced by the use of appropriate media. Media can be used to give routine information and instructions that can lay the groundwork for teaching–learning sessions. For media to be an asset to the teaching process they must be chosen carefully and used appropriately.

Various media can be used to facilitate learning; no one medium, however, is universally the best. Media must meet a specific purpose. Media must be used in such a way that they promote the accomplishment of behavioral objectives. Media must also be compatible with the type of instructional methods used. For example, a written description may not be the best way to teach facts and to stimulate the body's senses or promote psychomotor skills. Media must be chosen with the learner's needs and abilities in mind. A book giving factual information about a disease cannot meet the emotional needs of a learner. Moreover, media must be previewed and evaluated prior to use. Just because a booklet or film has been commercially produced does not ensure that it is appropriate for the intended audience or that it is up-to-date. Finally, media must be used under conditions that promote their usefulness. Crowded seating, a screen that is too small, too much interference, or bad lighting can distract from even the best media.

Prior to choosing or using any type of medium each nurse must ask:

- Is the medium accurate?
- Is the medium appropriate for the intended audience?
- Is the medium appropriate for the type of instructional methods chosen?
- Can the medium help the learner meet the behavioral objectives (Frantz, 1980)?

The multimethod approach for teaching seems to facilitate learning. Media can help to broaden methods of information delivery and to stimulate a variety of the learner's body senses.

Written Materials

Discharge instruction sheets, pamphlets, brochures, and booklets are commonly used in many health-care facilities as a means of providing information to clients and patients. Chapter 16 lists sources for commercial materials. All too often, however, these materials are not appropriate for the population they are given to and are of limited value. Although written information can serve as a reinforcer of oral interactions and can be used by individuals at home (Sharpe, 1974), written materials must be on a level that individuals can read and understand to be effective. Studies of public and patient populations have found average reading abilities do not exceed the eighth-grade level, (Berg & Hammitt, 1980; Doak & Doak, 1985; Northcutt, 1975; Boyd, 1988); yet the reading levels of patient education literature usually far exceed the eighth-grade reading level (Boyd & Brunner, 1982; Boyd, 1988; Boyd & Citro, 1983; Taylor et al., 1982; Michielutte, 1990). The last grade of formal schooling is not an accurate indicator of an individual's reading ability; many persons who have had some formal schooling may be illiterate (Doak & Doak, 1985). Persons who cannot read or who read poorly may not disclose this fact. This often leads the nurse to assume that the patient can read. Conversely, persons with low levels of formal schooling may read at higher levels. This is especially true for individuals such as secretaries who have jobs that require daily reading (Boyd & Feldman, 1984; Boyd, 1988).

Individuals who read on or below a fourth-grade level are classified as illiterate; those reading on a fifth- to seventh-grade level are considered functionally illiterate, that is, they can read but with limited competency and are not fully capable of carrying out everyday tasks that require reading. Persons who read on or above an eighth-grade level are deemed literate (Bormuth, 1973; Redman, 1988). On average, 25 percent of the adult population is functionally illiterate, with minorities and the elderly having higher levels of impaired literacy (Boyd & Wienrich, 1991).

When writing or choosing written material for the educationally disadvantaged as well as for more educated individuals, certain guidelines can be used. With many types of written information such as pamphlets describing a procedure, the question–answer format is best. This format allows the person to quickly scan the information and find the topic of particular interest. The questions should be short, to the point, and written in the first person; for example, "When will I get to eat and drink?" The answers, too, should be concise; for example, "Within 1 to 2 hours after you come back to your room." The pamphlet's information should not try to make the reader an expert on the topic but, rather, adequately inform him. The information should be patient or client centered—what the patient or client will experience and what the patient or client needs to know to satisfactorily understand and cope with the condition, disease, or procedure. Medical terms should be used but defined by using the lay person's language and analogies if possible (Boyd, 1981; Boyd & Wienrich, 1991).

Following are guidelines for developing written materials:

- Use boldface type, italicize, or underline words and ideas for emphasis.
- Begin with an introduction that states the purpose of the piece to orient the reader.
- Place appropriate visuals (charts, photos, etc.) next to the related idea as it appears in the text.

Paragraphs

- Use one idea for each paragraph.
- Start each paragraph with a strong topic sentence.
- Vary the length of the sentences.
- Space new concepts with the use of analogies or examples.

Sentences

- A sentence should be short, about ten words or less.
- Avoid complex sentence structures.
- Use the active rather than the passive voice.

Choice of Words

- Words of three or more syllables should be avoided. For example, use doctor rather than physician (see Table 11–3 for an exchange list of words).
- Abbreviations such as "MI," "SCAN," or "TRP," should be avoided.
- Shorter words should be substituted for longer ones, for example, "give" versus "administer" or "wipe clean" versus "thoroughly cleanse" (U.S. Dept. of Health and Human Services, 1982).

Choice of Type

- 8 to 10 point type should be used for patients with normal vision. 12 to 14 point type should be used for patients with failing vision and for children.

  this is 8 point type

  this is 10 point type

  this is 12 point type

  this is 14 point type

- Lines should be no more than 50 to 70 characters.
- White space should be used to rest the eyes (double spacing and margins).
- Upper and lower case letters should be used; ALL CAPS makes text harder to read.
- Serif type (letters with horizontal strokes at the bottoms and tops of letters) should be used; it is easier to read (Felker, 1982).

TABLE 11–3. EXAMPLES OF FREQUENTLY USED POLYSYLLABIC WORDS AND THEIR MORE SIMPLE SYNONYMS

accompany—go with	identical—same	qualified—suited
accomplish—carry out	illustration—picture	
acquire—gain	inadvertent—careless	recapitulate—sum up
alternative—choice	inadvisable—unwise	recognize—know, accept
annually—yearly	incision—cut	recuperate—get well
apply—put on, use	incorrect—wrong	rehabilitate—restore
attempt—try	indication—sign	
available—ready	inhibit—check, hinder	salient—main
	initial—first	segment—part
cessation—stop, pause	instrument—tool	similar—like
compassion—pity	intention—aim	similarity—likeness
competent—able	interrupt—stop	situated—placed
conclusive—final		stimulate—excite
concrete—real	laceration—cut, tear	sustenance—support
confront—meet		
conversion—change	manifest—clear, plain	tertiary—third
correspond—agree	minimal—smallest	transcription—copy
	modification—change	
delete—strike out		ultimate—last, final
detrimental—harmful	observe—note	uncommonly—rarely
disconnect—undo	obvious—plain	unequivocal—clear
disintegrate—break up	occurrence—event	unfounded—groundless
	opportunity—chance	unnecessary—needless
formulate—draw up		utilize—use
fundamental—basic	palatable—pleasing	
	penetrate—pierce	vacillate—waver
gratify—please	perforation—hole	validity—truth
guarantee—backing, promise	permission—consent	visualize—picture
	pharmacist—druggist	voluminous—bulky
hazardous—risky	present—give	
humid—damp	principal—main, chief	

Adapted from The short for the long, *Division of Health Education, South Carolina Department of Health and Environmental Control, 1977. Used with permission.*

This is serif type
This is sans-serif type

When determining the reading abilities of individuals, the nurse can use two guidelines: (1) in general, persons do not read above the eighth-grade level, and (2) individuals will probably read two to five grade levels below the last grade completed in formal schooling. When considering the potential reading abilities of the educationally disadvantaged, the nurse must also consider the person's general vocabulary deficiency.

The reading level of patient–health education materials can be determined by using various readability formulas. These formulas are based on an analysis of the grammatical components of the material versus the content. Various language elements such as the number of syllables, sentence structure, and sentence length are

TABLE 11–4. SMOG GRADING

Step 1. Count 10 consecutive sentences near the beginning, middle, and end of the material (total = 30 sentences). A sentence is any list of words ending in a period, question mark, or exclamation point.

Step 2. Count every word of three or more syllables in the 30 sentences. If a word is repeated count the repetition also.

Step 3. Obtain the nearest square root of the number of three or more syllabic words.

Step 4. Add three to the square root. This gives you the SMOG Grade.

Example

Step 1. 10 sentences (beginning)	*Step 2.* 21
10 sentences (middle)	23
10 sentences (end)	23
30 sentences total	67 total
Step 3. $\sqrt{67} = 8$	
Step 4. 8 + 3 = 11th grade	

Adapted from McLaughlin, G. H. SMOG grading—a new readability formula. Journal of Reading, *May 1969, 12, pp. 639–646.*

counted and used in mathematical equations or plotted onto graphs (Dale & Chall, 1948; Flesh, 1948; Fry, 1968). A simple, yet reliable formula for assessing readability is the SMOG Grading Formula, which requires less than 10 minutes to use for each piece of literature (McLaughlin, 1969). Table 11–4 outlines the steps for obtaining the reading level of materials by using the SMOG formula. Table 11–5 shows a fast conversion table.

TABLE 11–5. SMOG CONVERSION TABLE

Total Polysyllabic Word Counts	Approximate Grade Level (+ 1.5 Grades)
0–2	4
3–6	5
7–12	6
13–20	7
21–30	8
31–42	9
43–56	10
57–72	11
73–90	12
91–110	13
111–132	14
133–156	15
157–182	16
183–210	17
211–240	18

Developed by McGraw, Harold C. Office of Educational Research, Baltimore County Schools, Towson, Maryland.

TABLE 11–6. SAMPLES OF DIFFERENT READING LEVELS

College Reading Level
With the onset of nausea, diarrhea, or other gastrointestinal disturbances, consult your physician immediately.

12th Grade Reading Level
If you experience nausea, diarrhea, or other stomach or bowel problems, call your physician immediately.

8th Grade Reading Level
If you start having nausea, loose bowel movements, or other stomach or bowel problems, call your doctor immediately.

4th Grade Reading Level
If you start having an upset stomach, or loose bowel movements, call your doctor right away.

Reading level assessment can aid in predicting the general difficulty that persons may have in reading a particular piece of literature. Reading level assessment can assist in helping nurses choose or write materials that are more appropriate for patients and clients. But reading level assessment when used as the primary criterion for materials selection may not in itself promote ease of reading (Meade & Smith, 1991). For example, although the word "void" is a one-syllable word and would contribute to a low reading level in a piece of patient education material, it may not be understood by the public. It would be appropriate to use more words or a polysyllabic word that is well known and increase the reading level slightly. For examples of various reading levels consult Table 11–6.

Displays: Chalkboards, Bulletin Boards, and Flannel Boards

Display boards can serve several purposes in health education. They can advertise upcoming events such as health fairs, prepared childbirth classes, or exercise sessions. They can inform by presenting health messages such as why car seats are important for children and why washing hands can decrease the transmission of germs. They can also serve as reinforcers of other health education efforts. Display boards are usually inexpensive, easy to construct, and a stimulus to an individual's visual sense.

Display boards should not be crammed with information. Rather, they should convey one idea or theme. The layout of pictures and lettering should draw attention to the most important element of the display. If the elements of the presentation need to be viewed or read in a given order, arrows or numbers can be used to help the viewer to properly progress through the display.

Pictures and lettering should be large enough to be easily discernible by the intended audience at a distance of 4 feet for small groups and at distances of 8 to 12 feet if the display will be used for a large class. To increase the legibility of the display, you can use high-contrast backgrounds and lettering as well as ample spacing between lines of print.

Although displays can be used as one form of information delivery, they are not universally helpful. Displays should not be the medium of choice when a great deal of information needs to be presented, when the learning involves psychomotor skills, or when several movements need to be shown, such as how to clean a wound. Flip charts can show movement in sequenced pictures, but the pictures must not leave out any part of the sequence. Learners may not be able to mentally construct a sequence of movements from A to C if B is not provided (Booher, 1975; Brown, 1989).

Graphics

Graphics consist of the nonlanguage elements of print such as graphs, flow charts, line drawings, and illustrations. The use of graphics in health education can add variety, condense facts and figures, show relationships, and draw attention to specific aspects of a presentation. For example, pictures are better than words when concrete concepts are involved, whereas words are better when dealing with abstract concepts (Booher, 1975; Felker, 1980). Although a picture can be "worth a thousand words," simple line drawings can be just as effective as actual pictures for learning when illustrating, for example, anatomy or machinery (Borg & Schuler, 1979; Dwyer, 1972). When depicting settings like the operating room, actual pictures may best provide the full scope of the information you wish to convey. Research has found that pictures can stimulate interest and help readers to comprehend and remember content (Brown et al., 1973).

Graphics can aid health educators to stimulate interest and promote learning but to do this they must be chosen carefully. Individuals who have low educational levels may not learn well from a graph but will get the concept quickly from a picture. Graphics may not be useful for persons with poor vision.

Overhead Transparencies and Slides

Overhead transparencies and slides can be used to augment an oral presentation. These teaching aids have many of the advantages of displays and graphics. They are easy to develop, of low cost, and add a visual dimension to the presentation. Transparencies can readily be made by hand, by thermofax, or by a photocopy machine. Transparencies and slides can also be easily up-dated or rearranged. In addition, they are easily stored and transported.

Overhead transparencies and slides should be clear and convey one idea or theme in each. Pictures and lettering should be easily readable. The background and subject matter (pictures, lettering, etc.) should have a high contrast. When preparing transparencies and slides, color can be used to attract attention, produce psychological effects, facilitate retention, and create an atmosphere (Turnbull & Baird, 1975). Primary colors (red, blue, and yellow) have been found to appeal strongly to children, secondary colors and light colors appeal to adults. In addition, warm colors (red, yellow, and orange) are more eye-catching than cool colors (violet, blue, and dark green) (Broekuizen, 1973). Color can also facilitate recall; for example, "Remember the red vessels—what were they called?"

Transparencies and slides can help get your message across, but they do take time to prepare and proper equipment must be available to use them (Cooper, 1990). Also, these teaching aids may not be appropriate for the vision impaired.

Audio and Audiovisual Materials

Audio and audiovisual materials include cassette tapes, films, and videocassettes. Cassette tapes can be used to present basic information, reinforce instructions, and as a step-by-step guide. Audiocassettes are especially beneficial for individuals who are vision impaired. These cassettes can also be used with programmed instructional workbooks. Audiocassettes are commercially available and can be easily and economically made. They are easy to transport and store and only require a tape recorder for their use. Individuals can use audiocassettes at home, for example, for practicing biofeedback and stress reduction techniques. Audiocassettes are the most valuable teaching aid for vision-impaired learners and for those individuals who have poor information-recall abilities.

Films and filmstrips are becoming more common as teaching aids in health education. This medium can depict real-life drama, promote cognitive learning, and encourage attitude change. Films are especially helpful when teaching psychomotor skills and are useful for the hearing-impaired individual (provided they are closed captioned) and for the illiterate individual (Boyd, 1983).

Filmstrips are relatively inexpensive but 16-mm films can cost several hundred dollars. The equipment necessary for using filmstrips is relatively inexpensive compared to movie projectors. Another drawback for these media is that they are often quickly outdated. Before using a commercially prepared filmstrip or film, it must be previewed for accuracy and appropriateness. Chapter 16 lists several sources for audio and audiovisual materials.

Video and Television

The use of videocassette players and television in health education has grown in recent years. Many clinics and hospitals use videocassette players and television to present a wide range of health information. Closed Circuit Television (CCTV) systems are a common teaching aid. Videocassettes and CCTV can present facts, promote attitude change, and demonstrate psychomotor skills. For example, a video player can be brought to a patient's bedside to present routine pre- and postoperative care. The same information might be presented by CCTV to individual patients or to groups (Burge et al., 1982). Health programming through CCTV may be continuous or it may be requested by patients or a health-care provider.

Programs for video players and CCTV can be made, providing you have the proper equipment, or they can be obtained commercially. Commercial programs must be closely previewed for accuracy and appropriateness. These teaching aids are especially helpful for the illiterate learner or those who have short attention spans.

COMPUTER-ASSISTED INSTRUCTION

Computer-assisted instruction (CAI) is perhaps the newest educational strategy available to health teachers. There is clear evidence that CAI can promote learning (Armstrong, 1989; Bell, 1986; Hulse, 1990; Heermann, 1988). CAI has been in limited use since the 1980s in patient education; because of the newness of the technology, cost, and unavailability, its use was not wide spread. In recent years, the availability of personal computers has increased, the cost has decreased, and the availability of patient education-oriented software has increased leading to a wider use of CAI for health teaching. Software programs are now available, for example, for general health assessments, nutrition, pregnancy, cardiovascular disease, surgery, diabetes, and arthritis self-care.

CAI offers many advantages in health teaching for both the learner and the teacher. For the learner, CAI is self-paced allowing the learner to move at his or her own speed. The computer is not impatient nor does it have time constraints. It will progress through content as quickly or as slowly as the learner dictates and reviews of material can be done as frequently as necessary to master the content. In addition, before the learner can move through the program, mastery must occur. CAI offers privacy for learning. There is no pressure to perform for the teacher, no peer pressure, and mistakes are a private matter. The computer-assisted learner must participate to move through the program. Feedback for learning is immediate and individualized with computer instruction. CAI is a new and novel way of presenting health content and many patients find it entertaining and fun. Finally, CAI helps promote independence and self-responsibility in learning.

Teacher-oriented advantages in using CAI include time efficiency allowing the nurse teacher more time to spend with teaching tasks such as psychomotor skills. The teaching content is consistent for all learners, nothing is changed or left out from learner to learner. Well-designed CAI uses up-to-date educational strategies and technology to best promote learning. CAI also helps document learner progress and helps evaluate how well they have learned. Special learners such as the hearing impaired, those with expressive or receptive aphasia, or those with learning disabilities may respond better to CAI than to more traditional methods.

Although CAI offers a new avenue to providing health content, it does have disadvantages and must be evaluated for its usefulness. At this point in time, perhaps the biggest disadvantage is the cost. Depending on the type of computer, printer, and software, one unit can cost $3,500.00 or more. Obviously, one unit would not be sufficient to meet the health-teaching needs of most settings and many institutions may not have the budget necessary to adequately provide CAI. Likewise, more than one software package would be needed. Even if someone in the health-care setting had the skills to develop software, it can take up to 500 hours of development time to produce 1 hour of instructional material. Although there has been an increase in software programs being developed for health teaching, there still are relatively few and those available may not be suitable to meet all learning objectives or for many patient populations. CAI is best used to promote learning in the cognitive domain. At present, software programs are limited in their usefulness to promote change in the affective domain. Most programs require literacy for use. In addition, computers "scare" many people—the computer illiterate, those with impaired literacy, and many of the elderly. Another disadvantage of CAI is that a computer is impersonal, lacks compassion, and cannot provide the human touch, which can be a facilitator to learning. The computer may not be suitable to poorly motivated or nondirectional learners.

In addition to cognitive concerns, the nurse must consider physical limitations of learners that can preclude the use of CAI. Use of a computer key pad may be difficult for learners with arthritis, Parkinson's disease, or partial paralysis. Key pads have multiple keys that are small and closely spaced; in addition, many of the keys are not used and can prove to be distracting and confusing. In the future, simplified keyboards with larger keys may eliminate this problem. Learners with impaired vision may find the use of CAI difficult. Many learners in tertiary care centers may not be able to take advantage of the CAI because pain, symptoms, and general fatigue make it difficult for them to sit for long periods of time in front of a computer screen.

CAI, as with other instructional methods, must not replace one-to-one interactions with health-care providers but rather serve as an adjunct to personal interactions. The use of CAI can be appropriate after a thorough assessment, which indicates that the learner can benefit from using the software program and that the CAI is appropriate to meet the learner's needs and abilities. CAI can be used to provide basic information, to augment, and to reinforce oral health teaching.

Three-Dimensional Teaching Aids

Three-dimensional teaching aids such as equipment, models, or displays can help learners grasp abstract thoughts more quickly and provide them with an opportunity to use all their senses—sight, smell, touch, taste, and hearing. The use of actual equipment is essential when teaching psychomotor skills, such as injections, wound care, or blood glucose monitoring. Learners must have the opportunity to handle, examine, and try out equipment before they use it in self-care activities.

Models help to provide the third dimension when the real object is not, or cannot be available. Models are especially useful when the nurse is teaching anatomy, physiology, the birth process, or cardiopulmonary resuscitation, for example. Frequently used models include hearts, breasts, testicles, and stomas as well as resuscitation dolls. Many models can be obtained free from medical equipment and pharmaceutical companies. Models can also be purchased from commercial vendors, and the prices vary greatly. Many nurses use their ingenuity and creativity to develop models. For example, one nurse knitted a large balloon-shaped stocking and used it with a doll to illustrate the birth process. Models need not be elaborate to get the point or concept across.

Displays are particularly helpful when several pieces of equipment must be used or when choices or alternatives are available. Displays can be used to help individuals who want to lose weight or who are on a diabetic diet to choose appropriate foods. For example, one nurse cut out pictures of a variety of foods from magazines and laid them on a table. She then gave each patient a paper plate and told them to go through the "paper buffet" and choose a well-balanced dinner, low in salt and cholesterol. After selecting their dinner, the patients evaluated each other's choices and shared their reasons for their choices.

Games, Simulations, and Demonstrations

Games, simulations, and demonstrations can stimulate interest, increase involvement in learning, offer the opportunity to put knowledge into practice, and rehearse problem solving and psychomotor skills (Davidhizar, 1982; Lewis et al., 1989). These teaching aids and methods promote better retention of information and add variety to learning. Games can be bought or they can be developed. Flash cards or pictures can be made, existing games like Bingo, checkers, or card games can be modified, or crossword puzzles can be developed.

Before developing a game, the nurse should be sure that it will help the learner meet certain behavioral objectives and that the learner has sufficient ability and background information to play the game (Walts, 1982; Cooper, 1989). A game that is too easy or overused can dampen interest and lead to boredom. A game that is too difficult for the learner can cause frustration and avoidance of the learning situation.

Games are especially useful when teaching children. Children often use games in school as a learning tool and respond well to the format and challenge. For example, a pediatric nurse developed a card game about cast care. The game could be used in one-to-one teaching or for groups. For each correct response to a question about cast care each child received a token. The accumulated tokens could then be used to purchase small toys, comic books, or stationery from the hospital gift shop.

Simulations and demonstrations are essential teaching techniques for promoting problem solving and psychomotor skills. Simulations can present a potentially threatening situation in a nonthreatening way. An example would be developing an angina attack scenario for a group of patients who have cardiovascular disease, then helping them discuss what causes angina, the signs and symptoms, and how they should handle the problem. Another example of simulations frequently used in health education involves pregnant women who practice prepared childbirth techniques.

Role playing can also serve as a method for developing psychomotor and affective skills. Family members can, for example, try on the role of the wheel chair bound or bedridden or try to experience the environment from the perspective of the hearing or vision impaired. Role playing can help family members develop greater empathy and understanding.

Demonstrations and return demonstrations provide a concrete, realistic learning experience. Demonstrations as compared to simulations involve using actual equipment. Demonstrations should reproduce the real situation as closely as possible (Cooper, 1982). Common examples of the use of demonstrations include crutch walking and cardiopulmonary resuscitation.

When you decide to use the demonstration as a teaching technique it is important to plan on plenty of time. Doing takes longer than telling. The learner must be prepared ahead of time about what to expect and what he or she will be required to do. Provide encouragement and coaching for the learner, especially the first few times that the skill is done. Also, plan to have an evaluation or closure session following the learner's practice sessions to provide immediate feedback.

SUMMARY

In this chapter, the implementation tools for health teaching have been presented. It is important that the nurse use several methods, if possible, with each learner to better facilitate learning. Educational, behavioral, and instructional strategies provide the nurse with a large repertoire of tools to choose from in her efforts to assist the learner in mastering teaching content. It is important to keep in mind that teaching strategies are chosen after individual assessment of the learner and must match the learner's abilities, the content to be taught, and the time and materials available to the teacher.

REFERENCES AND READINGS

Armstrong, M. L. Orchestrating the process of patient education: Methods and approaches. *Nursing Clinics of North America*, 1989, *24*(3):597–604.

Ausubel, D. *The psychology of meaningful verbal learning: An introduction to school learning*. New York: Grune & Stratton, 1963.

Bell, J. A. The role of microcomputers in patient education. *Computers in Nursing*, 1986, *4*(6):255–257.

Berg, A., & Hammitt, K. B. Assessing the psychiatric patient's ability to meet the literacy demands of hospitalization. *Hospital and Community Psychiatry*, 1980, *31*, 266–268.

Bigelow, G., Stickler, D., Leisbon, I., & Griffiths, R. Maintaining disulfiram ingestion among outpatient alcoholics: A security-deposit contingency contracting procedure. *Behavioral Research and Therapy*, 1976, *14*, 378–381.

Bille, D. A. A study of patients' knowledge in relation to teaching format and compliance. *Supervisor Nurse*, 1977, *8*, 55–62.

Bloom, B. S. (Ed.). *Taxonomy of educational objectives: The classification of educational goals. Handbook I: Cognitive Domain*. New York: D. McKay, 1956.

Booher, H. Relative comprehensibility of pictorial information and printed words in procedural instructions. *Human Factors*, 1975, *17*, 266–277.

Borg, W., & Schuler, C. Detail and background in audiovisual lessons and their effect on learners. *Educational Communication and Technology*, 1979, *27*, 31–38.

Bormuth, J. Reading literacy: Its definition and assessment. *Reading Research Quarterly*, 1973, *9*, 7–66.

Boyd, M. D. How to write a teaching aid that patients will actually read. *RN*, October 1981, 90, 94.

————. Patient education literature: A comparison of reading levels and the reading abilities of patients. *Advances in Health Education: Current Research*, 1988, Vol. I., 101–110.

————. An emergency room teacher's guide. *Nursing Management*, February 1983, 65–67.

————, & Brunner, C. Reading levels of systemic lupus erythematosus literature. *Arthritis and Rheumatism*, 1982, *25*, 82. (Abstract)

————, & Citro, K. Cardiac patient education literature: Can patients read what we give them? *Journal of Cardiac Rehabilitation*, 1983, *3*, 513–516.

————, & Feldman, R. H. L. Information seeking and reading and comprehension abilities of cardiac patients. *Journal of Cardiac Rehabilitation*, 1984, *4*, 343–347.

_____, & Hollander, R. B. Patient education: A study of registered nurse's attitudes, time spent teaching and their administrative support. *Advances in Health Education: Current Research,* 1988, Vol. I., 91–100.

_____, & Wienrich, S. P. The literacy impaired older adult: Assessment strategies for effective teaching. (Unpublished manuscript, 1991)

Broekuizen, R. T. *Graphic communication.* Ft. Lauderdale, Fla.: McKnight Publications, 1973.

Brown, J. W., Lewis, R. N., & Harcleroad, F. F. *AV instruction: Technology, media and methods* (4th ed.). New York: McGraw-Hill, 1973.

Brown, S. How to create patient education tools. *RN,* 1989, *52*(2):77–78.

Burge, S., Boyd, M. D., & Rudoff, L. *Getting ready for surgery.* Alexandria, Va.: Medvision, 1982.

Cahill, M. (Ed.). *Nurse reference library: Patient teaching.* Springhouse, Pa.: Springhouse Corp., 1987.

Cline, R. T. Interpersonal communication skills for enhancing physician–patient relationship. *Maryland State Medical Journal,* 1983, *32*(4):272–278.

Coleman, J. S., Walker, T. S., & Barkership, L. E. The Hopkins games program: Conclusions from seven years of research. *Educational Researcher,* 1973, *2*(8),3–7.

Cooper, S. S. Methods of teaching revisited—the demonstration. *Journal of Continuing Education in Nursing,* 1982, *13*(3),44–45.

_____. Teaching tips: Creative teaching strategies. *The Journal of Continuing Education in Nursing,* 1989, *20*(2):95–97.

_____. Teaching tips. One more time: The overhead projector. *The Journal of Continuing Education in Nursing,* 1990, *21*(3):141–142.

Cosper, B. How well do patients understand hospital jargon? *American Journal of Nursing,* 1932–1934, 1977.

Dale, E., & Chall, J. S. A formula for predicting readability. *Educational Research Bulletin,* January 21, 1948, 11–20, 37–54.

Davidhizar, R. E. Simulation games as a teaching technique in psychiatric nursing. *Perspectives in Psychiatric Care,* January–March 1982, *20*(1):8–12.

Dinoff, M., Rickard, N. C., & Colwich, J. Weight reduction through successive contracts. *American Journal of Orthopsychiatry,* 1972, *42*, 110–113.

Doak, C. C., Doak, L. G., & Root, J. H. *Teaching patients with low literacy skills.* Philadelphia: J. B. Lippincott Co., 1985.

Doak, L. G., & Doak, C. C. Patient comprehension profiles: Recent findings and strategies. *Patient Counseling and Health Education,* 1980, *2*, 101–106.

Dunbar, J. M., Marshall, G. D., & Hovell, M. F. Behavioral strategies for improving compliance. In R. B. Haynes, D. W. Taylor, & D. L. Sackett (Eds.), *Compliance in health care.* Baltimore: Johns Hopkins University Press, 1979.

Dwyer, F. *A guide for improving visualized instruction.* State College, Pa.: State College Learning Services, 1972.

Felker, D. (Ed.). *Document design: A review of the relevant research.* Washington, D.C.: Carnegie Mellon University and Siegal & Gale for the American Institutes of Research, 1980.

Fitzpatrick, J. J., Taunton, R. L., & Benoliel (Eds.). Annual Review of Nursing Research, Vol. 6, 1988.

Flesh, R. F. A new readability yardstick. *Journal of Applied Psychology,* 1948, *32*, 221–233.

Fry, E. A. A readability formula that saves time. *Journal of Reading,* 1968, *2*(7):513–516.

Frantz, R. A. Selecting media for patient education. *Topics in Clinical Nursing*, July 2, 1980, *2*, 77–85.

George, G. If patient teaching tries your patience, try this plan. *Nursing '82*, May 1982, 50–55.

Green, L. Educational strategies to improving compliance. In R. B. Haynes, D. W. Taylor, & D. L. Sackett (Eds.), *Compliance in health care*. Baltimore: Johns Hopkins University Press, 1979.

Hallburg, J. C. Teaching patients self-care. *Nursing Clinics of North America*, 1970, *5*, 223–231.

Haynes, R. B., Sackett, D. L., Gibson, E. S., et al. Improvement of medication compliance in uncontrolled hypertension. *Lancet*, 1976, *1*, 1265–1268.

Heermann, B. *Teaching and learning with computers*. San Francisco: Jossey Bass, 1988.

Hulse, S. F. Is computer-assisted instruction for you? *Radiation Therapy*, 1990, *61*(3):227–229.

Joyce, C., Joyce, L., Ellis, K. C. et al. Quantitative study of doctor–patient communication. *Quarterly Journal of Medicine*, 1969, *38*, 183–194.

Klausmeier, H. J., & Ripple, R. D. *Learning and human abilities: Educational psychology* (4th ed.). New York: Harper & Row Pub., 1975.

Knowles, M. S. *The modern practice of adult education*. New York: Associated Press, 1970.

Larsen, K. M., & Smith, C. K. Assessment of nonverbal communication in the patient–physician interview. *Journal of Family Practice*, 1981, *12*(3):481–488.

Lewis, D. J., Saydak, S. J., Mierzwa, I. P., & Robinson, J. A. Gaming: A teaching strategy for adult learners. *The Journal of Continuing Education in Nursing*, 1989, *20*(2):80–84.

Ley, P., & Spelman, M. S. *Communicating with the patient*. London: Staples Press, 1967.

Ley, P. Primary rated importance and recall of medical statements. *Journal of Health and Social Behavior*, 1972, *13*, 311–317.

_____. The measurement of comprehensibility. *Journal of the Institute for Health Education*, 1973, *11*, 17–20.

_____. The use of techniques and findings from social and experimental psychology to improve doctor–patient communications. In *Health Education and Primary Care: Conference Report* (pp. 14–35). Leeds Department of Community Medicine and Leeds Polytechnic. Leeds, England, 1975.

_____. Towards better doctor–patient communications: Contributions from social and experimental psychology. In A. E. Bennett (Ed.), *Communications between doctors and patients*. London: Oxford University Press, 1976, pp. 75–98.

_____, Bradshaw, P. W., Eaves, D., & Walker, C. M. A method for increasing recall of information presented by doctors. *Psychological Medicine*, 1973, *3*, 217–220.

Lindeman, C. A. Patient education. In Fitzpatrick, J. J., Taunton, R. L., & Benoliel, J. Q. (Ed.). *Annual Review of Nursing Research*, Vol. 6. New York: Springer Pub. Co., 1988.

MacMillan, P. Teaching and learning, insight and growth. *Nursing Times*, August 26, 1981, 1513–1514.

Mager, R. F. *Preparing instructional objectives*. Belmont, Calif.: Fearson Publishers, 1975.

Mahoney, M. J., & Thoresen, C. E. *Self-control: Power to person*. Monterey, Calif.: Brooks-Cole, 1974.

Maletzky, B. M. Behavior recording as treatment: A brief note. *Behavioral Therapy*, 1974, *5*, 107–111.

Maslow, A. *Motivation and personality*. New York: Harper & Row Pub., 1970.

McLaughlin, G. H. SMOG grading—a new readability formula. *Journal of Reading*, 1969, *12*, 639–646.

Mehrabian, A. *Nonverbal communication.* New York: Aldine-Atherton, 1972.

Meade, C. D., & Smith, C. F. Readability formulas: Caution and criteria. *Patient Education and Counseling*, 1991, *17*(1):153–158.

Michielutte, R., Bahnson, J., & Beal, P. Readability of the public education literature on cancer prevention and detection. *Journal of Cancer Education*, 1990, *5*(1):55–61.

Nelson, R. O., Lipinski, D. P., & Black, J. L. The relative reactivity of external observations and self-monitoring. *Behavioral Therapy*, 1976, *7*, 314–321.

Northcutt, N. *Adult performance study.* Austin, Tex.; Division of Extension, University of Texas at Austin, 1975.

Padberg, R. M., & Padberg, L. F. Strengthening the effectiveness of patient education: Applying principles of adult education. *Oncology Nursing Forum*, 1990, *17*(1):65–69.

Redman, B. K. *The process of patient teaching in nursing* (4th ed.). St. Louis: C. V. Mosby, 1980.

———. *The process of patient teaching*, 6th ed. Chicago: C. V. Mosby Co., 1988.

Roter, D. L., Hall, J. A., & Katz, N. R. Patient–physician communication: A descriptive summary of the literature. *Patient Education and Counseling*, 1988, *13*, 99–119.

Sharpe, T. R., & Mikeal, R. L. Patient compliance with antibiotic regimens. *American Journal of Hospital Pharmacy*, 1974, *31*, 479–484.

Steckel, S. B., & Swain, M. A. Contracting with patients to improve compliance. *Journal of the American Hospital Association*, 1977, *51*, 81–84.

Strauss, A. L., & Glaser, B. *Chronic illness and the quality of life.* St. Louis: C. V. Mosby, 1975.

Taylor, A. G., Skelton, J. A., & Czajkowski, R. W. Do patients understand education brochures? *Nursing and Health Care*, 1982, *6*, 305–310.

Thrush, R. S., & Lanese, R. R. The use of printed materials in diabetes education. *Diabetes*, 1962, *11*, 132–137.

Turnbull, A. T., & Baird, R. N. *The graphics of communication* (3rd ed.). New York: Holt, Rinehart and Winston, 1975.

U.S. Department of Health and Human Services. Pretesting in health communication methods: Examples and resources for improving health messages and materials. Bethesda, Md.: National Cancer Institute, NIH Pub. No. 83-1493, 1982.

Walts, N. S. Games and simulations. *Nursing Management*, 1982, *13*(2):28–29.

Weinrich, S. P., & Boyd, M. D. Teaching tools for the elderly: Evaluating for success. *Journal of Gerontological Nursing*, 1992, *18*(1):15–20.

Weintraub, W. *Verbal behavior: Adaptation and psychopathology.* New York: Springer-Verlag, 1983.

Weisman, C. S., & Teitelbaum, M. A. Women and health care communication. *Patient Education and Counseling*, 1989, *13*, 183–199.

12

Age-Related Factors Influencing Selection of Teaching Strategies

Nancy I. Whitman

A variety of teaching–learning strategies exists. These include stimuli based upon verbal communication, such as lectures, discussions, books, and audiotaped lessons; those based upon visual experiences, such as demonstrations, models, and pictures; and other that combine visual and verbal experiences, such as illustrated pamphlets, television, and slide-tapes. Timing, pacing and sequencing of content, practicing exercises, and reinforcement techniques are also important strategic considerations. It is up to the nurse–teacher, sometimes in conjunction with the learner and sometimes independently, to select the strategies that will best facilitate learning. An important factor to consider when individualizing strategies for each lesson is the development level of the learner.

Three general areas related to development are important considerations when choosing teaching–learning strategies. These include physical maturation and abilities, psychosocial development, and cognitive capacity. One of these areas may become more important than the others under certain circumstances or because of the nature of the content being taught. When the content relates to technical skills or manipulation of equipment, assessment of physical maturation will provide essential information for planning an approach to the psychomotor learning. It will help identify factors related to the amount of practice and supervision that will be needed to master the skill. Identification of physical impairment predetermines strategies that compensate for or are independent of the impairment. Psychosocial developmental assessment provides information about interpersonal factors. Determining the efficacy of group or individual instruction, the support systems that are available to reinforce learning, and life-stage-related motivational factors is helpful. Cognitive ability, including knowledge base about the topic under consideration, is an important determinant of the level for beginning the lesson, of pacing, and of the amount of repetition needed. This also helps to determine whether active participation, visual, verbal or visual–verbal learning experiences would be most useful.

Chapter 8 addressed assessment of developmental characteristics of learners. This chapter focuses on determining strategies for individuals based on the developmental assessment. General considerations will be introduced first and then specific implications for teaching children, adults, and the aged will be discussed.

CHOOSING MEDIA AND METHODS

Selection of teaching–learning strategies is based upon the content area being taught and the developmental level of the learner. The availability of teaching media and materials often influences the selection process as well. Developmental factors must be considered even when choosing from a limited supply of materials.

Content Area

The type of content to be mastered—cognitive, attitudinal, or psychomotor—must be determined as a prerequisite to considering teaching method alternatives. Although a variety of strategies may be employed for cognitive content (for example, learning the signs, symptoms, prevention, and treatment of hypoglycemia), a more limited list is available for psychomotor skill acquisition (learning to give an insulin injection) and attitudinal learning (acceptance of adherence to a diabetic regimen as important for health). Table 12–1 provides a list of often-used methods to stimulate learning. These were discussed in detail in the preceding chapter.

Typically, verbal, visual, and visual–verbal methods are used for cognitive content, although problem solving, role playing, games, and simulations may be used very successfully for higher level mastery. For example, once knowledge about diabetic management is mastered, role playing of the various situations commonly encountered by the diabetic facilitates mastering application of this knowledge. Field trips, games, and simulations may also be used to promote discovery learning.

Psychomotor learning usually necessitates an initial exposure to the skill components and an opportunity to perform the skill under supervision so that feedback can be obtained. Visual–verbal strategies such as pictures, posters, television, and narrated demonstrations thus work best in introducing the components of the skill;

TABLE 12–1. STIMULI TO FACILITATE LEARNING

Verbal	Spoken: Lecture, audiotape, discussion Written: Lists, books, pamphlets, posters
Visual–Verbal	Pictures, posters, diagrams, identified body outlines, TV, slide-tape, narrated demonstration
Visual	Pictures, posters, models, puppets, body outlines, slides
Active Participation	Return demonstration, role play, games and simulations, problem-solving exercises, field trips

a subsequent return demonstration with actual or simulated equipment facilitates mastery.

Attitudinal changes are the most difficult and usually are made slowly. Although there is still controversy about what strategies actually work best, many indicate that active participant experiences best promote attitude developments.

Developmental Implications for Lesson Planning

In planning health teaching, a variety of lesson components must be adapted to optimize the learning of individuals of different developmental levels. A list of these can be found in Table 12–2, and general implications of each will be described below. Specifics for each age group may be found in the discussion of the age groups which follow.

One of the first factors to enter into the planning of teaching–learning strategies is consideration of the amount of involvement that the learner should have in the planning. Although individuals will respond differently, generally speaking, adolescents and adults should be given the opportunity to assist in planning the approach to learning. The cognitive and experiential abilities and self-esteem needs of these older learners promotes active participation in planning. The participation also enhances the potential efficacy of the teaching–learning.

The location of a lesson, timing, number of sessions, pacing, and sequencing will vary significantly for learners of differing developmental levels. All learning is optimized when the environment is a secure one. For the adult, security may be developed in an unfamiliar learning environment through interpersonal interactions with the teacher and other learners. Security is not easily established for a child; thus, when possible, teaching–learning interactions should occur in an environment that the child already perceives as safe and secure. The home or familiar school room is the optimum, but it is usually not the place children are commonly seen by health-care providers. When other environments are to be used, they should be adapted for the age of the children who will be using them. Child-sized furniture and reachable places are helpful to keep a room from overwhelming the child. When selecting a teaching–learning environment in a health-care setting, it is imperative to select one that is not associated with painful procedures and, hence, anxiety provoking. (Refer to Chapter 5 for further discussion of the environment.)

When selecting lesson locations, consideration of individual versus group setting may be an alternative. Traditionally, most nurse teaching has been on a one-to-

---

TABLE 12–2. LESSON COMPONENTS TO VARY FOR LEARNERS OF DIFFERENT DEVELOPMENTAL AGES

Learner Participation in Lesson Planning

Lesson Structure: Location, group vs. individual, timing, number of sessions, pacing, sequencing

Content Considerations: Language level, stimuli: visual, visual–verbal, verbal, active participation

Enhancement of Learning: Practice, reinforcement

one basis. Currently, group teaching–learning interactions are being used to assist individuals with common health-care needs. Antepartal classes and cardiac life style change for risk reduction are two types of health content that commonly use a group setting. Although individual considerations are important in determining how effective a group setting might be, developmental factors also play a role. The key factors that can influence the effect of groups from a developmental standpoint are distraction and support. Distraction from the group may adversely affect younger learners—toddlers, preschoolers, and even some young school-age children. Older adults also may find other group members' activities and questions an impediment to their learning. Group support can, however, be a positive factor. This is true for those age groups that can profit from others' ideas and reactions—older school-aged children through adults.

The timing of a lesson also varies according to the developmental level of the learner. Whether the learning is to be short term or long term is also important. Short-term learning lasts temporarily, for example, only for the length of an event such as a diagnostic test. Long-term learning involves a lasting behavior change. For short-term learning, young learners and learners with short-term memory loss (as occurs with some aged individuals) need lessons that are timed to occur relatively close to the event involved. For example, if the nurse is preparing a preschooler for an x-ray procedure, the lesson about the procedure is best taught no earlier than several days prior to the procedure. This timing allows the preschooler to harness coping capacity but limits the time for fantasizing about the event. There is also sufficient time to reinforce learning and to clarify misconceptions. Older children and adults, on the other hand, have broader coping experiences and can use time between the teaching session and a procedure to invoke these as needed. Their more developed cognitive processes also help in distinguishing reality from imagination. When considering long-term behavior changes, the timing for beginning the teaching in relation to the event becomes important for ensuring that adequate coping has begun. Because the behavior change involved will need to be practiced for a long time after the initial learning, the change to be made and the causative factor, illness or trauma, must be accepted before effective learning begins. Because adolescents and adults are able to see future implications of events, coping often takes longer and hence teaching may need to be delayed.

The total number of sessions and sequencing of each lesson is dependent on the amount and type of content within the lesson. The length of sessions can be determined by the attention span of the learner, and the number of sessions tentatively determined by dividing single lesson time into the time estimated for total content. Variations will occur according to learning abilities. Sequencing of information is usually done from general to specific and from easier to more complex material. This can be done with learners of all developmental levels. Experiential learning involves acting, understanding the particular act, and then generalizing so that the action can be repeated in new circumstances. In order for this type of learning sequence to be effective, action and consequences must be recognized as related, and cause and effect must be understood. Experiential learning is not cognitively understood much before the age of 7 or 8. Experiential learning may be used for younger children to develop habit formation, that is, acts habitually formed but not necessarily understood.

The last lesson component to be considered is pacing. For the younger learner and the aged learner, pacing must usually be slower to allow time for cognitive processing. The nurse–teacher needs to observe any learner closely to determine if progress through the lesson is occurring at an appropriate rate for the learner.

Choosing the level and language of the stimuli is crucial for optimizing learning and is extremely dependent on the developmental level of the learner. Thorough assessment will help determine what scientific terminology is known to the learner. Younger clients and those with decreased cognitive abilities need simple, concrete words. The school-age child has a basic understanding of body parts and functions, so more scientific terms may be taught and used. A variety of stimuli may be used as a part of the learning experience. Active participation is best for younger individuals or those with decreased cognitive abilities. This can be accomplished through experiences using real or simulated materials. Cognitive abilities are normally incremental with age and, therefore, realistic visual and concrete verbal stimuli can be incorporated into the learning experience of older children. For types of experiences involving the higher level of cognitive abilities verbal stimuli can be used. Refer to Table 12–1 for examples of stimuli in each category mentioned above.

When the nurse is selecting learning experiences, it is wise to choose the simplest stimuli that will be effective, but use whatever visual, visual-verbal, or verbal stimuli that can be understood by the learner. A variety of stimuli can be used to facilitate learning. Indeed, it is suggested that using several different stimuli is beneficial to learning.

Exposing the learner to content is not enough to ensure learning. Practice and reinforcement are both essential. The developmental level of the learner can help predict the amount and type of practice needed. Younger children or older adults learning psychomotor tasks typically need more practice time to master skills. The lack of the development of fine motor coordination on the part of the younger child and the loss of some coordination in addition to visual changes in the elderly account for this. Adaptations in practicing cognitive content are also necessary for the same age groups.

All learners need reinforcement for learning. This may be internal (self-identified) or external (outside or other-identified). Young children usually require more immediate and external reinforcement in the form of visible symbols and parental approval. As children develop in the older school-age and adolescent years, other significant people play a part in their lives. These respected individuals, for example, teachers, ministers, and peers, can be helpful reinforcers for learning. Adults make much more use of internally motivated reinforcement. Since most learning is problem centered, satisfaction in finding solutions to handle or alleviate the initial problem is reinforcing in itself.

In the discussion above, a number of lesson components which must be adapted for different developmental levels were described. The remainder of this chapter presents detailed information about teaching–learning strategies for different developmental ages.

INFANT AND TODDLER

Implications for Health Learning

Participation in planning health teaching for the infant and toddler involves the parents, rather than the child learner. In addition, although the infant has a great capacity for learning, most of this learning is not health related. Thus, guidelines which follow are for the toddler. Since separation causes so much anxiety, parents should be present whenever possible and become involved with their child's learning activities as well. Because of the anxiety often shown with strangers, one nurse–teacher should establish a relationship with child and family, and then consistently be involved in teaching–learning activities with the child. Growth and developmental theory indicates that teaching–learning activities for this age group should involve active participation. Strategies that promote use of gross motor abilities and sensory and tactile experiences work very well. Reading stories and getting the child's response as well as using pictures, dolls, and puppets can stimulate learning. Any approach toward toddlers should include simple terminology and an honest and calm manner. The tone of voice heavily influences the type of attention and response from the child.

Whenever possible, health lessons for this age group should take place in a familiar environment. Wellness health habits can be taught in the home or familiar preschool environment. When a very young child is hospitalized, a safe and secure environment should be selected for teaching–learning sessions. Many institutions designate the child's bed as a safe place and all intrusive and hurtful procedures are done in the treatment room. Other times a "playroom" is identified as a haven from unpleasant hospital procedures. Since children of this age have not developed peer interactional behavior, individual instruction works best.

Because young children have no real sense of time, health teaching must occur in close proximity to the time of any event to which the teaching relates. For example, when preparing a toddler for the arrival of a new sibling, the teaching should begin only a week or two before the new baby is due. Owing to the limited attention span of this young age group, teaching should be done in very short 2- to 5-minute sessions. Several short sessions can be used to accomplish health teaching that necessitates more time. These sessions should also be clustered close enough together that the learning from one session is not forgotten but actually facilitates further learning. Pacing can be determined by observing the child's response and level of attention. If the environment is unfamiliar, anxiety may necessitate slower pacing.

Immature psychomotor skills and limited cognitive abilities necessitate ample practice to achieve learning. Young children respond best to their parents, thus one of the best reinforcers is a smile accompanied by warm encouragement and praise from a parent.

Strategies for Short-Term Learning

Preparing an individual for a procedure is a common nursing responsibility and involves using strategies for promoting short-term learning. For the toddler, this type of teaching should take place immediately prior to the event. As with any age group, it is important to know what the child has been told about the procedure. An explanation of what the child will feel should be presented in simple, concrete nonthreatening terms with associated visual and tactile experiences. Since a major concern is separation, the explanation should include a reassuring statement that accurately describes parental contact during and/or after the procedure. Providing some guidance on how the child can cope is also helpful. Telling the child to "squeeze your hands," "hold the Bandaid," or "cry when it hurts" helps channel the child's responses.

Strategies for Long-Term Learning

By the age of 2 to 3, children are able to stand steadily and manipulate large objects. With the development of these abilities, self-care activities related to hygiene can begin. Children can be taught to manipulate the toothbrush and to use a washcloth and soap. Because toddlers are able to understand simple language, safety rules can be taught as well—"Wait and pet the kitty after she finishes eating." A child of this age can also begin an "exercise program" through modeling of parents and may even be assisted to use mobility as a means for stress control.

Ritual, repetition, and imitation are strategies useful for long-term learning during toddlerhood. Games and skill development strategies are developmentally appropriate. Play is a method children use to learn about and test their thoughts of the world. The nurse–teacher should utilize playful strategies in health teaching for this age group as well.

Parental values of health and knowledge of health behavior will have an impor-

TABLE 12–3. IMPLICATIONS FOR THE TODDLER'S HEALTH LEARNING

Key Developmental Factors	Implications for Health Learning
Physical Maturation	
Motor: Upright mobility grossly coordinated	Able to learn simple activities: Dressing, washing, "exercise," tooth brushing
Hand–eye coordination: Manipulation of large objects	
Cognitive Development	
Sensorimotor (Piaget)	Learns from actual experiences and use
Distractible	of senses
Communication:	Short—2–5 minute—sessions work best
Vocabulary 500–1000 words	Use concrete, nonthreatening terms
Expression mainly through motor channels	relative to sensory experiences
	Approach honestly
Active fantasy life	Able to learn to pick out good "snacks"
Recognizes simple concrete objects	and body parts
Psychosocial Development	
Autonomy vs. shame and doubt (Erikson)	Involve parents and encourage
Separation anxiety	reinforcement of behaviors
Need for parental approval	Incorporate activity during learning or as
Utilizes mobility for coping	part of what is to be learned
Learning occurs largely through social interaction and modeling	Demonstrate, encourage parental modeling

tant influence on the child's health attitudes and behaviors (Pender, 1987). For this reason, it is important to work with parents as well as with children when assisting the toddler to learn self-care health behaviors. The older toddler can learn to perform many healthful self-care skills, such as buckling a car safety restraint or eating raisins instead of chocolate candy, but the reason for the persistence of the behavior in children of this age is initially parental modeling and reinforcement. Table 12–3 provides a summary of the key developmental factors of the toddler and associated implications for health learning.

PRESCHOOL

The preschool child, though still dependent upon the family, is expanding contact with the surrounding world. The child is usually able to interact with the nurse–teacher more comfortably and may participate in planning health teaching–learning sessions. Participation is limited, however, to selecting from between a small number of options (two or three choices). To facilitate the developing initiative of this age group, two choices should be given whenever possible. "Would you rather look at the pictures about the test you will be having or have me show your dolly about the test?" is a choice preschoolers can make. Preschoolers can also help determine when they would like a health-teaching session. When offering choices related to time, the nurse should use routines and daily events with which the child is familiar, "We can do this right after dinner or just before Sesame Street."

Parents continue to provide support for this age group and can be helpful participants in the teaching–learning session. When a preschooler is particularly reluctant to interact with the nurse, the parents may be taught first and then supervised as necessary while they teach the child. Since preschoolers have begun to interact with peers, some group teaching is possible. Group size is an important consideration. When the group becomes too large, actions of some participants may be distracting. Five to eight preschoolers is usually a good group size. If content is at all threatening, one-to-one interaction allows the nurse to assess an individual child's response, fears, and misconceptions more readily.

The use of play, active participation, and sensory experiences work well for this age group (Anderson, 1990). Physical and visual stimuli are better than verbal ones since the language ability of the preschooler is limited. When words are used, neutral, concrete, action-oriented ones should be chosen. The nurse must encourage children to put explanations in their own terms so misconceptions can be recognized and clarified. Fantasies and fears need also to be acknowledged and dealt with. Body outlines may be used since this age group knows external body parts and basically recognizes some internal body parts.

The location for the teaching–learning session, like that for the toddler, should be in an environment which the preschooler perceives as safe and secure. The preschooler is present oriented, so teaching sessions should be closely sequential to activities or events to which the teaching relates. Health-teaching sessions should be comparatively brief (no longer than 15 minutes) and spaced to prevent forgetting.

The nurse must be patient and use a rather slow pace. Material being presented should be related to activities and experiences with which the child is already familiar.

The preschool child may need a number of practice sessions in order to master skills or cognitive information. Through supervision of psychomotor skills and eliciting feedback from the child, the nurse can provide reinforcement, clarify or correct, and determine the need for further practice. Parental praise, approval, and tangible rewards are strong reinforcers for preschoolers. Tangible rewards that work especially well with this age include "badges" and seals or stars for a chart. Rewards should be given immediately upon successful completion of the learning task.

Strategies for Short-Term Learning

When preparing preschoolers for procedures, fear of bodily injury must be kept in mind and minimized. This can be done by showing equipment or replicas and allowing the child to manipulate it whenever practical, by specifying the body parts involved, and by calling attention to the safety of those parts the child often fears will be harmed (genitals are a special object of concern in this age group). Visual aids such as body outlines, dolls, and models are helpful for identifying body parts. Because of the vivid imagination of this age group, it is necessary and important to identify the sensory experiences the child will have and equally important to clarify that nothing else will be experienced. Because the coping mechanisms of this age group are still limited, it also helps to tell the child what he or she can do to help—"Hold very still"—and what you will be doing to help—"I will be there to hold your hand and to help you remember to hold still." A child of this age also needs to be taught the reasons—relative to the child—for procedures, and to understand that these are not a punishment for "bad" behavior or "bad" thoughts. Preschoolers do not understand causation, so information about cause and effect or process will not be understood. When preparing preschoolers for health care experiences, it is important to focus on describing sensations and the sequence of events according to the child's daily experiences (Betz, 1983).

Often in the health-care setting, little time is available before a procedure, and teaching is done only a day or some hours before the event. When preplanning is possible, the nurse–teacher should plan for teaching to begin several days, but not longer than a week, before the scheduled event. This provides time for the preschooler to use available coping mechanisms. It also allows the nurse time to clarify what is being learned and provide reinforcement.

Strategies for Long-Term Learning

Physical maturational skills and cognitive development are sufficient for the preschooler to be able to participate independently in a variety of self-care health behaviors such as dressing, toileting, and washing. Because orientation to time is still rudimentary and knowledge of cause and effect still lacking, preschoolers need reminding about doing these activities. Increasingly broad explorations of the environment necessitate expanding safety knowledge to include information about poisonous plants, actions with strangers, pedestrian safety, and use of public facilities. The preschool child can understand simple explanations of purpose (why) and should be given explanations that include perceptual experiences they have previously encountered. Because of the ability to count, this age group can help with simple skills requiring counting, for example, diabetic urine testing. Although they cannot assume complete responsibility, children on medication regimes can be taught when their pills are due in relation to daily events.

Modeling continues to be an important way the child learns. Although the

TABLE 12–4. IMPLICATIONS FOR THE PRESCHOOLER'S HEALTH LEARNING

Key Developmental Factors	Implications for Health Learning
Physical Maturation	
Motor: Runs easily, beginning ability to balance	Able to be quite independent with basic self-care, still needs reminders
Expands environment	
Well-developed bowel and bladder control	
Hand–eye coordination	
Manipulation of large pencils and crayons still results in a degree of imprecision	
Able to build fairly complicated block structures	
Cognitive Development	
Preoperational (Piaget)	Able to learn safety rules and rationale when explained simply and repeatedly
Communication:	
Vocabulary 1000–2000 words	Able to learn name, address, phone number
Still relies heavily on symbolism and mobility of play	
Vague understanding about bodily functions, interested in conception and childbirth	Learns from actual situations, visual symbols (drawings, dolls, pictures), and sensory experiences
Curious	Use simple, concrete, nonthreatening terms
Reality still not discriminated from fantasy	Elicit feedback through child's terms and play
Egocentric	
Limited attention span	Answer questions honestly and in an accepting manner without embarrassment
Relates time to common events in daily life	
	Focus on the positive in relation to the child
	Brief—15 minutes maximum—learning sessions
	Relate events to known daily habits
Psychosocial Development	
Initiative vs. guilt (Erikson)	Involve parents, remind of the role of parental modeling
Family remains of primary importance although other persons may be significant	Specify any body parts involved and sensory experiences
Imitation of same-sex parent role	
Fear of body injury	

family remains primarily responsible for modeling, the expanded environment of the preschooler brings the child into contact with others, for example, nursery school teachers, church school teachers, and parents of other children. This can be reinforcing as the child practices self-care behaviors in a variety of environments and receives positive feedback. This process facilitates the incorporation of habits.

It is common, though not desirable, when emphasizing self-care responsibilities to this age group, for adults to focus on the negative consequences. For example, the emphasis is on catching a cold after going outside without a coat, rather than the positive one—in this case, the beneficial effects of wearing a coat (Bruhn & Cordova, 1977). In order to incorporate self-care responsibilities, it is important to begin to emphasize the benefits of healthful practices in terms of the child's continuing pleasurable activities. Preschool children with chronic illness may not understand the illness. The nurse can assist the child to recognize body feelings and provide simple explanations of the illness, while reassuring the child that the illness is not caused by the child's actions (Reichenback, 1986). Table 12–4 provides a summary of teaching strategies for the preschooler.

SCHOOL AGE

Implications for Health Learning

Participation in activities is an important factor in the development of the self-image and self-esteem of the school-age child. This developmental need, coupled with increasing cognitive abilities, facilitates this age group's participation in planning for health learning.

A variety of teaching–learning strategies may be used with school-age children. Active investigation is effective in both increasing awareness and in aiding learning retention. Repetition and summarizing are useful methods for reinforcing learning. This age group also responds to modeling, peer group activities, and mass media. School-age children can assume a large responsibility for their own health care. They are able to make decisions based on simple scientific knowledge of cause and effect. Their objectivity and language abilities allow them to make observations about themselves and their health status and to share these. Although parents may provide support for the younger school-age child, older children may not need parental presence during learning sessions. Once a child reaches the age of 9 to 10, it is best to ask his or her preference about parental presence. Groups of mates of the same age become increasingly important and may therefore be useful to facilitate some health learning.

School-age children are used to learning in a school-like environment. There are often simulated classrooms in hospital settings which may be used for health teaching–learning sessions. Although safety and security issues become less important for the school-age child, during hospitalization the unfamiliar environment and discomfort of illness or treatments may cause these issues to be, at least temporarily, important again. The nurse must assess this carefully when choosing the teaching–learning setting. Although lessons can be comparably longer (15 to 30 minutes each) for the school-age child than for those who are younger, it is important to space lessons if a great deal of content will be covered.

It is especially important to listen to the school-age child. Exposure to an ever-expanding world brings the child into contact with a variety of experiences and terms, which may provide helpful foundations for learning or lead to misconceptions and confusion.

An expanded ability to use symbols and language allows school-agers to understand less visible events through diagrams, models, and pictures. They can be assisted to move from the concrete—how to do something—to the more abstract—why it is necessary to do something or the interpretation of results of actions. They still relate events best to their own experiences. A school-age child can deal with scientific and medical jargon, but often has misconceptions that need clarification. Time must be provided for the school-ager to clarify, validate, and expand health knowledge. Privacy is also increasingly important to the school-age child, who responds well to verbal reinforcement. Praise, especially from a respected individual, is very rewarding.

Implications for Short-Term Learning

School-age children need to be prepared for procedures far enough in advance to allow time to cope with the forthcoming event. They can understand the purposes of a procedure as it relates to them, and need to know what is expected, how they will feel, how they will participate, and about how much time a procedure will take. Coloring books and booklets written by other children are well received. Analogies of things with which children are familiar also help them understand ideas; for example, the heart can be likened to a pump, the ureter to a hose. Body outlines and drawings are useful teaching tools. These children are also interested in how equipment works and what it is for, and should be oriented to equipment whenever possible.

Implications for Long-Term Learning

Cognitive development, decision-making skills, and physical dexterity make it possible for school-agers to assume responsibility for their own health actions and to learn to value wellness. Information about body functions, stress control, exercise regimes, nutrition, sex education, basic first aid, environmental awareness, and safety can be introduced.

School-age children with therapeutic treatment regimens can usually assume responsibility for carrying these out with minimal assistance. For example, diabetic children with sufficient hand–eye coordination can be taught to give their own insulin, children with neurogenic bladders can be taught clean catheterization techniques. This age group can also be taught symptoms to report and simple actions to take when symptoms occur. A child this age also needs help in understanding that illness is caused by many factors and is not caused merely by the child's actions.

The school-age child has the capabilities to learn to be an active participant in maintaining well-being as well as preventing illness. Health actions to take, and what ones others can do for health, can be learned. Since attitudes are increasingly

TABLE 12–5. IMPLICATIONS FOR THE SCHOOL-AGE CHILD'S HEALTH LEARNING

Key Developmental Factors	Implications for Health Learning
Physical Maturation Motor: Moves energetically but with increasing grace and balance. Able to participate in skilled sports Hand–eye coordination: Control and timing of motor movements well developed by age 8–9	Can manage simple psychomotor tasks as young school-ager and manipulate more complex equipment such as insulin injections after age 8–9
Cognitive Development Concrete operations (Piaget) Communication: 　Extensive vocabulary Understands cause and effect Attention span expands to allow 2–3 hours work at a time Decision-making skills develop Develops orientation to past, present, and some future time	Able to learn about healthful eating, injury control, sexuality, basic first aid, exercise regimens Learns through language—verbal and some written—using known terms, diagrams, and models Often needs misconceptions clarified Should be given explanations of purpose and role in activity Lessons of 15–30 minutes work well Able to make simple decisions related to own health and illness Needs time to sort out new things
Psychosocial Development Industry vs. inferiority (Erikson) Expanding interaction with peers Competition, compromise, and cooperation develop Increased awareness of sexual self and own uniqueness Fears disability, loss of status, loss of control	Praise is a good reinforcer May learn well in group setting Privacy is important Allow control through some help in planning

influenced by those outside of the family, group activities are often useful strategies for enhancing learning of health behaviors and values. Table 12–5 summarizes implications for teaching–learning based on the development of the school-age child.

ADOLESCENT

Implications for Health Learning

The cognitive abilities of the adolescent allow participation in all phases of health learning, including planning what is to be learned and how. The advanced language capabilities facilitate the use of scientific jargon and rationale, and complex models and diagrams. Written information can also be helpful to the adolescent. These individuals can deal with outcome potentials of health actions or illness and should be given specific and detailed information to do this realistically. As with late school-agers, privacy is an important feature for the adolescent and can greatly influence attentiveness and response to health-learning situations. Because the adolescent relates well to the peer group, learning can be enhanced using group methods, providing the entire group is interested in dealing with the subject matter.

Adolescents may also have misconceptions about health—illness or wellness—that need clarification. Adolescents often react negatively when the self-image is threatened. An easygoing "that's a common thought, but . . ." is a much better approach to aiding the adolescent's learning than an outright contradiction.

Reinforcement for adolescents is provided by recognizing achievement. Peer recognition is especially important.

Implications for Short-Term Learning

Adolescents can be prepared for temporary health events and procedures in the same way adults are. Information on the purpose, general procedure, time involved, sensations experienced, participation necessary, and after effects are all important to emphasize. Because of the adolescent's great concern about peer relationships and body appearance, extra attention should be given to appearance or functional changes that will occur as a result of any procedure, how long the changes will last, and if and how they might affect the adolescent.

TABLE 12–6. IMPLICATIONS FOR THE ADOLESCENT'S HEALTH LEARNING

Key Developmental Factors	Implications for Health Learning
Physical Maturation	
Motor: near adult capacity	Able to learn complex self-care skills
Physical growth spurts may produce temporary clumsiness	Able to manipulate equipment for own medical treatments
Hand–eye coordination: very discrete	
Cognitive Development	
Formal operations (Piaget)	Able to learn about accident prevention,
Communication:	environmental safety, sexuality, and
Interprets language	health problems such as acne, obesity,
Understands satire and nuance	pregnancy, venereal disease, and
Understands complexities	substance abuse
Orientated to past, present, and future	Learns through verbal and written language
	Able to understand complex models and diagrams
	Can understand implications of health state on future outcomes
Psychosocial Development	
Identity vs. identity diffusion (Erikson)	Able to make own decisions related to
Struggles for independence and self-control	health
Group acceptance very important	Allow control through help with planning as much as possible
Compares own appearance and function to an ideal image	Adolescent and parents should be worked with separately
Exploring ideas for future life	Privacy extremely important

Implications for Long-Term Learning

The adolescent can benefit from a variety of teaching–learning strategies and appreciate a wide range of content areas. Topics such as environmental safety, stresses related to career choices, nutritional choices, exercise life styles, abortion, venereal disease, and substance abuse are important to introduce to the adolescent. Health-damaging behaviors, when learned and reinforced in childhood, are later much more difficult to change. Though positive health behaviors can be readily learned by children, the strong influence of societal and peer pressure on adolescents poses a greater barrier to learning health-promoting behaviors (Pender, 1987). This age group should be made aware of and given information about self-care behaviors. In addition, the adolescent should be challenged to evaluate the philosophy about the values related to these.

Adolescents have the ability to make their own decisions. Health learning can be enhanced by providing information to increase awareness of and knowledge about various life styles and their outcomes, by reinforcing existing healthful behaviors, and by supporting active participation in decision making about self-care behaviors. Adolescents who have chronic illnesses are developmentally able to manage treatment regimens quite independently, but often other developmental tasks and peer pressures may exert a negative influence. Adolescents can profit from problem solving and role playing to clarify values and behaviors related to illness management. Developmental implications for the adolescent's health learning are summarized in Table 12–6.

ADULTHOOD

Encouraging Adult Learner Participation

Cross (1981) suggests that six factors influence adult learner participation. These include self-evaluation, attitudes toward learning, life transitions, the importance of goals and the expectations of experiences for meeting goals, information related to learning opportunities, and perceptions of barriers toward using learning opportunities. All of these must be considered when planning health education for adults.

If either self-evaluation or the attitude toward learning are negative, these areas will need to be improved. Negative self-evaluations may be related to health status and difficulty in coping with health changes. Strategies related to facilitating coping would need to be employed before proceeding with teaching–learning strategies. Attitudes toward learning are more difficult to change. Often a simple learning program designed to guarantee a successful outcome can facilitate a more positive attitude.

Life transitions occur between life stages. In health, a transition stage can also occur between one health state and another. In either situation, transitions can both stimulate and curtail learning. Individuals often seek out learning experiences during transitional stages. The nurse can optimize health learning during transition stages by first increasing an adult's awareness of health content appropriate to the transition phase or to the next life stage or health state. Sometimes adults concentrate on specific concerns related to their self-identified life stage or health state and are not open to learning about other topics. The nurse must recognize when this is occurring and facilitate learning in the area of interest first.

The value an individual places upon goals and the expectations of experiences that facilitate meeting those goals is the fourth factor that influences adult participation in learning. Both illness and wellness health states affect goal attainment. When a goal is threatened, if the goal is valued, an adult may be motivated to participate in learning about health-related topics that will facilitate meeting the goal. For example, an individual who experiences cardiac arrhythmias and angina may be motivated to learn and practice stress control in order to maintain a top level management position and progress in the business world. Another individual in the same career position may have no illness but may recognize increased productivity is related to health promotion behaviors. This individual might seek learning experiences related to nutrition, exercise, and stress reduction for maintaining a wellness state.

Cross (1981) suggests that adults have to have information about the existence of learning opportunities in order to participate. While this is also true within the health field, it is more relevant in some situations than in others. When adults are hospitalized, the nurse–teacher has ready access to acquaint them with health-learning opportunities and begin the health-teaching process. Those adults with chronic illnesses, even when well managed outside a hospital, have the potential for being reached through clinic or physician appointments. It is the segment of the population without health problems that may not be aware of health-learning opportunities. This group offers a substantial population of learners. Nurses must develop better means of reaching this audience and communicating to them the variety of health teaching that nurses can offer.

Adult participation in health learning is influenced by the perception of the ease or difficulty of participation in teaching–learning sessions. Time and access are two important factors for the nurse to consider when planning for adult learners who are not already within the health-care setting. Barriers for learners in the hospital setting are related to health status. These are discussed in detail in Chapter 6.

Once the adult learner has agreed to participate in the teaching–learning experience, the nurse can use a variety of strategies to maximize learning. Strategies for adults will be discussed below and differing strategies for working with the older adult will be specified.

Implications for Adult Health Learning

The willingness of adults to pursue learning is positively correlated to beliefs that they have control over their lives. Adults may also stop learning activities if self-image is threatened. For both of these reasons, adults need to be involved in identifying the learning content and methodology.

A lecture format can be used for presenting content that stimulates the adult to seek more information and for augmenting basic knowledge levels. Discussion is appropriate to increase awareness about a health topic for problem solving and for consideration of health values. Charts, demonstrations, and models can also be useful for presenting content that is more complex or less well known to the learner. Varying resources facilitate adult learning. Self-directed learners use human resources, paid experts, and literature. Nurses can provide direction to accurate sources. Determining the adult's preferred type of resource will facilitate making suggestions that the adult learner will use.

The nurse should remember that the adult learner brings to the teaching–learning environment a variety of experiences. These need to be recognized and used when appropriate to provide foundations for new learning. Anderson (1990) notes that activities that improve self-esteem act as motivators to further learning and action, and that errors are seen as negatively impacting self-esteem. Thus, adults are often concerned about accuracy. This concern can contribute to positive self-esteem and enhance motivation, or it can limit willingness to try new behaviors and participate in new learning opportunities. When the adult is overly focused on error-free performance, the nurse needs to adjust the pace of the teaching–learning interaction and provide support for risk taking in learning. Gentle corrections and the notation that some errors are very common also help protect the self-esteem of the learner.

Adult learners need feedback about learning progress. Persistence and effectiveness are enhanced when the developing changes are recognized and they are told the level of competence they are exhibiting. Reinforcement of learning is internal. The pleasure and satisfaction of accomplishment and the ability to apply newly learned solutions to problems are rewarding for adults.

Specific Strategies for the Older Adult

Normal physiological changes associated with aging account for the major differences in the approach toward the older adult. Accurate assessment will help the nurse–teacher determine which of the strategies discussed below are appropriate for the individual older learner. To compensate for visual changes, the nurse–teacher should ensure that lighting is adequate and glasses, if used, are clean and available. In the hospital setting, obtaining glasses from the bedside table or the home is sometimes overlooked. If visual media are used, they should have large print and distinct, noncomplex configurations with high contrast colors. Speaking clearly at a normal rate is usually sufficient to compensate for losses of sound perception and discrimination. Since the elderly hear low pitch better than higher frequency sounds, deepening the pitch of the voice can be helpful. The intensity of the speaking voice can be raised as needed. Some older adults do not like to admit to a hearing problem. The nurse–teacher can help ensure being heard by seeking frequent feedback from the older adult learner. Having this older learner repeat information also promotes practice and aids retention.

Neurologic changes increase cognitive response time in the older adult. For this reason, it is especially important to allow adequate time for the learner to process information and new knowledge. Motor changes secondary to illness may also affect the rate of learning psychomotor skills. Short learning sessions with short-term, reachable goals increase the likelihood of success. When possible, the older adult should be assisted to self-pace learning. Distractions are disruptive. To

or family stresses; and prevention and management of changes in health status related to common health problems like upper respiratory infections, influenza, and periodontal disease.

Health-related areas of interest for individuals in middle adulthood relate to natural physical changes, increasing incidence of illness, and psychosocial changes commonly experienced. Both physical and psychological symptoms associated with the so-called change of life are also areas of concern. The changing basal metabolic rate leading to obesity provokes reexamination of diet and exercise patterns. Decreased endurance and energy may prompt evaluating the balance of rest, sleep, and exercise.

Cardiovascular disease and cancer in this population also generate interest in learning about frequency of health screening as well as life style habits that reduce

TABLE 12–7. IMPLICATIONS FOR THE ADULT'S HEALTH LEARNING

Key Developmental Factors	Implications for Health Learning
Physical Maturation	
Motor: During young adulthood systems function at peak	Able to be independent in all aspects of self-care and health decision making.
Some decrease in muscle tone during middle adulthood; outcome varies	Action may be influenced by economics, sociocultural practices,
Hand–eye coordination: at best during young adulthood, declines not seen until late adulthood	personal values
Energy: more quickly expended and more slowly recovered during middle adulthood	
Cognitive Development	
Full cognitive capacity	Can handle a variety of levels of difficulty
Flexibility, past experience, and confidence help with learning	Experiential as well as written and verbal methods are useful
Learning motivated when it is meaningful and applicable	Identifies own readiness to learn
	Content should be relevant to existing life needs
	Past knowledge and experience used as reference points
	Analogies useful to illustrate more complex ideas
Psychosocial Development	
Intimacy vs. self-isolation (Erikson— young adult)	Needs to be involved with planning and directing learning
Generativity vs. self-absorption and stagnation (Erikson—mature adult)	Can use learning to cope with role changes, developmental changes in
Life style choices—career, family important	career, life style alternatives; to prevent and manage illness
Self-sufficiency of early adulthood expands to include social and civic responsibilities	

TABLE 12–8. IMPLICATIONS FOR HEALTH LEARNING IN LATE ADULTHOOD

Key Developmental Factors	Implications for Health Learning
Physical Maturation	
Sensory changes:	Distinct, large configurations in visual
Decreased acuity and accommodation of vision	aids, glasses clean, accessible; good lighting; eliminate glare; use high-contrast colors
Loss of perception of high tone sounds and some sound discrimination	Speak clearly, at a normal rate, close to learner. Increase loudness and deepen
More easily fatigued, less able to sit for lengthy periods	pitch as needed
	Short learning sessions
Cognitive Development	
Affected by motivation, interest, sensory alteration	Present content at a slow pace or foster self-pacing
Decreased speed of response	Allow adequate response time
Less efficient short-term memory	Provide repetition, opportunities for recall
Simultaneous activities disruptive	Present smaller amounts of information at one time
	Environment should eliminate distracting sights and sounds
Psychosocial Development	
Ego integrity vs. despair (Erikson)	Establish reachable short-term goals
Well-developed life style habits	Encourage participation in decision
Changes in roles occur through retirement, loss of spouse (others) through death	making and planning for learning
	Integrate new behaviors with previously established ones
Changes in body image due to effects of aging	Family members should participate
	Apply to current situation

risks. In middle adulthood, individuals must also learn to cope with changes in role and self-concept as children grow up and leave home, retirement approaches, and visible physical changes continue. Most older adults maintain their independence as much as possible. Changing life style habits of long standing is extremely difficult. When teaching about new behaviors, more success is achieved when they are integrated with previously established ones. Alternatives, rather than total changes, should be discussed. Accident prevention; orienting (or reorienting) about early detection of illness and available health-care services; nutrition; elimination; changes in sleep patterns; and management of conditions such as arthritis, osteoporosis, and glaucoma are examples of content areas of interest to the older adult.

The adult can profit from a variety of teaching strategies and learning experiences. Promoting a climate of respect and identifying mutually agreed upon goals are essential for promoting adult learning. Tables 12–7 and 12–8 summarize key developmental factors and implications for health learning for adults in general (Table 12–7) and for the older adult (Table 12–8).

SUMMARY

Nurses are involved in teaching–learning situations with clients of all ages. Developmental characteristics related to physical maturation, cognitive development, and psychosocial development influence strategies for teaching and learning. The learner's participation in lesson planning, various components of the lesson structure, considerations related to the level and presentation of content, and practice and reinforcement techniques all vary according to the developmental age of the learner. Selecting strategies based upon developmental considerations enhances teaching effectiveness and hence increases the potential for successful learning.

REFERENCES AND READINGS

Ager, C. L. Teaching strategies for the elderly. *Physical and Occupational Therapy in Geriatrics,* 1986, *4*(4),3–14.

Alywahby, N. F. Principles of teaching for individual learning of older adults. *Rehabilitation Nursing,* 1989, *14*(6),330–333.

Anderson, C. *Patient teaching and communicating in an information age.* Albany, NY: Delmar Publishers Inc., 1990.

Ashby, L., & Travis, S. Teach yourself how to teach an older patient. *RN,* 1988, *51*(4), 25–26.

Austin, B. A., Atwater, C., & Waage, M. A preoperative teaching booklet for pediatric patients. *Today's OR Nurse,* 1986, *8*(6),24–33.

Banks, E. Concepts of health and sickness of preschool- and school-aged children. *Children's Health Care,* 1990, *19*(1),43–48.

Berger, K. S. *The developing person through the life span.* (2nd ed.) NY: Worth Publishers, 1988.

Betz, C. L. Teaching children through play therapy. *AORN Journal,* 1983, *38*(4),709–720, 724.

Bruhn, J., & Cordova, F. A. A developmental approach to learning wellness behavior. Part I: Infancy and early adolescence. *Journal of Health Values,* 1977, *1*(6),246–254.

Canam, C. Developing a peer-helping program for adolescents. *Canadian Nurse,* 1984, *80*(7),41–44.

Clarke, J. H., MacPherson, B., Holmes, D. R., & Jones, R. Reducing adolescent smoking: A comparison of peer-led, teacher-led, and expert interventions. *Journal of School Health,* 1986, *56*(3),102–106.

Cohen, L. J. Bibliotherapy: Using literature to help children deal with difficult problems. *Journal of Psychosocial Nursing,* 1987, *25*(10),120–124.

Crider, C. Children's conceptions of the body interior. In Bibace, R., & Walsh, M. E. (Eds.). *New directions for child development: Children's conceptions of health, illness and bodily functions.* San Francisco: Jossey-Bass, 1981, pp. 49–66.

Cross, K. P. *Adults as learners.* San Francisco: Jossey-Bass, 1981.

Elsberry, N. L., & Sorensen, M. E. Using analogies in patient teaching. *American Journal of Nursing,* 1986, *86*(10),1171–1172.

Fielo, S. B., & Rizzolo, M. A. Handle with caring: Meeting elderly clients' special learning needs. *Nursing and Health Care,* 1988, *9*(4),192–195.

Fox, V. Patient teaching: Understanding the needs of the adult learner. *AORN,* 1986, *44*(2),234–238.

Gratz, R. R., & Pilivin, J. A. What makes kids sick: Children's beliefs about the causative factors of illness. *Children's Health Care,* 1984, *12*(4),156–162.

Gessner, B. A. Adult education: The cornerstone of patient teaching. *Nursing Clinics of North America,* 1989, *24*(3),589–595.

Gilman, C. M., & Frauman, A. C. Use of play with the child with chronic illness. *ANNA Journal,* 1987, *14*(4),259–261.

Kick, E. Patient teaching for elders. *Nursing Clinics of North America,* 1898, 24(3),687–693.

Kim, K. K. Response time and health care learning of elderly patients. *Research in Nursing and Health,* 1986, *9*(3),233–239.

Knight, R. W. Herkimer helps us teach . . . an easy-to-make robot. *MCN,* 1982, *7*(5), 332, 334.

Knowles, M. *The adult learner: A neglected species* (2nd ed.). Houston, TX: Gulf Publishing, 1984.

Lempers, C. Adult education strategies important for nurses. *AARN Newsletter,* 1989, *45*(1),14–15.

Padberg, R. M., & Padberg, L. F. Strengthening the effectiveness of patient education: Applying principles of adult education. *Oncology Nursing Forum,* 1990, *17*(1),65–69.

Pender, N. J. *Health promotion in nursing practice.* Norwalk, CT: Appleton & Lange, 1987.

Perry, S. E. Teaching tools made by peers: A novel approach to medical preparation. *Children's Health Care,* 1986, *15*(1),21–25.

Picariello, G. A guide for teaching elders. *Geriatric Nursing,* 1986, *7*(1),38–39.

Pidgeon, V. Children's concepts of illness: Implications for health teaching. *Maternal-Child Nursing Journal,* 1986, *15*(3),23–35.

Porterfield, L., & Harris, B. Information needs of the pregnant adolescent. *Home Healthcare Nurse,* 1985, *3*(6),41–43.

Pridham, K. F., Adelson, F., & Hansen, M. F. Helping children deal with procedures in a clinic setting: A developmental approach . . . competence and self-esteem. *Journal of Pediatric Nursing,* 1987, *2*(1),13–22.

Reichenback, M. B. A framework for the nature and development of health beliefs in children. *Maternal Child Nursing Journal,* 1986, *15*(3),119–127.

Steward, M. S., & Steward, D. S. Children's conceptions of medical procedures. In Bibace, R., & Walsh, M. E. (Eds.). *New directions for child development: Children's conceptions of health, illness and bodily functions.* San Francisco: Jossey-Bass, 1981, pp. 67–83.

Vessey, J. A. Comparison of two teaching methods on children's knowledge of their internal bodies. *Nursing Research,* 1988, *37*(5),262–267.

Vessey, J. A., Braithwaite, K. B., & Weidmann, M. Teaching children about their internal bodies. *Pediatric Nursing,* 1990, *16*(1),29–33.

Waidley, E. K. Show and tell: Preparing children for invasive procedures . . . a picture book. *AJN,* 1989, *85*(7),811–812.

Weinrich, S. P., Boyd, M., & Nussbaum, J. Continuing education: Adapting strategies to teach the elderly. *Journal of Gerontological Nursing,* 1989, *15*(11),17–20.

13

Strategies for Teaching Health Values

Carol J. Gleit

Assisting an individual to change behavior may or may not be easy. Health professionals often assume that the learner is well educated, well motivated, and interested in ensuring a reasonable level of bodily functioning and generally preserving health. The ideal patient profile is a person who believes he or she is susceptible to the diagnosed or possible illness and that it can cause harm. This individual believes in the treatment offered by the health professional and that the benefits exceed the disadvantages and cost. Many learners need assistance in integrating content learned from health professionals into their life styles in a manner acceptable to them. Miller et al. (1982), in a study of 27 cardiac patients, found that although the subjects knew the effects of smoking on the heart, the continued instruction to stop smoking only led to irritation. The authors concluded that other approaches were needed to help change smoking behavior. This includes an awareness and clarification that certain health attitudes, feelings, and values need to be negotiated to newer values more contributive to healthful living. In other words, the learner needs help in translating and practicing health-generating behaviors.

TEACHING AND LEARNING IN THE AFFECTIVE DOMAIN

Teaching in the affective domain involves emotional learning outcomes and feeling tones expressed in attitudes, beliefs, values, or interests. The domain has its own defined limits yet interacts with the cognitive and psychomotor domains. Although lip service has been paid to the affective domain in health teaching, there is more need for legitimizing its place in health education. Currently, our knowledge about learning attitudes and values is limited. A further complication of teaching in this area is that teaching may involve this domain solely, such as assisting in raising self-esteem, or it may be a part of teaching involving other domains, for example, assisting in raising self-esteem so that the client will work on ileostomy care. Feeling states may need to be considered, whether the primary teaching involves the cognitive, affective, or psychomotor domain. We know that anxiety, for example, affects learning, attention span, and retention of facts. A high level of anxiety impairs retention of facts, reduces capacities to attend, and therefore can impair learning a cognitive or psychomotor skill.

KRATHWOHL'S HIERARCHICAL LEVELS OF LEARNING IN THE AFFECTIVE DOMAIN

Although Krathwohl et al. published the Taxonomy of Educational Objectives in the Affective Domain in 1964, the use of the domain is limited in health education and fraught with difficulties. Difficulties surrounding the affective realm were identified as a general lack of clarity in affective objectives in the literature, a lack of a readily identifiable ordering principle on which to build a taxonomy, and a general perception that such a taxonomy would not be useful. Krathwohl (1964) has pointed out that giving learners appropriate experience in the affective domain is as important for changing behavior as giving experience in the cognitive domain. Affective objectives may encompass behaviors ranging from simple awareness to demonstration of complex and internally consistent qualities of character and conscience, expressed as interests, attitudes, values, and appreciations.

Krathwohl (1964) has identified five hierarchical levels in the affective domain for the process of internalizing values. The levels of this taxonomy help teachers to identify values and sequence the behaviors leading to internalization of the values. The five levels are listed in Table 13–1.

Krathwohl's taxonomy, developed for the field of childhood education, illustrates a hierarchical arrangement of levels of complexity in the affective domain that can be used for health behaviors. Generally, one would expect to find the lower

TABLE 13–1. FIVE LEVELS FOR INTERNALIZING VALUES

Level	Steps in Level
1. Receiving stimuli	Passive attending, active attending, awareness developing
2. Responding to stimuli on request	Willingly responding, taking satisfaction in responding
3. Valuing an activity	Voluntarily responding and seeking ways to respond
4. Conceptualizing values	
5. Organizing values	Prioritizing these into a system of values, behavior consistently representative of internalization of value

Adapted from Krathwohl, D., Bloom, B. S., & Masia, B. B. Taxonomy of educational objectives: Handbook II: Affective domain. *New York: Longman, Inc., 1964. Reprinted with permission.*

levels used in patient and client teaching, if for no other reason than time limitations. The higher levels of complexity take a substantial amount of time, perhaps years, to reach. The higher levels also involve an increasing amount of self-responsibility. Each level is discussed further.

Attending

The least complex level has to do with attending to stimuli received in regard to attitudes, values, and feelings. In the health arena, beginning self-awareness, or consciousness-raising activities may be related to attitudes regarding abortion, over-eating, or smoking.

Responding

At the next higher level, responding to stimuli, health-related behaviors include expression of feelings, attending to distorted perceptions, and exploring responses to emotional reactions with which the client has been unable to deal, such as grief or change in body image. Objectives that Krathwohl cites for this level include: willingness to comply with health regulations, personal satisfaction in carrying out sound health practices, and acceptance of primary responsibility for making major life choices.

Valuing

The third level, valuing, is illustrated by a client choosing to learn assertiveness training. As another example, a values clarification process such as Rath and Simons' (described in Chapter 7) may be used to arrive at well-thought-out values related to stands on various health issues. Examples of objectives Krathwohl has listed are: desires to attain optimum health, deliberate examination of a variety of viewpoints on controversial issues with a view of forming opinions about them, and active involvement in a daily stress management program.

Conceptualization

The fourth level, conceptualization of a value, relates to some internalization and follow-through of a valued stance. Krathwohl (1964) further differentiates internalization as multidimensional, having a simple to complex aspect, conscious to unconscious aspects, and external to internal control. The latter aspect is consistent with the use of the terms *locus of control* by Rotter and the Wallstons (see Chapter 7). In conceptualization, three processes, compliance, identification, and internalization, are on a continuum. Compliance corresponds to a beginning level of internalization where the individual complies with expectations without commitment to them. In identification, the person gains satisfaction from the response and accepts the values implied in the behavior. The use of internalization refers to one's acceptance of certain values, attitudes, and interests into one's own system, whereby one is guided by these, regardless of external input, such as from a teacher or other health professional.

It is possible to remain at the beginning level of the conceptualization in compliance. If the above definition of compliance is accepted, the idea of doing what the health professional suggests or demands may be appropriate for some individuals, perhaps those "externals," to use Rotter's phraseology. Problems would arise at the point where the health professional is no longer available to keep reinforcing the client to conform to the prescription. If the client can gain satisfaction from engaging in the behavior or, further, freely choose and prize those health-generating behaviors independently, a behavior could be lasting. This would be exemplified by an externally oriented individual transforming to become internally oriented. Examples such as choosing and engaging in wellness practices, such as physical fitness, stress management, nutritional awareness, and environmental sensitivity, incorporate self-responsibility and can lead to achieving a high level of wellness. Diabetic or arthritic patients who understand their illness and practice exercises, nutrition, and illness management can learn to live with being diabetic or arthritic. Krathwohl has listed objectives relating to health care as: developing a plan for regulating one's rest in accordance with the demands of one's activities; beginning to form judgments concerning the type of life one wants to lead.

Organizing
At the highest level, organizing a value system having priorities encompassing a single whole might be like Rogers' description of the self-actualizing person or Ardell's description of high-level wellness. Although health professionals usually do not incorporate teaching at this level, encouraging or facilitating self-responsibility is within the nursing role. It may be that at this level of learning the individual's philosophy of wellness–illness as incorporated in his or her life style is one of independence and self-responsibility, and that the locus of control is internal. Krathwohl's examples of health-related objectives are: the readiness to revise judgments and to change behavior in light of new evidence; the viewing of problems in objective, realistic, and tolerant terms; and the confidence in one's ability to succeed.

It is apparent that achieving objectives developed from the lowest level, receiving and "attending" to new (affective) material, may not require much time and effort on the part of the client. Through a variety of learning experiences, a client can gain increased self-awareness by becoming aware of and willing to receive new material. With the second level of responding, gaining satisfaction and rewards can also be accomplished without a great deal of time and effort. Once the third level of valuing is attempted, learning experiences tend to require much more time, effort, and complexity than nurses usually provide. Generally, the higher the level at which the objective is stated, the more time and effort are required to achieve it. The highest levels may take years to reach and may require repeated emphasis and reinforcement on the part of the learner. The caveat is to recognize the ordering of affective objectives and to realistically deal with them in terms of time and effort. It is usually necessary to achieve less complex objectives before attempting those requiring more internalization. For example, newly diagnosed diabetic patients must go through changes in their self-concept, self-awareness, and attitudes. They must also achieve higher level objectives in the psychomotor and cognitive domains to reach the internalization of a set of values. Through this process they are incorporating the personal meaning of being a diabetic. And, as new developments and changes come about in the diabetic arena, the whole topic may need reworking in new areas of content and skills.

STRATEGIES FOR CHANGE

In health situations requiring a major reorganization of attitudes and feelings, the patient must examine actual practices and responses to the topic, openly discuss them, compare them with alternatives, and move from an intellectual awareness to commitment and practice of the new behavior. Much effort, as well as time, usually is needed to accomplish this major reorganization. There are a variety of strategies to facilitate this process.

PLISSIT MODEL

A model illustrating a hierarchical approach, developed by Annon (1976) for use with sexuality concerns, is the PLISSIT model. The first step is P, permission giving. The teacher gives "permission" for client expression of feelings. This matches the first two levels of Krathwohl's hierarchy, receiving and responding. LI refers to providing limited information, and SS, specific suggestions, consistent with the third level, valuing. IT refers to intensive therapy, congruent with the higher levels of the hierarchy. Mims (1980) has adapted the model for nursing, again for use with clients having sexuality concerns. As can be seen from the Mims–Swenson model (Fig. 13–1), hierarchical levels prevail for client need and nurse teaching. Mims mentions that practitioners who operate exclusively from the life experience level may provide haphazard sexual health care. Nurses need the basic facts about themselves and their clients, admitting that emotions and values affect the care (teaching) provided. For the intermediate level, Mims acknowledges that many sexual concerns are alleviated simply by "giving permission" for the learner to engage or not engage in specific behaviors. Permission may be given verbally or nonverbally. Mims identified a preoperative patient's needing to discuss fears of rejection about losing a body part, or a handicapped client needing to acknowledge sexual needs although not able to have intercourse. Other examples the author mentions are a client's need of permission to acknowledge an increased or decreased libido during situational or developmental crises or that some clients need permission to enjoy oral–genital sex, masturbating, or homosexual activities in which they are participating. Others need permission to feel comfortable about life style choices such as celibacy, heterosexuality or autosexuality (Mims, 1980). The advanced level of this model includes suggestion giving, therapy, educational programs, and research projects. Mims points out that specialized knowledge is needed for the nurse to operate at this level. More recently, Fogel, Forknou, and Welch (1990) and Chapman and Gughrue (1987) identified the current usefulness of the model.

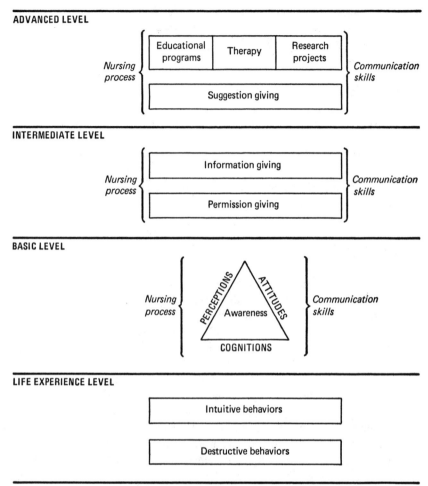

Figure 13–1. Sexual health: A model for nursing education and nursing practice. (*From Mims, F. H., & Swenson, M.* Sexuality: A nursing perspective. *New York: McGraw-Hill, 1980, p. 5. Reprinted with permission*).

Krathwohl (1964) points out that age is an important factor in attempts to reorganize whole sets of values. He reports more goal achievement in value restructuring in children than adults. This is because there is more structuring than restructuring.

VALUES CLARIFICATION

Values, beliefs, and attitudes have been traditionally taught through modeling, persuading, limiting choices, imposing rules, and appealing to conscience (Kozier & Erb, 1985; Egan, 1990). In each there is an imposition of values that the health professional thinks the client should attain. A very different approach for learning values development is values clarification, proposed by Raths in 1966. Values clarification is a process by which individuals find their own answers (values) to situations (Raths et al., 1966). Raths asserts it is not a transmission of the values of the health professionals, nor an imposition of values, but a process whereby the individual arrives at his or her own freely chosen values. The principle is that no one set of values is right for everyone. For example, the learner may select a more health-generating behavior than the health-damaging choice in which the learner was engaging. The assumption is that the individual can arrive at values by a cognitive process of choosing, prizing, and acting. Within these three categories are the following seven subprocesses (Raths, 1966, p. 30):

Choosing:	1. Freely
	2. From alternatives
	3. After careful consideration of the consequences of each alternative
Prizing:	4. Cherishing, being happy with choice
	5. Willing to offer the choice publicly
Acting:	6. Doing something with the choice
	7. Repeatedly, in some pattern of life

Choosing freely indicates that the values chosen are not adapted from others without much thought.

Choosing from alternatives involves individuals considering options before committing themselves to one choice.

Choosing after consideration of consequences means considering the significance of the choice. A person could reject or confirm the choice because of or in spite of the consequences.

Prizing and cherishing is a continuous process in which the individual asks: Do I cherish, prize my position, belief? Unprized beliefs still influence behavior but are not considered values.

Publicly affirming, when appropriate, is sharing the quality of the individual's value. If one feels strongly about an issue he or she may share the value with others.

Acting on a value involves action, incorporating the value into behavior.

Acting with a pattern shows consistent behavior over time.

A belief, attitude, or feeling becomes a value when all seven steps have been satisfied. The learner applies each of the seven steps to an emerging or already held belief, behavior pattern, or attitude. Because values are derived from one's experience and are learned, the essence of the process is skill in decision making. The nurse–teacher can help learners identify conflict areas, examine and choose from alternatives, set goals, and act.

Decision making involves choosing, sorting through alternatives, examining consequences, and selecting alternative approaches. Another way of stating the steps in a decision-making process is: (1) identifying and defining the concern or problem; (2) stating alternative solutions; (3) evaluating each alternative; (4) choosing a solution; (5) deciding how to implement a solution; and (6) evaluating the results. If this is the case, inferences about values cannot be made from behavior itself. The client as learner is a part of determining whether values teaching is in order. Furthermore, it is apparent that learning values teaching also involves the cognitive domain. Raths et al. (1966) emphasize the process of valuing, not the values themselves. They list 30 clarifying responses teachers can employ to discuss the various subphases of the valuing process (Raths, Harmin, & Simon, 1978). These are:

1. Is this something that you prize?
2. Are you glad about that?
3. How did you feel when that happened?
4. Did you consider any alternatives?
5. Have you felt this way for a long time?
6. Was that something that you yourself selected or chose?
7. Did you have to choose that; was it a free choice?
8. Do you do anything about that idea?
9. Can you give me some examples of that idea?
10. What do you mean by _____: can you define that word?
11. Where would that idea lead; what would be its consequences?
12. Would you really do that or are you just talking?
13. Are you saying that . . . (repeat in statement)?
14. Did you say that . . . (repeat in statement)?
15. Have you thought much about that idea (or behavior)?
16. What are some good things about that notion?
17. What do we have to assume for things to work out that way?
18. Is what you express consistent with . . . (Note something else the person said or did that may point to an inconsistency)?
19. What other possibilities are there?
20. Is that a personal preference or do you think most people should believe that?
21. How can I help you do something about your idea?
22. Is there a purpose for this activity?
23. Is that very important to you?
24. Do you do this often?
25. Would you like to tell others about your idea?
26. Do you have any reasons for saying (or doing) that?
27. Would you do the same thing over again?
28. How do you know it's right?
29. Do you value that?
30. Do you think people will always believe that?

Values, then, are not imposed on learners, but assistance with a rational approach to deciding on values is undertaken. Christen (1984) uses Raths' seven-step value clarification process as a model for developing positive dental health values.

Choosing or selecting options on a conscious level is the first step in the process. Raths acknowledges that if this first step is not taken, if choices for values are not made, behaviors such as apathy, inconsistency, hesitancy, overconformity, overdissension, or unproductive role playing result. It appears that the nurse as teacher could enter into this process by facilitating the process with the learner. Raths et al. (1966, pp. 38–39) suggest the following ways that a teacher could assist the learner in the development of values:

1. Encouraging the learner to make choices and make the choices freely.
2. Assisting in the discovery and examining of available alternatives when faced with choices.
3. Assisting the client in weighing alternatives thoughtfully, reflecting on the consequences of each.
4. Encouraging learners to consider what it is they prize and cherish.
5. Giving opportunities to make public affirmations of the choices.
6. Encouraging action, behavior, and living in accordance with choices.
7. Assisting clients to examine repeated behaviors or patterns in their lives.

By helping clients in these ways, the process of valuing is encouraged. Learners can clarify for themselves what they value. This is very different from persuading clients to accept some predetermined set of values. The assumption is that people can learn to make their own decisions. Egan (1990) stresses the importance of challenging clients to clarify their values, carefully insuring not to impose teacher values.

Krathwohl's taxonomy and Raths' process are complementary. Raths' work assists in looking at the process of developing values, while Krathwohl's work delves into the process of internalizing the values when developed.

INCREASING SELF-RESPONSIBILITY

Strategies useful in the affective domain involve assisting clients in their responsibility for personal development for their own health actions, reorganizing their feelings, and achieving a sense of increasing self-esteem. From the humanistic perspective, the definition of learning is the discovery of personal meaning. The role of the teacher is more of a facilitator than a purveyor of information, more nondirective and less structured. The relationship between the client and nurse–teacher is a partnership. Instead of the nurse directing "you ought to . . . ", there is an encouragement of expressing feelings about, for example, hypertension, exercise, or stress management. When feelings are explored, perceptions can be clarified. A client and nurse mutually work on identifying needed changes. This is not to say that in some instances, such as an acute life-threatening illness like a heart attack, persuasion from those with expertise is negated. In preventive activities and many long-term illnesses, the problem of compliance has led health professionals into partnering with clients. Once tried, it can be seen to be much more effective than making the client a dependent person who is to follow directions of the nurse. Egan (1990) sees client self-responsibility as a core value of the helping process.

NONDIRECTIVE (COUNSELING) STRATEGY

A facilitative environment encouraging self-responsibility would encompass warmness and responsiveness to clients and a kind of permissiveness for the expression of feelings. The client is not judged. The nondirective strategy, similar to a counseling model, deals with three areas: (1) present feelings; (2) distorted perceptions; and (3) alternatives that are unexplored because of an emotional reaction to them. Elements from Rogers (1969) and Fromm (1957) undergird this approach.

If a client feels he or she cannot learn, opportunity for expression is provided. Perhaps an adult learner's prior experience with teaching was 20 years ago and there was substantial unpleasantness connected with teaching. In this situation, a nurse attempting to teach stump care to a person with an above-the-knee amputation may first work with client's hesitancy to learn by facilitating expression and exploration of feelings. This approach can also be useful with children. Winch (1981) reports exploring attitudes and feelings of school-age children at a summer camp for diabetics through pictures, drawings, and use of puppets. Open-ended discussions were also found helpful in identifying feelings. Many instances of distorted perceptions exist in the health arena, and nurses have many opportunities to become skillful in assisting individuals.

Many of the difficulties preventing cognitive or psychomotor learning can be eliminated by dealing with feelings before attempting to teach ileostomy care or diabetic foot care, for example. Dealing with the emotional content of decision making and thought processes can enhance learning. Practice in identifying and expressing feelings may be an end in itself. Identifying distorted perceptions may assist the client in general, or for future health actions. Heckel (1981) exemplifies this approach with patients who have psoriasis through the use of role playing in explaining psoriasis to others. In order to become comfortable talking about their disease, these individuals participate in small group sessions to share their secret anxieties and receive a buildup of self-esteem. Lastly, they are encouraged to use affirmation techniques, such as "I'm a beautiful person and free of psoriasis," 20 times a day.

When content has personal meaning, and when exploration of feelings about self and self-competence are undertaken, there may be movement toward acceptance of illness. A patient may feel helpless after surgery. A nurse could state as an objective: the patient will verbalize decreased feelings of helplessness. The nurse would spend time with the patient and help vent the feelings of helplessness. Active listening would lead to acknowledging and reinforcing growth-oriented behaviors. Patient strengths would be emphasized, rather than limitations. In this strategy, the nurse shows acceptance, by reflecting client feelings and paraphrasing content. There is a limited structure, although leads like "What do you think of . . . " or "Can you say more about . . . " are used. Initiative remains with the client rather than the nurse giving explanations or information such as "Don't you think it would be better if . . . " or in other ways attempting to convince the client.

Joyce and Weil (1980, p. 155) have divided this strategy, which they call the counseling method, into five phases. These are summarized and adapted for nursing situations:

Phase One: Defining the helping situation; encouraging free expression of feelings.

Phase Two: Client is encouraged to define the problem and express positive and negative feelings; the nurse accepts and clarifies the situation.

Phase Three: Insights are developed through discussing the problem and the nurse supporting the client. The client sees new meaning in the experience.

Phase Four: Client plans initial decision making with clarification by the nurse.

Phase Five: Client develops more positive actions with support of nurse.

The content dealt with is personal, centering on the individual's own feelings, experiences, insights, and solutions. In the use of this strategy, the nurse must accept the fact that the client can cope with feelings and has the capacity for self-direction. The teacher does not judge, advise, reassure, or respond in any other way that indicates a lack of confidence in a patient's ability. It is not easy to develop this frame of reference!

Developing self-assertiveness is helpful as part of learning more self-responsibility. With assertiveness training, decreased feelings of helplessness and frustration can ensue, which may lead to an increased sense of self-responsibility. Assertiveness can be learned and practiced. Practice in handling positive or negative feelings, setting limits, and initiating activities can eventually help an individual in goal achievement and energy conservation while promoting good feelings about self and others. Role playing or role reversals of situations may be used to practice assertive stances. Heppner (1989) strongly urges helpers to assist clients with their decision-making and problem-solving skills, in that the majority of clients need this kind of assistance.

AWARENESS TRAINING

Awareness training, as originally put forth by Schutz (1967) can also be used to build self-assurance and self-responsibility. This is another nondirective strategy used in small groups to assist the client in being more in touch with feelings. Experiential exercises or games in encounter groups are frequently used to increase self-awareness and to understand self-responsibility. There is much variation in the use of awareness training. Lewis & Streitfeld's (1980) *Growth Games* contain examples. Davis et al. (1980), while citing others, point out that much body tension is not felt because awareness is directed to the outside rather than the inside world.

Locating and exploring one's body tension is important in recognizing and reducing stress. The authors give examples to help identify areas of tensions. To see the purpose of being self-aware as the interrelationship of all people and the part the individual plays in his or her own growth and development and also that of others can be inordinarily useful (Girdano & Dusek, 1988).

SELF-AFFIRMATION

Self-affirmation is another example of increasing self-responsibility, whereby a person chooses a positive goal stated in the present tense to influence healing. "I enjoy feeling physically strong." "I am a confident person." The individual may say the one-sentence affirmation 20 times a day or write it on a 3" × 5" card and look at it several times a day. The idea is that the person's mental imagery will evoke emotions that will motivate achievement of the affirmation. DuBrey (1982) and Girdano and Dusek (1988) both describe in detail how positive affirmation can be successful. There are growing numbers of self-help books on this topic; for example, Shaef's (1991) *Affirmations for Women Who Do Too Much*. Girdano and Dusek (1988) illustrate the use of affirmations for those with irritable bowel syndrome and insomnia, among other entities.

LOCUS OF CONTROL FOCUS

A final related aspect of self-responsibility is locus of control (described in Chapter 7). In considering examples such as stopping smoking, handling emergencies, coping with overeating, self-responsibility is an important dimension. Many studies report that "internals," those who believe health and illness to be within their control and caused by their own behavior and efforts, are more likely to be alert for health information and to take steps to solve their health problems. Assessing client locus of control may be useful in determining whether health-generating behaviors will be tried. The idea is that someone who believes he has some control over his health is more likely to engage in health-generating behaviors. Hussey and Gilliland (1989) reported that locus of control is important in determining behavioral change in incorporating new medications, diet, or other life style choices.

Arakelian (1980) summarized a large number of studies that concluded behavior change could be modified toward an internal locus of control. Quoting MacDonald, she identified three major methods for promoting increased internality or internalization training. These are (1) reconstrual of stimuli, (2) action-oriented approach, and (3) counseling techniques (1980). The first, reconstrual of stimuli, involves reinterpretation or reorientation of a particular life situation. For example, if a diagnosis or treatment is viewed as a punishment, the negative event could be reinterpreted as a challenge, a potential growth experience. The action-oriented approach emphasizes the adoption of new behaviors, rather than attitude change. Behavior rehearsal or role playing can be used to eliminate self-defeating behaviors.

Practice in self-reliance for asthmatic children and clarifying self-management problems for hypertensive patients can be used to increase self-confidence.

Counseling techniques involve the teacher's challenging externally oriented verbalizations, such as "I can't learn to catheterize myself," and rewarding internally oriented choices. In this method, the individual recognized the difference between being influenced by others and by the self as a source of control (Arakelian, 1980). The author admits that more experience with these techniques is needed, but that the need for nursing therapies in this area is important.

Research in this area is not conclusive (Arakelian, 1980). Rosenblum et al. (1981) found no significant difference between internally and externally controlled mothers who had their children immunized and those who did not. Arakelian (1980) points out that when locus of control is used as the only predictor of achieving objectives or outcomes, the results may not reach statistical significance. Although many health behaviors are complex and multidimensional, locus of control is one important focus to consider. Girdano and Dusek (1988) again emphasize that locus of control determination is important for those in weight management, smoking cessation, essential hypertension and irritable bowel programs.

CONTRACTING

Another way of helping clients to take charge of their own health actions is through contracting (Janz et al., 1983; Armstrong, 1989; Egan, 1990; Rankin & Stallings, 1990). A contract is a working agreement, continuously renegotiable between the nurse, client, and family (Sloan & Schommer, 1975). A contract can establish congruence among the purposes and priorities of clients and nurses. The client is perceived as a responsible partner in self-care. A health contract is mutually developed with the clinician contributing expertise and knowledge in health-care assessment and decision making. The client contributes knowledge, priorities, insight, and coping strategies related to the health needs to the contracting process (Hayes & Davis, 1980). Hayes and Davis (p. 84) use Raths' values clarification process in their five steps to health-care contracting:

1. Problem identification and priority ranking.
2. Contract development, including a description of the responsibilities and expected activities of the individuals involved.
3. Contract implementation.
4. Contract evaluation and periodic renegotiation of contract terms as necessary.
5. Contract termination upon achievement of established goals.

Herje (1980), a nurse who used contracts with people from 6 to 87 years of age, reported using contracts in school settings, on Indian reservations, in senior citizen high-rise developments, as well as in hospitals and outpatient facilities. In her view, individuals who pose difficulties with the contracting process are those who are in life situations in which they manifest denial, confusion, or grief, and are temporarily immobilized. Herje suggests that for these people the nurse can be an active listener and referral source and can offer a concerned follow-up. At a later time contracting may be of positive value.

Herje (1980) lists those patients who never would be able to contract as:

1. Those who have minimal cognitive skills.
2. Those who are unwilling to try being more active in their own health care.
3. Those who see the place of authority and control for health matters outside rather than within themselves.
4. Those who, because of medical emergencies, cannot make decisions regarding their treatment.

Many benefits have been identified from the use of contracting. Among them are: (1) the client becomes a participant in the decision-making process regarding the treatment plan and makes a commitment to behavior change; (2) an opportunity is provided to discuss potential problems and solutions; (3) the contract fosters accountability through written specification of each party's share of the responsibility for the client's health care; (4) the signatures of all partners involved create formal commitment; (5) the document provides an instrument of communication for others involved in the client's care and facilitates evaluation of the progress by permitting comparison of activities and outcomes with the precise terms of the contract; (6) the contingency component provides additional incentive through reinforcement of the desired behaviors (Janz et al., 1983; Rankin & Stalling, 1990; Anderson, 1990).

The following basic elements included in a nurse–client contract include goals, time frame, client responsibilities, nurse responsibilities, intervals for evaluation, reward, dates for contract to begin and terminate, and signatures of nurse and client. Guidelines for contracting and a sample contract are found in Chapter 11 (Table 11–2).

Both nurse and client retain copies of the contract. Essential to the concept of contracting is agreement by both that the goals are appropriate and realistic. Contracting allows clients a sense of success and control over their actions. Steckel and Swain (1977) along with many others have reported successful research results when contracting is used.

Egan (1990) indicates that the preferred contract may be the self-contract or a contract in which the person self-administers the reward and the helper is available for support and encouragement. Rankin and Stallings (1990), Kirkenold, Gruder, and Mermelstein (1991) point out that this type of contract is less costly, enhances the self-control skills of the individual, and increases levels of self-responsibility. Egan (1990) avers that self-contracts are especially helpful for more difficult aspects of client programs, in that they help focus client energies.

Janz et al. (1983) summarized the result of 15 research studies using contracting with individuals for weight change, smoking cessation, alcoholism, drug abuse, renal disease regimens, and hypertension regimens. The majority of studies revealed at least positive short-term results for people with a variety of conditions and health-generating behaviors in both hospital and community settings. More recent authors continue to document the usefulness of contracting.

SUMMARY

Teaching clients in the affective domain may be done by itself or in combination with the cognitive and psychomotor domains. Levels of complexity range from helping clients become aware of topics in specified areas to developing abilities to explicate values on their own. The time involved may be quite long, especially when higher level objectives are met. Dalis and Strasser (1977, pp. 74–75) identify 14 affective abilities that values awareness and clarification strategies can help with:

1. Awareness that the decisions they make are based in part on the values they hold.
2. Awareness of the role of data in decision making.
3. Awareness of the processes they or others use during a discussion and the effects of those processes on others.
4. Awareness of some of the values they hold.
5. Ability to systematically explicate their own values.
6. Ability to systematically infer the values of others.
7. Ability to analyze the source of data as one way of judging validity of those data.
8. Ability to weigh possible/probable consequences before implementing a course of action.
9. Ability to recognize when they or others in a discussion are shifting topics.
10. Ability to use language patterns that enable them to disagree with others while maintaining open lines of communication.
11. Ability to interact effectively with others whose values differ.
12. Ability to communicate their feelings, opinions, and attitudes effectively.
13. Ability to explicate the conditions that affect (1) the successful implementation of a course of action or (2) the prioritization of one's values.
14. Awareness of the role of conditions in decision making.

Health teaching, to be effective, must focus on helping clients gain insight into themselves and their values as well as giving information and explanations. The strategies mentioned in this chapter provide methods for nurses to facilitate a client's discovery of personal meaning and acceptance of responsibility for growth.

REFERENCES AND READINGS

Anderson, C. *Patient teaching and communicating in an information age.* Albany, N.Y.: Delmar Publishers, Inc., 1990.

Annon, J. The P-LI-SS-IT model. *Journal of Sex Education Therapy,* 1976, 2, 1–15.

Arakelian, M. An assessment and nursing application of the concept of locus of control. *Advances in Nursing Science,* September/October 1980, 25–42.

Armstrong, M. L. Orchestrating the process of patient education. *Nursing Clinics of North America,* 1989, 24(3),605–610.

Becker, M. H. (Ed.). *The health belief model and personal health behavior.* Thorofare, N.J.: Charles B. Slack, 1974.

Chapman, J., & Gughrue, J. A model for sexual assessment and intervention. *Health Care of Women International*, 1987, *8*, 87–99.

Christen, A. G. The development of positive dental health values. *Health Values: Achieving High Level Wellness.* January/February 1984, *8*(1),5–12.

Clark, C. C. *Enhancing wellness: A guide for self-care.* New York: Springer-Verlag, 1982.

Dalis, G. T., & Strasser, B. B. *Teaching strategies for values awareness and decision making in health education.* Thorofare, N.J.: Charles B. Slack, 1977.

Davis, M., McKay, M., & Eshelman, E. R. *The relaxation and stress reduction workbook.* Richmond, Calif.: Harberger Publications, 1980.

DuBrey, R. J. *Promoting wellness in nursing practice: A step by step approach to patient education.* St. Louis: C. V. Mosby, 1982.

Egan, G. *The skilled helper* (4th ed.) Pacific Grove, Calif.: Brooks/Cole Publishing Co., 1990.

Fogel, C. I., Forknou, J., & Welch, M. B. Sexual health care. In Fogel, C. I., & Lauver, D. *Sexual health promotion.* Philadelphia: W. B. Saunders Co., 1990, 39–53.

Fromm, E. *Man for himself.* New York: Holt, Rinehart & Winston, 1957.

Girdano, D. A., & Dusek, D. E. *Changing health behavior.* Scottsdale, Arizona: Gorsach Scarisbrick Publishers, 1988.

Hayes, W. S., & Davis, L. L. What is a health care contract. *Health Values: Achieving High Level Wellness,* March/April 1980, *4*(2),82–89.

Heckel, P. The unshared disease: Teaching patients to cope with psoriasis. *Nursing '81,* June 1981, 49–51.

Heppner, P. P. Identifying the complexities within clients thinking and decision-making skills. *Journal of Counseling Psychology,* 1989, *36,* 257–259.

Herje, P. A. Hows and whys of patient contracting. *Nurse Educator,* January/February 1980, 30–33.

Hussey, L. C., & Gilliland, K. Compliance, low literacy, and locus of control. *Nursing Clinics of North America,* 1989, *24*(3),605–610.

Janz, N. K., Becker, M. H., & Hartmen, P. E. Contingency contracting to enhance patient compliance. *Patient Education and Counseling,* 1983, *5*(4),165–178.

Joyce, B., & Weil, M. *Models of teaching* (2nd ed.). London: Prentice-Hall International, 1980.

Kirkenald, S. E., Gruder, C. L., & Mermelstein, R. J. Compliance-enhancement in a group based smoking cessation program. Poster presented at the Twelfth Annual Meeting of the Society of Behavioral Medicine, Washington, D.C., March 1991.

Kirschenbaum, H. Clarifying values clarification: Some theoretical issues and a review of research. *Group and Organizational Studies,* 1976, *1,* 100–114.

Kozier, B., & Erb, G. *Fundamentals of nursing* (3rd ed.) Menlo Park, Calif.: Addison-Wesley, 1987.

Krathwohl, D. R., Bloom, B. S., & Masia, B. B. *Taxonomy of educational objectives: Handbook II: Affective domain.* New York: D. McKay, 1964.

Lewis, H., & Streitfeld, H. *Growth games.* San Diego, Calif.: Harcourt, Brace & Jovanovich, 1972.

Miller, S. P., McMahon, M., Garrett, M. J., & Johnson, W. L. Values of regimen compliance as perceived by ischemic heart patients. *Health Values: Achieving High Level Wellness,* August 1982, *6*(4),7–12.

Mims, F. H., & Swenson, M. *Sexuality: A nursing perspective.* New York: McGraw-Hill, 1980.

Rankin, S. H., & Stallings, K. D. *Patient education* (2d ed.) Philadelphia: J. B. Lippincott Co., 1990.

Raths, L. E., Harmin, M., & Simon, S. B. *Values and teaching: Working with values in the classroom.* Columbus, Ohio: Chas. E. Merrill, 1966.

Rogers, C. *Freedom to learn.* Columbus, Ohio: Chas. E. Merrill, 1969.

Rosenblum, E. H., Stone, E. V., & Skipper, B. E. Maternal compliance in immunization of preschoolers as related to health locus of control, health value, and perceived vulnerability. *Nursing Research,* November/December 1981, *30*(6),337–342.

Rotter, J. B. *Social learning theory and clinical psychology.* Englewood Cliffs, N.J.: Prentice-Hall, 1954.

————. Generalized expectancies for internal versus external control of reinforcement. *Psychological Monographs,* 1966, 80 (Whole No. 609).

Schaef, A. W. *Affirmations for women who do too much.* New York: Harper & Row, 1991.

Schutz, W. J. *Expanding human awareness.* New York: Grove Press, 1967.

Sloan, M. R., & Schommer, B. T. The Process of Contracting in Community Health Nursing. In B. W. Spradley (Ed.), *Contemporary Community Nursing.* Boston: Little, Brown, 1975, 221–229.

Steckel, S. B., & Swain, M. A. Contracting with patients to improve compliance. Hospitals (JAHA) December 1, 1977, *5*, 81–83.

Winch, A. E. Learning about diabetes can be fun. *Diabetes Educator,* Spring 1981, 34–41.

14

Teaching Populations with Special Needs

Marlyn Duncan Boyd

Patient and client education, like other health education efforts, is usually geared toward meeting the needs of the "average" person. The exceptional individual, such as the non-English–speaking, illiterate, mentally or physically handicapped person, is often disadvantaged beyond obvious impairments because nurses are not accustomed to meeting their educational needs. In fact, research studies have found that nurses do not feel confident caring for persons from an ethnic or cultural background different from their own (Holtz & Barian, 1990). The educationally, culturally, mentally, or physically handicapped person can learn; their learning needs, however, may be more complex and the teaching methods needed to accomplish the education more challenging than those to which the nurse is accustomed.

Learning is a complex process. As discussed in Chapter 4, most learning in health education requires that the person be able to understand, remember, and reason, then use these mental processes to change physical behavior. Learning how to self-administer insulin requires that the person "know" how and, just as importantly, be able to "do" the skill as well. Many factors may influence how well the patient or client learns both mentally and physically. Two factors that make learning more difficult are learning disabilities and handicapping conditions. Learning disabilities are defined as:

> a generic term that refers to a heterogeneous group of disorders manifested by significant difficulties in the acquisition and use of listening, speaking, reading, writing, or mathematical abilities. These disorders are intrinsic to the individual and presumed to be due to central nervous system dysfunction. Even though a learning disability may occur concomitantly with other handicapped conditions (e.g., sensory impairment, mental retardation, social and emotional disturbances) or environmental influences (e.g., cultural differences, insufficient/inappropriate instruction, psychogenic factors), it is not the direct result of those conditions or influences. (Hammill et al., 1981, p. 336)

As noted by this definition, many factors can contribute to learning problems. The nurse cannot correct these learning problems but teaching methods can be accommodated to ensure that the teaching is efficient and learning is maximized. This chapter addresses some of the more common learning disabilities and handicaps encountered by nurses, as well as strategies to more effectively meet the learning needs of these special populations.

THE EDUCATIONALLY DISADVANTAGED

There are two basic forms of educational disadvantages: lack of formal schooling and lack of social learning. In the latter case, the individual has not had opportunities to interact within a wide range of social situations. Patients or clients who have not had the opportunity of one or both forms of learning are at a disadvantage within the health-care system. Individuals who feel inferior to health-care professionals, both socially and educationally, do not request or receive the same amount of information as those patients who are well educated and of the same social class as their health-care providers (McIntosh, 1974; Yankelovich et al., 1979). In addition, the educationally disadvantaged may have more difficulty understanding commonly used medical jargon (Cosper, 1977; Wright & Hopkins, 1977). Nurses, however, have an advantage in communicating with the educationally disadvantaged because their patients and clients tend to use them as a frequent source of health information (Boyd & Feldman, 1984; McIntosh, 1974).

The person who has had little (less than 8 years) or no formal schooling presents a challenge to the nurse–teacher. The lack of formal schooling may indicate a limited vocabulary and an inability to read. Poor vocabulary and reading skills do not necessarily reflect on one's intelligence; the majority of the people of the world are illiterate (Hemler & Chabot, 1974). Low levels of formal schooling and restricted vocabularies indicate the importance of simplifying both written and oral instructions. Chapter 11 provides specific guidelines for developing effective written materials and for promoting successful oral communication.

It is important that nurses not underestimate the learning potential of the educationally disadvantaged person; the educationally disadvantaged do not have subnormal intelligence, but below average educational preparation. The amount of information retained is often not related to intelligence but it is related to the person's levels of interest and motivation to learn (Ley & Spelman, 1967; Doak et al., 1985). Because of limited vocabularies the educationally disadvantaged often cannot accurately articulate their needs, describe bodily functions, or emotions (MacMillan, 1981). In addition, because of their lack of formal schooling, they may not have a basic understanding of anatomy and physiology and may have difficulty with abstract concepts. The nurse must start at a more concrete level of information with these persons than with the educationally advantaged. It is important that nurses not overestimate the amount of understanding of the basic sciences even by the well educated; doctoral preparation in economics does not prepare a person to understand the intricacies of the functioning of the human body any more than a degree in nursing prepares the nurse to understand macroeconomics (Boyd, 1981). Each individual learner presents a challenge to the nurse.

The educationally disadvantaged or literacy-impaired individuals comprise a large segment of the U.S. population. An average of 25 percent of any given patient population is functionally illiterate or illiterate (Bormuth, 1974), meaning, that they cannot read or comprehend written language well enough to follow the directions on a bottle of aspirin, order from a menu, or use the telephone book. The percentage of the literacy-impaired individuals increases within minority groups, in rural areas, and in certain geographical areas. Virtually every nurse will be called upon to teach patients with below average literacy skills.

Often, when asked to describe the average illiterate person, the nurse will describe the typical skid-row scenario. Nothing could be more wrong. Persons with impaired literacy are found in all geographical areas of the United States and among all economic strata. Some common characteristics of the literacy-impaired individuals that nurse educators need to be aware of when teaching include:

1. Difficulty organizing thoughts. Putting things in chronological order, most important to least important or in categories is very difficult.
2. Slower comprehension, particularly with new or abstract concepts.
3. A limited vocabulary. Their vocabulary is limited to everyday occurrences. Nuances of terms are nonexistent (most vocabulary is gained through reading).
4. Not asking questions or seeking information. They often feel uncomfortable trying to articulate questions and do not want to appear "dumb."
5. Poor problem-solving skills.
6. A perspective limited to everyday experiences; abstract concepts have to be dealt with through concrete examples.
7. Difficulty interpreting graphs, charts, and diagrams (Doak et al., 1985).

How can you tell if your patient cannot read? Asking him or her is not the way to find out. Most people who cannot read will try to hide the fact. There is a great social stigma involved in being illiterate. Three good, in the ball park type of assessment questions might include: "How far did you go in school?" People tend to read three to five grade levels below the last grade that they completed. So, if a patient has completed less than the tenth grade he or she is probably functionally illiterate at best. The second question is, "What kind of work do you do (did)?" If their job requires reading, then they probably can read on an eighth grade level or better. The third question, "What kinds of things do you read in an average week?" People who can read well enough to glean information or enjoyment out of the material, usually read. If the patient reads the newspaper, *Readers Digest,* grocery store tabloids, or romance novels, he or she can probably read on an eighth grade level or better. If you are still uncertain about whether or not the patient can read and understand the material you plan to give him or her, have the patient read it and tell you what he or she learned. Chapter 11 details how to develop and critique materials for low literacy reading levels.

TEACHING PERSONS OUTSIDE THE MAINSTREAM CULTURE

In all cultures, health-care practices are an integral component of daily living. How an individual views health, illness, disease, and death is helpful information about values and beliefs that reflect the person's cultural environment. Culture is defined by Taylor as "that complex whole which includes knowledge, belief, art, law, morals, custom, and any other capabilities and habits acquired by a man as a member of society" (Paul, 1955, p. 462). The nurse who has an understanding of an individual's cultural background can be a more effective teacher. How individuals perceive events on the continuum of health and illness, and how they perceive health-care providers, will have an impact on the effectiveness of the teaching–learning interaction (Tripp-Reimer, 1989). When health-care providers are from a different culture or subculture than that of the patient or client, communication problems can arise. Health-care providers may not fully understand patient or client behavior or may misinterpret responses to treatment or teaching. In addition, the health-care professionals representing the dominant culture tend to think that their ways of thinking and acting are the correct and logical ones. They tend to regard the beliefs and actions of the subculture, particularly if they are very different, as perplexing and strange (Asante et al., 1979; Tripp-Reimer, 1989).

The nurse who strives to effectively communicate with persons of other cultural origins is aware that communication is both verbal and nonverbal, and that it is value laden. Verbal communications consist of both oral and written means of communication. Obviously verbal communication can be a problem with different languages and different cultural perspectives; nonverbal communication can either facilitate or impede verbal learning as well. Nonverbal behavior, or body language, can be used to accentuate verbal behavior, show acceptance, and interpret verbal behavior. Eye contact, touching, posture, and distance are all used differently among various cultures. By learning the meaning and restrictions of their use within a particular cultural group the nurse can communicate more effectively and can help prevent barriers to communication. Chapter 11 provides more information about nonverbal communication.

Values are often expressed through nonverbal behavior and the way in which people communicate is influenced by the values they hold. How the nurse communicates with a person of another cultural heritage is very important, since it is not only a way to transfer information but also a way to show caring and respect as well. Differences in values can cause gaps in communication or result in miscommunication (Anderson, 1990). It is typical for people to consider their value system, their culture, and their health beliefs superior to others. To effectively communicate with patients and clients of other cultures, nurses can explore the particular health issue from the client's perspective. When two people of different value systems interact, the communication becomes intercultural and communication patterns must be adapted. Assumptions about the patient or client from a different culture cannot be based on the health-care provider's cultural belief and values.

Dr. Tripp-Reimer, a nurse specializing in cross-cultural nursing, recommended that when a nurse is faced with a cross-cultural interaction that she first do a cultural assessment. She defines a cultural assessment as a systematic appraisal of the patient's beliefs, values, and health-care practices, which is done to determine the patient's needs and determine nursing interventions. A cultural assessment involves first doing a general assessment to determine how much the patient identifies with his or her ethnic group, religion, and patterns of communication. Next, the nurse elicits information regarding why the patient is seeking care, his or her perspective about why the problem exists, and tried and anticipated treatments for care. Finally, the nurse must detail information about how cultural influences may impact on projected treatment strategies. The nurse educator should be aware that preferred methods of learning are often culturally based. For example, some cultural groups have a strong tradition of oral teaching, others have strong traditions in the use of peer educators. How the patient prefers to learn should be part of the assessment (Tripp-Reimer, 1989).

Another factor that can inhibit teaching and communication in intercultural settings is stereotyping. Stereotyping is setting a standard expectation of other peoples' behavior and setting a value upon them as persons. Stereotyping blocks effective communication and teaching—each client is a unique individual and must be viewed as such. Stereotyping can inhibit trust, rapport, and understanding in teaching (Asante et al., 1979). The nurse needs to approach an intercultural teaching session with an open-minded, accepting, and accommodating manner, and to accurately assess cultural barriers to communication and incorporate the client's beliefs with those of Western health care.

The federal government recognizes as disadvantaged, in addition to the poor, four minority groups. Minority groups are considered disadvantaged for a variety of reasons: low incomes, low educational levels, and sociocultural disadvantages. This discussion primarily focuses on the cultural and health-care disadvantages of these groups.

The four disadvantaged groups are: (1) Asian and Pacific Islander Americans, including peoples of Japanese, Filipino, Samoan, Korean, Chinese, Cambodian, Laotian, and Vietnamese descent; (2) American Indians; (3) Hispanic Americans, including people of Spanish, Central or South American, Mexican, and Cuban descent; and (4) black Americans, including peoples of African Caribbean, and Haitian descent. Minority groups account for 24 percent of the United States population (Table 14–1). In general, these minority groups tend to have lower incomes and less education than the general American population (U.S. Bureau of the

TABLE 14–1. PERCENT DISTRIBUTION OF THE UNITED STATES POPULATION BY ETHNIC GROUP

Ethnic Group	Percent
White	84
Black (Jamaican, Black Puerto Rican, Haitian, Nigerian, West Indian)	12
Spanish origin (any race)	8
Other races	3
Asian & Pacific Islander	3
American Indian, Eskimo, and Aleut	1

From U.S. Bureau of the Census, 1990, p. 8.

Census, 1990). These factors, low income and low educational levels, in addition to the differences in cultural backgrounds, offer a challenge to the nurse. The nurse can better understand the entry level of minorities into the Western health-care system by having an understanding of their cultural and health-care beliefs.

ASIAN/PACIFIC PEOPLES: CULTURE AND HEALTH-CARE PRACTICES

Beliefs

In many areas of the United States, especially the West Coast region, there are large groups of Asian/Pacific peoples. The states with the greatest concentrations of Asian/Pacific people are New York, New Jersey, Washington, California, and Texas. Each of these states has over 100,000 persons of Asian descent (1990 Census). Many people in the western regions are descendants of Asians who came to America during the great gold rush in California. Others are recent immigrants who entered the country following the Korean and Vietnam Wars. Over 700,000 persons of Asian/Pacific origin have relocated to the United States since 1975. Regardless of whether they are first-, second-, or third-generation Americans, language barriers can be a primary problem in teaching. Even when language barriers are overcome, the health-care professional is still confronted with the effects of culture and religion on health-care practices.

The Asian/Pacific peoples represent a wide variety of ethnic, religious, and language backgrounds. Four philosophies dominate the backgrounds of most Asian/Pacific peoples: Buddhism, Confucianism, Taoism, and Phi. Within these philosophies are several recurrent themes: (1) the dominance of male authority, (2) pride or "saving face," and (3) strong family structures. To help the nurse better understand these philosophies and beliefs and how they can affect health care the basic premises of these beliefs will be discussed briefly.

Buddhism's fundamental belief is that life is suffering. Through doing good deeds and other acts of generosity, the believer can attain a higher station in the next life. Reincarnation is a fundamental concept in Buddhism.

Confucianism focuses on the development of moral qualities of the personality: humaneness and moral duty and obligation toward oneself (Kubota & Matsuda, 1982). Confucianism gives the following guidelines for interpersonal interactions. Based on patterns of obligation and status, authority runs from inferior to superior.

- Subject to ruler (emperor)
- Wife to husband
- Child to father
- Junior to elder
- Pupil to teacher (Asante et al., 1979)

These authority patterns dictate social interactions and family decision making. Traditionally, women have been subservient to men at all times. The need for individuals to be in harmony with the universe is another belief of Confucianism. People are between heaven and earth and must be in harmony with the two elements. In addition, ancestor worship is an intrinsic component of daily living and the observance of burial and mourning rituals is very important.

Taoism is drawn from Chinese beliefs in the Yin (negative) and the Yang (positive) forces of nature. Taoism stresses the need for humankind to be in harmony with nature, that is, to have the Yin and Yang in balance. Illness is thought to be caused by an imbalance in the forces and is a curse from heaven.

Phi is a religion founded on the belief that there are a variety of spirits that can be good or bad. These spirits can be housed in objects, the earth, or in the elements (Kubota & Matsuda, 1982).

Health-Care Practices

The Asian/Pacific health-care system is a combination of Chinese and Vietnamese folk medicine and Western medicine intermingled with the various religious beliefs. Traditionally, Asian/Pacific health care has been based on using family members, sorcerers, healers, and monks in treating illness. Folk medicine is considered "slow" and Western medicine is viewed as "fast." The culturally transplanted Asian/Pacific Islander may first try family cures, then consult a healer or sorcerer within the community, before going to a Western medicine site such as a physician's office or an emergency room (Mechanic, 1972). Because they seldom seek Western medical care unless they are very sick and traditional methods have failed, their symptoms may be severe or their disease far progressed. Initial teaching, therefore, may need to be confined to acquainting them with their surroundings and any impending procedures.

Common forms of traditional medical practices for the Asian/Pacific peoples include the use of herbs, maintaining a balance between hot and cold, spiritual practices, and dermabrasion. Homegrown herbs are often used as the first attempts to rid the sick person of symptoms. If herbal treatment fails a spiritual leader is often consulted. Ailments and diseases are typically classified as hot or cold and home remedies are used to help restore a balance in the Yin and Yang. Foods and beverages are also classified as hot or cold and are used to help restore the balance. For example, if an ailment is considered cold in origin, the proper treatment entails eating hot foods or drinking hot beverages. Although the classifications vary somewhat from group to group, the following are common categories:

Hot	Cold
Red meat	Fruits
Sugared or sweet foods	Vegetables (rice)
Coffee	Fish
Spices such as garlic, onion, and ginger	Shrimp
	Oysters
	Clams
	Duck

In addition to the above, drugs and natural elements are also classified as hot or cold. A similar concept is that of defining an ailment or disease as internal or external (Brink, 1976). For example, a fever may be defined as internal in origin and would be treated by an ointment applied to the skin.

Dermabrasion is a frequently used home remedy often misunderstood by Western health-care practitioners. It is used to treat a variety of ailments including chills, loss of consciousness, dermatitis, headaches, muscle pains, cold symptoms, diarrhea, and fever. Placing the rim of a heated cup on the skin, pinching or rubbing the skin until welts appear, or burning a small area of skin just enough to produce a blister are common practices. The belief is that such practices help to remove poisons from the body and restore its balance (Branch & Paxton, 1976; Kubota & Matsuda, 1982). By itself, dermabrasion actually causes little physical harm and may provide a great psychological comfort for the patient. It is extremely important that the nurse does not reprimand the family for such practices nor should dermabrasion be mistaken for child abuse. Rather, the family member can be told that other treatments are available and that the dermabrasion is probably not necessary.

The first barrier to overcome when teaching peoples of Asian/Pacific heritage is the language barrier: interpreters can help facilitate interactions. Family members or friends who are bilingual cannot only help with translation, but they can also help reinforce information or instruction at home. During initial contacts, the nurse can help to educate the family about Western health care, identify any particular concerns, help to dispel any fears, and clarify misconceptions. In addition, the nurse can learn more about their beliefs and values about health. The assessment phase of the teaching–learning process is especially important with people of other cultures. How to do a complete assessment is covered in Chapter 10.

When approaching the non-English–speaking person, a quiet, knowledgeable, and purposeful stance will be reassuring because these qualities project wisdom and dignity—qualities that are very important and valued in Asian/Pacific cultures. Obtaining eye contact may be difficult and may be perceived as inappropriate and confusing for the individual because of the superior–inferior hierarchy of their culture. The person may not ask questions because this would also be considered disrespectful. Because of the formality of their social interactions, they need to be assured that it is all right to ask questions. The nurse should also try to anticipate possible questions or concerns and volunteer the information.

Typically more than one family member will accompany the individual to the health-care setting. The initial conversation should be addressed to the eldest person or to a man, if one is present. This shows respect for their elders and is especially important because the eldest person or the man will be the one to make any decisions—even if the health concern is a female issue such as what type of birth control to use. Another reason to address men in such interactions is that usually they are better educated than the women. This is not to say that the women are to be ignored, but rather that more can be accomplished if the initial interaction is one that conforms to the patient's values and beliefs about social encounters, especially in showing an understanding of the concern for honor and "saving face." Every precaution should be made not to embarrass the patient or family.

Common areas of concern and potential embarrassment for Asian/Pacific people include the fear of language barriers, of giving blood, of surgery, and invasion of privacy. Language barriers can be overcome with the use of an interpreter. Laboratory tests, particularly giving blood, are a concern because of a common belief that removing blood makes one weak and the blood may not be replenished. Other fears are that blood that is taken will be magically used against them or sold to their enemies. The patient may be comforted by explaining how blood is replenished in the body, why the blood is needed, and how it will be used and disposed of (Shultz, 1982). Fears of surgery and mutilation are common and stem from the belief that souls inhabit various parts of the body. Detailed explanations help to reduce fears of surgery. The fear of loss of privacy is common, particularly in hospitals. The genital area is virtually never exposed even in private in Asian/Pacific societies. The use of hospital gowns, which expose patients when they are turned, being catheterized or bathed, can contribute to a great deal of embarrassment and humiliation, especially among unmarried women. Every precaution should be taken to protect their privacy.

Few assumptions can be made when teaching persons from other cultural backgrounds; thinking and beliefs may be totally different from the dominant Western culture. The nurse can encourage questions and assess the person's understanding of information and procedures. To avoid misconceptions, the nurse can have patients or clients describe in detail what they will be doing (self-medication, a dressing change, etc.) and demonstrate the procedure. The nurse can assess if any folk medicine or magic will be used. If so, the nurse can then decide whether there is a possibility of a drug interaction or if other adverse effects such as infection can occur. An example would be the common practice of placing a coin over the umbilicus of a newborn infant and binding the abdomen with cloth (Perry, 1982). As with other learners, specific instructions are very important. To facilitate understanding, instructions can be individualized; this communicates that the person is the focus, not the disease or condition. For example, before instructing the person to take a drug with meals the nurse needs to assess how many meals the person usually eats and at what times. Otherwise, the person may take the medicine only once a day or as often as six times a day.

Tailoring patient and health education for people of Asian/Pacific origin can be challenging, but with patience, ingenuity, and an awareness of cultural differences the nurse can be an effective teacher.

THE AMERICAN INDIAN: CULTURE AND HEALTH-CARE PRACTICES

Beliefs

The 1990 Census reports that close to 1.7 million American Indians live in the United States. They are found in each state but predominantly populate the west. The Bureau of Indian Affairs recognizes over 500 tribes; the largest of these are the Navajo, Cherokee, Sioux (Dakota), Chippewa, and Pueblo. The degree to which

American Indians have integrated into Anglo culture and Western health-care practices varies. Although there is a great diversity in the Indian subcultures, some commonalities can be found.

The nurse–educator must recognize that the present-day American Indian has characteristics that set them apart ethnically and culturally from the non-Indian. These include: a strong pride in being Indian and a desire to remain Indian in language and culture; a spiritual attachment to the land; sharing with others; strong familial ties; a lack of strong materialism; a belief in the supernatural for both animate and inanimate objects and sharing with others (Mail et al., 1989).

The American Indian culture is steeped in centuries of tradition. The family is important and extended families are the norm (Mail et al., 1989). Many Indian tribes are matriarchal: the women or mother is the central figure; in the Navajo tribe, descent is traced through females. In many Indian tribes, it is the grandmother who gives permission for medical care and procedures for the children of the family. In addition, a child may have more than two grandmothers. These "extra" women have all played an important role in caring for the child and slight nuances of terms differentiate between them (Kneip-Hardy & Burkhardt, 1977; Mail et al., 1989).

In many tribes, to be poor is to have few or no relatives; it is therefore an expected show of family unity to have many relatives visit the hospitalized family member. The relatives may not exchange words for hours; it is their presence that is important (Branch & Paxton, 1976). This tradition can cause problems when visiting hours and the number of visitors are limited. It is very important to explain the rules governing visiting hours to both the patient and the family.

Decision making is also a family effort (Hosey, 1990). It may be necessary to wait until key family members are present before decisions can be made about hospitalization or related health measures. This time delay may be misinterpreted by health professionals as a sign of an inability to make decisions or a lack of understanding of the severity of the health problem. A physician working on a Navajo reservation described efforts to obtain a consent for surgery for a child as an all-day affair. The patient's mother agreed to the surgery but said that the child's grandmother had to be consulted. After spending more than an hour discussing the need for surgery with three different "grandmothers," the physician finally met and obtained the consent from the eldest woman in the family. As evidenced in the previous example, the elders—especially the women—are looked to for wisdom and guidance.

Although the Indian family is close, the American Indian holds privacy and individual rights highly. A fundamental concept of Indian culture is that no person has the right to make decisions for another (Primeaux, 1977). This belief seems to be in direct conflict with the belief in matriarchal decision making but it is not. This belief can impede gathering information from family members about a client or patient's health; health information is personal. Another problem is language. The tribal languages do not have terms comparable to the technical and medical jargon used when describing Western medicine's concepts or procedures. Family members or friends who are bilingual are necessary to facilitate communication and teaching.

Health-Care Practices

Within the Indian culture, illness is viewed as a sign that disharmony exists between the person and nature. Cure of this disharmony involves herbs and religion. Medicine, health care, and religion are closely integrated (Shoemaker, 1981; Mail et al., 1989). This poses a problem when the Indian confronts Western medicine, because religion and belief in the supernatural are not a part of the treatment. Various rituals for the sick or injured are viewed as essential. The use of specific foods, herbs, necklaces, and amulets is common and can often be integrated into the practice of Western medicine. A place can also be made for the tribal medicine man or shaman in the treatment. Obviously, there must be cooperation between the tribal healers and the Western health-care team. Treatments by medicine men often involve a sing, a ritual involving chanting and sand painting as well as providing objects for the person to wear or place nearby. Accommodating the medicine man is as logical and therapeutic for the American Indian as allowing a priest, minister, or rabbi to visit and pray with a person of the Catholic, Protestant, or Jewish faith.

When teaching American Indians, it is important for the nurse to be aware that they are a proud, cooperative, stoic yet sensitive people who value their dignity, family, and tribal affiliations. Eye contact is often considered a sign of attention getting and is viewed by some tribes as disrespectful. It is further avoided so that another person may not view the Indian's soul (Kneip-Hardy & Burkhardt, 1977). This behavior can be misunderstood during teaching as a lack of interest. Colors, too, have special significance; some are good, others are bad. This belief can pose a problem with medication. Making sure that the Indian understands that a particular colored capsule is "good" even though it is a "bad" color can be a challenging task for the nurse. In general teaching, large groups may not be the best method to use because many Indians may feel uncomfortable in groups when discussing personal information. Asking questions in groups may also be difficult since this calls attention to oneself and is considered showy. Another reason for one-to-one teaching is the language problem (Primeaux, 1977). Courtesy, respect, patience, and a willingness to include the family are educational musts (Mail et al., 1989). By becoming acquainted with the cultural and religious beliefs of American Indian groups, the nurse may be better able to understand their health behaviors and facilitate healing and learning.

HISPANIC AMERICANS: CULTURE AND HEALTH-CARE PRACTICES

Beliefs

There are over 19.4 million Hispanic Americans in the United States (U.S. Bureau of Census, 1990). Although Hispanics are found in all areas of the United States, the largest concentrations are found in California and Texas (which have one half of the Hispanic population), Arizona, New Mexico, and Colorado. The cities of Los Angeles, New York, Chicago, and San Antonio are home to 21 percent of the U.S. Hispanic population. As with other minority groups, Hispanic Americans come from several origins. The largest group of Hispanic Americans (63 percent) are of Mexican origin. The next largest group are from Puerto Rico (12.7 percent), followed by Central and South America (11.5 percent) and Cuba (5.3 percent). Other Hispanic origins account for 8 percent. As far as geographic distribution, 45 percent of all Hispanic Americans of Puerto Rican descent live in New York City; whereas, about two thirds of Cuban Americans live in the Miami area. About 75 percent of Mexican Americans live in Texas and California (Bureau of the Census, 1990; Westburg, 1989). Needless to say, although Hispanic Americans may share many characteristics, each subgroup has cultural subtleties unique within their own group. Although they originate from a variety of geographic locations and ethnic backgrounds, they share some commonalities, primarily language and religion. Within Hispanic culture, kinship, interpersonal relationships, and independence are very important. The people in general are proud, sensitive, and expressive both in their joy and in their grief. Tradition is very important, and health-care practices represent the continuity of practices initiated by their ancestors. Men typically are the head of the household and are expected to be macho, or strong, brave, and independent. It is the man's responsibility to take care of his family. Because of this belief, the Hispanic male may deny signs and symptoms of illness and resist seeking medical assistance (Mechanic, 1972). Many men may be reluctant to take the sick role because they fear a loss of respect by their family and friends (Branch & Paxton, 1976). These beliefs are of particular concern when teaching about rehabilitation or chronic diseases. Teaching may therefore be difficult because the Hispanic male may deny his illness and resist continued signs of a loss of manliness such as daily medication, rest, or frequent checkups.

It is acceptable for Hispanic women to exhibit signs and symptoms of illness, and it is a woman's place to deal with the ill or injured. There is a very strong bond between mothers, daughters, and sisters. This cultural norm is most evident in childbearing and childrearing. Many Hispanic women feel more comfortable with a female relative, rather than their husbands, at their side during labor and delivery. The typical Anglo set-up, which encourages the father to be in the labor and delivery rooms, could make both the wife and husband uncomfortable (Griffith, 1982).

Health-Care Practices

The modern system of health care used by many Mexicans, Latinos, and Mexican Americans is *curanderismo*, a folk medicine. Curanderismo is a blend of medical practices from a variety of Hispanic origins. It views disease as an imbalance of "hot" and "cold" within the afflicted person. Some diseases are "hot" while others are "cold," and remedies or cures are brought about by restoring a balance. Cures are usually brought about by the use of "hot" or "cold" herbs and foods. The source of a disease can also be considered magical, emotional, caused by dislocated body parts, or of Anglo origins. In contrast, health is often viewed as a gift from God and something that individuals have little control over. Optimal health is the state that allows the person to go about activities of daily living independently and without discomfort (Twaddle & Hessler, 1977).

Some practical areas of belief and tradition of curanderismo that can clash with the Western health-care system are: (1) the belief in and treatments of ailments of magical origin, (2) the belief in hot or cold causes and cures of illness, and (3) expectations of health-care professionals and treatment of illness. The belief in magic can be very strong. One of the most common beliefs about physical or emotional illness is that a hex or magical spell has been put on the person. A common form of hexing has its origins in voodoo; pins are put into the areas of vital organs in a wax doll representing the hexed person. The only way to remove the hex is to have a medicine man, or curandero, take the hex upon himself (Twaddle & Hessler, 1977). The nurse can assess the person's belief in what has caused the illness and use this information in planning teaching.

Hot or cold ailments are treated by the use of opposing hot or cold treatments. Cold foods include lamb, cow's milk, and oatmeal, and are used to treat hot ailments, such as bleeding or certain skin disorders. Hot foods include goat's milk, pork, rice, and beans, and are thought to help cold ailments, such as measles or ear infections. There seems to be no rationale for what constitutes hot or cold, save tradition (Branch & Paxton, 1976; Twaddle & Hessler, 1977). In most cases the traditional hot or cold foods can be used in conjunction with Western medical treatment.

The *curandero,* who is the healer in the curanderismo health-care system, is analogous to a physician. Coming from a background of being treated by the curandero, the Hispanic American may find it difficult to adjust to Western health care. The curandero typically spends a great deal of time with his patients and does a complete (total body) examination regardless of the complaint. The Western physician who only checks a patient's ears for a complaint of an earache may be viewed as lazy, incompetent, or uncaring. The amount of time spent by health-care providers with Hispanic Americans is very important. The nurse will want to try to structure an unhurried teaching session to gain the confidence of the Hispanic learner.

The curandero charges what he thinks his patients can afford to pay and often accepts payments of food or handicrafts. In comparison, the treatment provided by a curandero is much less expensive than Western medicine (Mechanic, 1972; Twaddle & Hessler, 1977). This fact alone may keep many Hispanic Americans from seeking Western medical care or may inhibit them from keeping return or routine appointments. In a survey of Hispanic Americans, 33 percent reported that they thought home remedies could best treat illness—better than prescription medicine (Anderson, 1986). This further illustrates their use of and belief in home remedies. When teaching the Hispanic American, the nurse can acknowledge this but also encourage the person to maintain contact with the Western medical system.

Westburg (1989) offers several suggestions for the health teacher when educating persons of Hispanic origin:

1. Include family members. Family members are a necessary part of decision making and support for decisions made.
2. Plan for enough space when teaching. Typical examination rooms and

some semiprivate rooms are not big enough to hold multiple family members.

3. Religion is important. The Roman Catholic Church and its doctrines influence the majority of Hispanic Americans. This should be taken into consideration when discussing family planning topics and as a source of spiritual support and hope.

4. Be sensitive to health beliefs. Because a large group of Hispanic Americans do believe in the efficacy of treatments from home remedies and other health-care sources outside Western medicine, their health beliefs are crucial to health teaching and treatment.

5. Modesty. One of the most frequent complaints of Mexican Americans about health-care treatment is that it proves embarrassing. Make every effort to provide privacy for both physical matters and sensitive topics like sexuality and bowel habits.

6. Be courteous and warm. Many Hispanics expect relationships to follow social protocol and interactions to be friendly. Do not rush and dismiss with formalities.

7. Provide written and audiovisual materials in Spanish. When choosing materials, try to use those that are culturally relevant and not just literal translations of English materials.

8. Try to learn to use a few words of Spanish. This will help increase rapport.

9. Speak slowly and clearly. For those who have difficulty with English, take time with teaching, use an interpreter if necessary, and remember that people usually understand a language better than they speak it.

10. An affirmative head shake does not always mean comprehension. Have patients review essential information and how to use it.

A helpful booklet, *Delivering Preventive Health Care to Hispanics,* can be obtained by writing the National Coalition of Hispanic Health and Human Services Organizations listed in the Chapter 16 Resources of this book.

The nurse can successfully use the cultural values of close family support, pride, and an appreciation of good health to facilitate the teaching. As with other cultural groups, the more aspects of Western health care that are integrated with the existing cultural beliefs the more successful the treatment will be. The nurse who understands and appreciates the cultural heritage of the Hispanic Americans can become a more effective teacher.

BLACK AMERICANS: CULTURAL AND HEALTH-CARE PRACTICES

Beliefs

Black Americans, because of their many origins, may speak a variety of languages including English, black English, British English, French, Spanish, or African dialects. Their cultural heritages are varied. Because of this, black Americans offer a particular challenge to the nurse. Generalizations about subcultural groups are

difficult. Those first-generation black Americans from African and Caribbean is-
lands may continue to carry on some tribal customs and a belief in voodoo. Tribal
customs vary greatly among various tribes. On the other hand, black Americans
who are descendants of colonial America may have integrated the majority of the
beliefs and practices of Western health care.

Some sociological and anthropological similarities have been found among
black Americans of African descent, especially the importance of the extended
family and belief in the supernatural cause of disease. Extended families, which
may comprise several households and usually are under elderly leadership, are
common. The extended family provides a network of emotional support and is used
to combine emotional, physical, and financial resources in times of crisis. The
structure is very evident during times of illness.

Respect for elders and ancestors is a common value (Shimkin et al., 1978). It is
not uncommon for the black American of African descent to be accompanied by and
consult the mother or father when making decisions. A client may ask to wait until a
health issue is discussed with an elder before agreeing to a change of diet or
exercising. In addition, a special family tie is found between grandchildren and
grandparents. For example, grandmothers may view it as their responsibility to stay
with their hospitalized grandchildren.

In many black cultural groups religion, illness, and health are still closely
intertwined. These beliefs are brought with the person into the Western health-care
system. Voodoo, a primary folk religion, developed as a result of African slaves
interacting with native Haitians on Haitian plantations, and was brought to the
United States through slave trade. Voodoo practices are widespread and diverse.
Believers see the world as inhabited by spirits. The physical environment is made up
of centers of spiritual energy such as cemeteries, Africa, and the seas. The majority
of voodoo spirits are believed to live in Africa but travel back and forth. All living
and inanimate objects possess spirits, some good and some bad. A priest or medicine man can help call forth or appease angry spirits.

In voodoo, illness is thought to be caused by not following one's duty to gods
or ancestors, breaking some taboo, or by a hex or spell placed by another person.
Relief from illness is found by identifying the causes and finding someone with
more power or greater magic to take countermeasures. This person is usually a
priest or witch doctor (Laguerre, 1980). Witchcraft, voodoo, magical healing,
omens, and ghosts can all be part of the beliefs of some black Americans, depending upon their cultural origin.

Health-Care Practices

The black American of colonial descent, although well accustomed to Western
health care, may continue to use selected home remedies that have been passed
down through the family and the black community for generations. Some health-
care practices steeped in tradition, magic, and ritual include mustard poultices
placed upon the chest of a person with a bad cough, a tarred rope worn to cure
rheumatism, nutmeg worn around the neck for neuralgias, and the use of various
herbs and teas to cure a wide variety of ills (Levine, 1977). The nurse can inquire if

the patient or client is using any home remedies and assess whether they are impeding treatment. If possible, folk medicine and religious practices should be integrated with the Western health-care treatment.

Subcultural Groups

Traditionally, only the four minority groups mentioned above have been explicitly identified as such within the United States; a wide variety of subcultures, however, are apparent in health-care settings. The astute nurse is aware of subtle differences in cultural backgrounds and their implications for teaching and health care.

Differences within the dominant Western culture have been found in the way Americans of Irish and Italian descent respond to illness. The Irish are more stoic in response to the same symptoms as compared with Italians (Mechanic, 1972). Differences in responses to illness have been found among families with similar cultural backgrounds and between the sexes. Higher socioeconomic groups, which can be a cultural subgroup, are more likely to obtain health care than lower socioeconomic groups (Aday & Anderson, 1975; Aday & Eichorn, 1972).

In a study of variations in the interpretation of health behavior of Appalachian clients, Appalachian and non-Appalachian health-care professionals identified five areas of client behavior. How behaviors were interpreted depended upon whether the health-care professional was from the Appalachian culture. Appalachian health-care professionals viewed the behaviors as positive while non-Appalachians saw the behaviors as negative or neutral. For example, when interpreting the tendency of Appalachians to have large families, the non-Appalachian health-care professionals stated, "Appalachians don't seem to care how many children they have. Children do not mean increased responsibility. You just start having children when you are between 16 and 20." The Appalachian health-care professional interpreted the tendency to have large families as "Children are important to Appalachian families. Appalachians love children. To have a child is to produce something of value; that's why it's difficult to get them to practice family planning. If a man has 10 children, it shows that he is really a man; for a woman, it means she also has a lot going for her" (Tripp-Reimer, 1982, p. 185).

As with minorities, subcultural groups can practice health-care regimes that differ from those of the dominant culture. The nurse can teach more effectively if aware of even slight cultural differences. Effective strategies would include the nurse's incorporating the client's particular health beliefs when they can cause no harm.

THE MENTALLY AND PHYSICALLY HANDICAPPED: MENTALLY RETARDED, APHASIC, BLIND, AND DEAF

Mental retardation can be caused by a variety of factors. Regardless of its etiology, over 3 million persons under the age of 21 in the United States suffer from some degree of impaired intelligence. Approximately 100,000 children born each year will be added to these statistics. There are three broad classifications of mental retardation:

1. *Mildly retarded* but educable, indicating an IQ between 51 and 75. These persons reach a mental age of 8 to 12 years.
2. *Moderately retarded* but trainable persons have an IQ between 21 and 50 and reach a mental age of 3 to 7 years.
3. *Severely retarded* are those persons with an IQ between 0 and 20 and reach a mental age of 0 to 2 years.

The nurse in the community and hospital settings will probably be involved in teaching persons in the first two groups. Persons in the first group—the mildly retarded—may be taught self-catheterization, pulmonary hygiene, or exercises, for example. Many of the general teaching strategies outlined for children in Chapter 12 are appropriate for this group. Mildly retarded persons can be taught to perform health functions that do not require abstract or complex problem solving.

Aphasia is often the result of the most common cause of brain damage in adults—stroke. Over 2 million persons in the United States have residual learning problems because of strokes, and another one-half million have cerebral vascular accidents each year. There are two basic types of aphasia: expressive and receptive.

Expressive aphasia is evidenced by an inability to speak, write, or gesture in ways that can be understood. Problems remembering words and proper sentence composition are common. Abstract words or concepts are particularly difficult for the aphasic person (Blanco, 1982). In contrast, receptive aphasia is exhibited as a difficulty understanding written and oral communication. What aphasic persons hear (as deciphered by the brain) is unintelligible (Dreher, 1981). Aphasic persons in general have problems with memory, retention of learning, and recall. These functions may, however, improve with time.

When teaching aphasic patients or clients, it is important to remember that their difficulties with learning are caused by aphasia and not by limited intelligence. Early teaching should be brief and center on explanations of procedures or routines. Later, when planning for discharge or when teaching in the home, teaching sessions may be lengthened depending upon the individual patient's or client's tolerance.

Teaching sessions should occur in an environment that is quiet and relaxed. Tension and frustration can decrease the aphasic person's ability to understand what is said. Nurses should assume that a person can understand even if he or she says nothing or talks unintelligibly. Information needs to be presented in short, simple sentences. Content should be as concrete as possible and any "nice to know" information eliminated. Questions should be phrased so that they can be answered by a yes or no, or by nodding the head; the nurse should be sure that verbal responses and nonverbal cues match. The person with expressive aphasia may say yes and mean no. When the aphasic person responds, the nurse must be patient; it may take several minutes for such a person to adequately articulate one thought. The nurse's nonverbal cues are very important. If the patient or client becomes aware that the nurse is hurried or frustrated, this will impair communication all the more.

The person needs time to respond and the nurse should not interrupt or try to second guess what is being said (Dreher, 1981; Jennings, 1981).

With receptive aphasia all these strategies apply; the nurse will want to slow her speech even more and speak each word distinctly—especially key words. Common words are better, for example, "Do you want something to drink?" or "Would you like water to drink?" instead of "Do you want a different beverage today?" Repeating a sentence can help the person have a second chance of deciphering it. Keeping the conversation simple and oriented in the present is better than trying to have the person remember something in the past. It is sometimes helpful to combine oral messages with written or gesture messages. The receptive aphasic person may be able to decipher one better than the other.

When teaching aphasic persons, it is important to treat them as adults and as persons of normal intelligence. Condescending baby talk or attitudes can only further frustrate individuals and compound communication problems. Also, normal speech tones are usually the rule unless there is a documented hearing impairment. Signs that a person is becoming fatigued can include an increase in slurring and changes in mood such as increased irritability, laughing, or crying.

Teaching the person with expressive or receptive aphasia may be more time consuming but the rewards can be great. Teaching can help decrease the patient's or client's anxiety, elevate self-esteem, and promote independence. The nurse who modifies the teaching methods to meet the learning needs of the aphasic person can better facilitate learning.

Blindness is defined as a visual acuity of 20/200 or less after maximal correction and can be congenital or caused by disease or trauma (Marlow, 1977). The person who has been blind for several years may have learned to read braille. If so, teaching strategies of both oral and written information can be used. Specific information or instructions can be typed in braille for the person to use as a reference. Many service organizations, libraries, schools, and universities will volunteer to prepare braille information.

If the individual has not learned braille, learning can be facilitated by oral and tactile approaches. When teaching blind persons, the nurse may find that their memory and recall are better than sighted persons. This ability can be used to maximize learning. The usual strategies for effective oral communication as outlined in Chapter 11 can be used with some modifications. Before touching blind persons, always speak to them first and identify yourself by both your name and title. "Knowledge" information can be presented as with other individuals. The teaching can be taped and the patient or client can listen to it until it is memorized, or the tape can be taken home to be listened to as often as needed. With psychomotor skills, tactile learning is important. Identifying pills by shape and size is useful. Capsules of a particular shape can be glued to the bottle cap to help the person identify various medications. When explaining procedures or treatments, the nurse needs to be as descriptive as possible and let the patient touch and handle the equipment. The nurse also needs to explain the origin and cause of noises associated with treatment or equipment.

Some individuals are not completely blind but their vision is so impaired that they cannot use their sight to accurately distinguish colors or shapes. These individuals can benefit from augmented oral and tactile teaching as well. Blindness or a severe vision loss affects only one method of information transfer—sight. By capitalizing on the vision-impaired individual's hearing and touch sensitivities the nurse can facilitate learning.

Deafness and hearing impairments, like blindness, can be congenital or caused by trauma or disease. Approximately 14 million Americans (1 out of 16) suffer from some degree of hearing impairment. Of this number, 1,800,000 are deaf (DiPietro, 1979). Hearing loss is a communication problem. Deaf or hearing-impaired persons may be unable to speak, have limited verbal abilities or poor vocabularies. Reading and writing skills may be poor, as well. It is estimated that 30 percent of deaf children are functionally illiterate; that is to say, their reading skills are not sufficient for them to function in a literate society. Although the illiteracy rates are high for deaf individuals, many deaf or hearing-impaired individuals are independent in activities of daily living. Most of these individuals will need health care and health-care teaching at some point in their lifetimes.

Different types of deafness lead to different skills and needs. If individuals have been deaf since birth (or before language acquisition), they may have little or no understandable speech, poor reading skills in English (English is a second language for this group), and limited knowledge of health vocabulary. They will often use sign language. If the deafness occurred after language acquisition, they may have fairly understandable speech, some ability to read and write in English, and fair lip-reading skills. Finally, if the deafness is a product of aging there may be poor lip-reading skills (visual impairments also contribute to this) but good reading and writing skills. In fact, hearing loss is the major communication problem of the elderly.

Sign language has been learned by most persons who have been deaf or severely hearing-impaired since birth or early childhood. If an individual uses sign language, a staff person or family member can serve as a translator. If no one is immediately available who can translate, translators are available. Section 504 of the Rehabilitation Act of 1973 (PL 93-112) states that:

> no otherwise qualified handicapped individual in the United States . . . shall solely by reason of his handicap, be excluded from participation in, be denied benefits of, or be subjected to discrimination under any program or activity receiving federal assistance.

This law, followed by the set of regulations for its implementation by the Department of Health, Education, and Welfare (HEW), has improved the quality of health care received by hearing-impaired persons. In addition, the HEW regulations specifically speak to emergency care:

> A recipient hospital that provides health services or benefits shall establish a procedure for effective communication with persons with impaired hearing for the purpose of providing emergency health care. (Subsection 84.52 (C)

TABLE 14–2. SIGN FOR COMMON HOSPITAL SITUATIONS

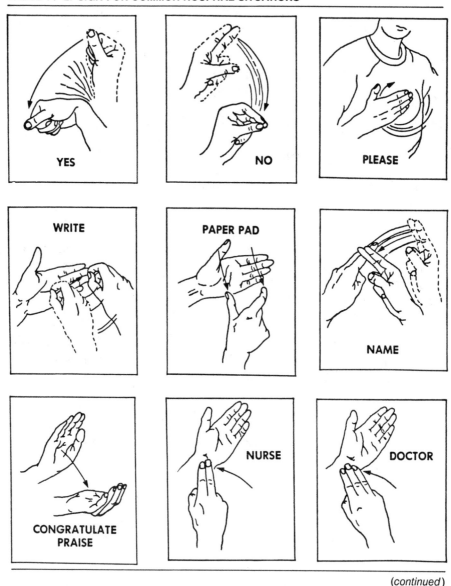

(continued)

The American Hospital Association has further expanded this mandate to include all aspects of patient care. Nurses working in hospital settings need only to contact the Registry of Interpreters for the Deaf (RID) and a skilled translator will be made available to the patient. Interpreters should be used wisely, maximizing the time that they are available. Such high priority times would be on admission (to describe to the patient what to expect, to describe normal routines, and to find out if there are any particular questions or concerns); during the history and physical

TABLE 14–2. (Continued)

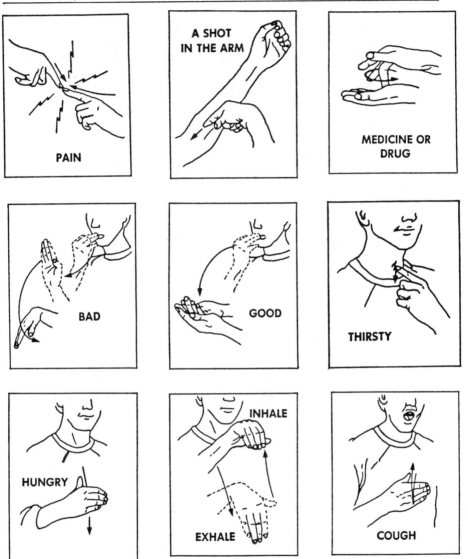

exam; during preoperative teaching; at times when informed consent is needed; and for discharge teaching.

To facilitate rapport, communication, and teaching it is helpful if the nurse can use some sign language. Table 14–2 shows "sign" for common hospital situations and Table 14–3 lists the sign alphabet.

Regardless of whether the nurse is using sign language, is teaching the patient

TABLE 14–3. MANUAL ALPHABET

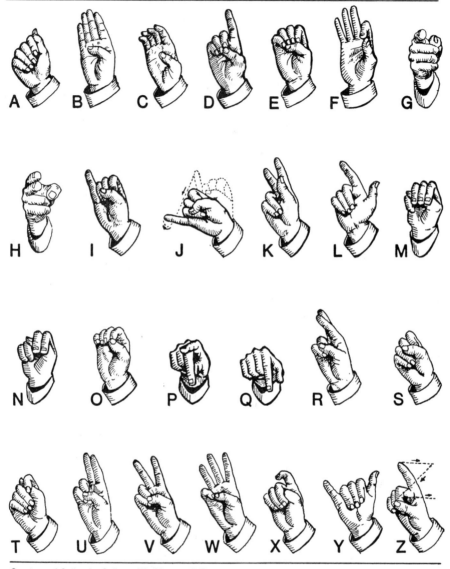

Courtesy of Gallaudet College, Washington, D.C.

through an interpreter, or is speaking to the hearing-impaired, the following guidelines apply:

- Allow adequate time for communication.
- Remember all communication is visual.
- Get the deaf person's attention by approaching from the front—try not to walk up from behind.

- Position yourself within 4 feet of the person and on the same visual level (this is especially important with children).
- Position yourself with light on your face.
- Keep your full face visible.
- Do not attempt to overarticulate your speech.
- Speak at a normal pace.
- Use simple sentences and words.
- If you are demonstrating something, sign or speak first and then do the demonstration.
- Do not overdo gestures or other nonverbal messages, but consider that pantomime can be helpful.
- Do not chew gum, eat, or cover your mouth when talking.
- Write out key words or phrases and have a pad and pencil handy.
- If the person uses sign, avoid inserting an intravenous line in the "sign" hand. (DiPietro, 1979; Navarro & LaCourt, 1980; Harrison, 1990).

If the nurse is using sign language, the words should be said as they are signed. Try to avoid excessive phrases, words, or gestures. If a patient is lip-reading it is very important for the nurse to add sign or writing, because only about 40 percent of the English language is visible on the lips and many of the visible letters look the same (DiPietro, 1979).

If the person is hearing-impaired or deaf in only one ear, the nurse can sit on the side of the "good" ear. Shouting should be avoided; speech should be slowed and adequate time given to the patient to interpret and give a response. Appropriate verbal or nonverbal cues can indicate that the person understands. If the person is wearing a hearing aid, it must be working properly with a good battery and be properly positioned before a teaching session can begin. To augment a one-to-one teaching session, closed-captioned audiovisuals and written materials can be used.

Teaching the hearing-impaired individual requires that the nurse modify teaching methods to facilitate learning. The outcome can be a knowledgeable and self-sufficient individual.

REFERENCES AND READINGS

Aday, L. A., & Anderson, R. *Access to medical care.* Ann Arbor: Health Administration Press, 1975.

Aday, L. A., & Eichorn, R. L. The utilization of health services: Indices and correlates—a recent bibliography, 1972. HEW Publication No. [HSM] 73–3003. Washington, D.C.: National Center for Health Services Research and Development, 1972.

Anderson, J. M. Health care across cultures. *Nursing Outlook,* 1990, *38*(3),136–139.

Anderson, J. M., Giachello, A. L., & Aday, L. Access to Hispanics to health care and cuts in services: A state-of-the-art overview. *Public Health Report,* 1986, *101*(3),238–262.

Asante, M. K., Newmark, E., & Blake, C. A. (Eds.). *Handbook of intercultural communication.* Beverly Hills: Sage, 1979, chaps. 8, 9, 21.

Blanco, K. M. The aphasic patient. *Journal of Neurosurgical Nursing,* 1982, *14*(1),34–37.

Bormuth, J. R. Reading Literacy: Its Definition and Assessment. *Reading Research Quarterly* 1(1973–1974),7–66.

Boyd, M. D. How to write a teaching aid that patients will actually read. *RN,* 1981, *44*(10),90–91.

_____, & Feldman, R. H. L. Information seeking and reading and comprehension abilities of cardiac patients. *Journal of Cardiac Rehabilitation,* 1984, *4,* 343–347.

Branch, M. F., & Paxton, P. P. *Providing safe nursing care for ethnic people of color.* New York: Appleton-Century-Crofts, 1976.

Brink, P. J. (Ed.). *Transcultural nursing: A book of readings.* Englewood Cliffs, N.J.: Prentice-Hall, 1976.

Cosper, B. How well do patients understand hospital jargon? *American Journal of Nursing,* Dec. 1977, 1932–1934.

DiPietro, L. *Deaf patients, special needs, special responses.* Washington, D.C.: Gallaudet College, 1979.

Doak, C. C., Doak, L. G., & Root, J. H. Teaching patients with low literacy skills. Philadelphia: J. B. Lippincott, 1985.

Dreher, B. Overcoming speech and language disorders. *Geriatric Nursing,* September/October 1981, *2,* 345–350.

Griffith, S. Childbearing and the concept of culture. *Journal of Obstetric, Gynecologic, and Neonatal Nursing,* May/June 1982, *11*(3),181–184.

Hammill, D. D., Leigh, E., & McNutt, G. (Ed. Larsen, S. E.) A new definition of learning disabilities. *Learning Disability Quarterly,* Fall 1981, *4.*

Harrison, L. L. Minimizing barriers when teaching hearing-impaired clients. *Maternal Child Health Nursing,* 1990, *15*(2),113.

Hemler, A., & Chabot, A. Sickle cell counseling in a children and youth project. *American Journal of Public Health,* 1974, *64,* 955–997.

Holtz, C. & Bairan, A. Personal contact: A method of teaching cultural empathy. *Nurse Educator,* 1990, *15*(3),13, 24–28.

Hosey, G. M., et al. Designing and evaluating diabetes education material for American Indians. *Diabetes Educator,* 1990, *16*(5),407–414.

Jennings, S. Communicating with your aphasic patients. *Journal of Practical Nursing,* April 1981, *4,* 22–23, 39.

King, S. H. *Perceptions of illness and medical practices.* New York: Russell Sage, 1962.

Kirk, S. A., & Winifred, D. K. On defining learning disabilities. *Journal of Learning Disabilities,* January 1983, *16*(1),20–21.

Kneip-Hardy, M., & Burkhardt, M. Nursing the Navajo. *American Journal of Nursing,* January 1977, 95–96.

Kubota, J., & Matsuda, K. J. Family planning services for Southeast Asian refugees. *Family and Community Health,* 1982, *5*(1),19–29.

Laguerre, M. S. *Voodoo heritage.* London: Sage, 1980.

Levine, L. W. *Black culture and black consciousness.* New York: Oxford University Press, 1977.

Ley, P., & Spelman, M. S. *Communicating with the patient.* London: Staples Press, 1967.

MacMillan, P. Teaching and learning, insight and growth. *Nursing Times,* August 26, 1981, 1513–1514.

Mail, P. D., McKay, R. B., & Katz, M. Expanding practice horizons: Learning from American Indians. *Patient Education and Counseling,* 1989, *13,* 91–102.

Marlow, D. R. (Ed.). *Textbook of pediatric nursing* (5th ed.). Philadelphia: Saunders, 1977, chap. 18.

McIntosh, J. Processes of communication, information-seeking, and control associated with cancer: A selected review of the literature. *Social Science and Medicine,* 1974, *8,* 167–187.

Mechanic, D. Social psychological factors affecting the presentation of bodily complaints. *New England Journal of Medicine*, 1972, *286*, 1132–1139.

Navarro, M. R., & LaCourt, G. Helpful hints for use with deaf patients. *Journal of Emergency Nursing*, November/December 1980, 26–28.

Paul, B. (Ed.). *Health, culture, and community.* New York: Russell Sage, 1955, p. 10.

Perry, D. S. The umbilical cord: Transcultural care and customs. *Journal of Nurse–Midwifery*, 1982, *27*(4),25–30.

Primeaux, M. Caring for the American Indian patient. *American Journal of Nursing*, January 1977, 91–94.

Shimkin, D. B., Shimkin, E. M., & Frate, D. A. (Eds.). *The extended family in black societies.* Chicago: Mouton Publishers, 1978.

Shoemaker, D. M. Navajo nursing homes: Conflict of philosophies. *Journal of Gerontological Nursing*, September 1981, *7*(9),531–536.

Shultz, S. L. How Southeast–Asian refugees in California adapt to unfamiliar health care practices. *Health and Social Work*, 1982, *7*(2),148–156.

Tripp-Reimer, T. Barriers to health care: Variations in interpretation of Appalachian client behavior by Appalachian and non-Appalachian health professionals. *Western Journal of Nursing Research*, 1982, *4*(2),179–191.

Tripp-Reimer, T. Cross-cultural perspectives on patient teaching. *Nursing Clinics of North America*, 1989, *24*(3),613–619.

Twaddle, A. C. & Hessler, R. M. A sociology of health. St. Louis: C. V. Mosby, 1977.

U. S. Bureau of the Census, 1990. United States Population Estimates, by Age, Sex, Race, and Hispanic Origin: 1980–1988. Series p-25, No. 1045. Washington, D.C.: U. S. Printing Office.

U. S. Department of Health, Education, & Welfare. Public Health Service, Resources Administration, Office of Health Resources Opportunity. *Health of the disadvantaged chart book.* Washington, D.C.: U. S. Government Printing Office, 1977.

Westburg, J. Patient education for Hispanic Americans. *Patient Education and Counseling*, 1989, *13*, 143–160.

Wright, V., Hopkins, R. Communicating with the rheumatic patient. *Rheumatology Rehabilitation*, 1977, *16*, 107–118.

Yankelovich, Skelly, & White, Inc. Family health in an era of stress. In *General Mills American family report*, 1978–1979. Minneapolis: General Mills, 1979.

15

Strategies for Group Teaching

Barbara A. Graham

A working knowledge of group process is essential to the teaching role. On a day-to-day basis, nurses interact with individuals and families, other nurses and other health-care personnel. They attend patient conferences, committee meetings, conduct health education classes, etc., all involving groups of people. In the current health-care environment, cost-containment issues and new forms of health-care organizations require that group process becomes increasingly central to the work day world of the health professional. Health-care personnel work in teams, are interdependent, and issues raised in the practice arena must be resolved with skilled negotiations (Sampson & Marthas, 1990).

Even though it is a common practice to conduct group teaching sessions, nursing literature has been heavily weighted on the side of patient education. In acute care institutions, clinics, schools, the work place, and other community settings, nurses identify groups of individuals in need of health teaching. They may initiate teaching with existing groups, and/or assist in organizing new groups for the purpose of health education. Several graduate education programs in community health nursing prepare nurses to assess learning needs at the aggregate and community level.

Whether an educational activity is planned for an individual or group, the principles of teaching and learning apply. In group teaching, however, there are more individual differences to consider. The level of motivation and the ideas and beliefs that are held about health vary among individual group members. The extent to which clients are attracted to a group also influences teaching and learning. Another consideration is the skill and knowledge of the nurse–teacher. Nursing education programs may include group teaching concepts in their curricula, but opportunities to apply the theory may be limited. Group teaching has received little emphasis in patient education textbooks. Consequently, some nurses may feel ill equipped by education and experience to be teachers and leaders of groups.

Importance of a Group Approach to Teaching

There are several good reasons for a group approach to teaching. One of the more obvious is simply that of efficiency. More people can be reached at less cost than in individually focused teaching. As health-care costs continue to escalate, finding more efficient modes of delivery is a priority. The current trend in health care for services to be community rather than hospital based supports the role expansion of nurses as leaders and teachers of small groups. Group teaching provides an opportunity to draw on the knowledge and life experiences of group members. Group membership offers the chance to learn new skills and behaviors in a supportive environment. Through group discussions, members can experience life situations such as peer pressure and the need to conform (Posthuma, 1989). By sharing with one another, individuals feel that they are important to group functioning. Group members receive positive reinforcement from one another, which enhances their self-concept and contributes to group cohesiveness. Group interaction helps to promote enthusiasm and motivation among group members. A spirit of "We're in this together," or "If others can do it, so can I" can provide the stimulus for individuals to take part in an exercise program or other health promotion activity. The success of many self-help and support groups is based on the idea of sharing common concerns. There are many individuals who would benefit from the teaching and support gained through a group experience. For example, groups to assist in coping with the natural losses encountered with aging and with the tasks that the aging person needs to do to prepare for death are becoming as important as groups to help new parents or the adolescent client (Wilson, 1985). The type of group participation and interaction described here is not likely to occur unless it is built into the teaching plan. Thus, a teaching plan must provide opportunities for group members to grow through their interaction with one another.

Definition of Group

Sampson and Marthas (1990) define group as "two or more individuals who share an interdependent relationship with one another." Seaman (1981) describes a group as a collection of individuals linked by some common identifiable characteristics. These definitions imply that group membership is more than a casual encounter. There is the expectation of accomplishment as a result of the group's interaction.

Group Size

In group teaching, size is a major consideration (Anderson, 1990). The larger the group the greater the personal resources, such as abilities, knowledge, and skills. In smaller groups of three or four persons, there is less diversity. The larger the group the less it is likely to accomplish, and the less likely it is that individual needs will be met. Active participation is more likely to be equal in small groups, while in larger groups several individuals may dominate the discussion. The purpose or task of the group can be used to determine group size. If the purpose of the group is a high level of interaction it may not be achieved in a large group. As group size increases, channels of communication also increase. Figure 15–1 depicts the possible number of communication channels among groups of three and four individuals.

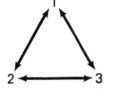

3-PERSON COMMUNICATION
= 6 CHANNELS

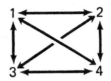

4-PERSON COMMUNICATION
= 12 CHANNELS

Figure 15–1.

As the number of participants exceeds the small group size, the frequency of communication for each individual declines, as does the overall discussion in the group.

Larger groups may be broken down into smaller units of six to eight individuals to facilitate interaction. In groups with fewer than five members, the interaction may be limited or tend to be leader focused. A group of six to eight members is large enough to have diverseness of opinion, yet small enough to permit interaction among all members (Arnold & Boggs, 1989). An advantage of small groups is that there are opportunities for individualized attention and skill development. In a diabetic clinic, for example, clients may learn about food exchanges and how to administer an injection of insulin. Clients are more likely to participate in the discussion and be comfortable practicing a skill in the presence of a smaller group. It is common for group teaching in health-care settings to be directed to families and/or small groups of clients–patients. The guiding consideration in determining group size is the nature and purpose of the group experience.

Group Process

A process is an identifiable sequence of events taking place over time (Johnson & Johnson, 1987). In a teaching context, process refers to assessment, planning, implementation, and evaluation. In other words, the process is how the teaching is accomplished.

TABLE 15–1. GROUP ROLES

Task Roles (Formal Purpose)	Maintenance Roles (Informal Purpose)
Initiator: Suggests new ideas/ways to solve problems. *Clarifier:* Interprets and elaborates, seeks understanding of group goals. *Informer:* Shares information from personal experience and/or knowledge. *Evaluator:* Measures group progress in relation to stated goals.	*Gatekeeper:* Helps keep communication channels open and group members actively involved. *Compromiser:* Seeks acceptable decisions or actions, is willing to yield or admit error. *Encourager:* Friendly and accepting, praises individual effort or morale booster.

Understanding group development facilitates teaching. Sharan and Sharan (1976) have described three stages in group development. In stage one, group members are beginning to establish a sense of belonging and to identify goals. The teacher promotes this stage of development by creating an open and accepting atmosphere. Having a specific plan will help allay anxiety and provide direction to group work. In stage two of group development, members have begun to participate in group activities and assume different roles. In stage three, there is a sense of belonging and identification with the group; the group becomes more independent. Group development is an ongoing process; there is overlap between stages and group behavior shifts back and forth between stages.

Group process is especially important in the development of a support group. Activities can be designed to help the participants become acquainted and to share ideas and concerns. Another strategy to promote cohesiveness and a sense of belonging is by making references to shared experiences among group members. Arranging for each member to have a companion who is similar in some respect, such as in age, sex, and educational level will also facilitate group interaction.

Much has been written about the development of role structures within groups. It is important to understand the various roles and how they might be used to facilitate teaching and learning. According to Bales (1953), all groups must develop role structures if they are to be successful in group member relations and in accomplishing group work. Task roles and maintenance roles refer to the types of communication used by group members. Several roles have been described in the literature. Those that are more relevant to the teaching–learning process are presented in Table 15–1. Task roles or functions refer to aspects of leadership in accomplishing group work. Maintenance roles are those that foster emotional support among group members.

Roles provide cues to group functioning. Assessing how group members function in task and maintenance roles facilitates teaching and learning. In teaching a family how to increase independent functioning in a family member who has suffered a stroke, positive communication patterns can be identified and reinforced. Acknowledging a family member who performs in the role of encourager, or suggests a new idea (initiator), reinforces positive behavior. Group members learn role behavior from the leader/teacher and from one another.

Teaching Tips

Being an effective teacher requires keeping current in new health information and having the motivation to perform well. Skilled teachers evaluate the teaching–learning process and look for new ways to be creative and improve their teaching performance. A common error is presenting too much material in the time allotted. There are no hard-and-fast rules for determining the amount of content to be presented in relation to time allotted. Practicing in a simulated teaching session is helpful. Another approach is to divide the allotted time according to the amount of content in each objective and distinguishing between what is essential versus that which would be "nice" to know. Allotting time for discussion and answering questions is an important consideration when developing the teaching plan.

If possible, teaching sessions are scheduled when the learners are fresh. In a setting where clients have long waiting periods, teaching sessions are scheduled when the clients first arrive rather than at the end when they have other matters to concern them. Home visits to teach infant care are planned for the same time a mother is to bathe her baby. A home visit provides an opportunity to assess the learning needs of all family members. The objectives and conveying of health information must be clearly presented; the subject matter organized and in logical sequence. Key points such as the side effects of certain drugs and when to seek medical care are reinforced. Nurses are careful to avoid the use of medical terms and abbreviations that clients do not understand. Another pitfall to be avoided is "telling" rather than "teaching." Such practice leads to little interaction and therefore little involvement between the teacher and learners. If clients are "told" rather than taught, their learning potential is not reached. The use of advance organizers help set the stage for individuals to become mentally receptive to a teaching session: statements like "Today we are going to talk about foods that have different amounts of sodium in them" or "At the end of the class I'm going to show pictures and ask you to choose foods that are high or low in sodium." Advance organizers are especially important when individuals are unfamiliar with the subject matter. Ausubel proposes that learning may be disorganized and ineffective if advance organizers are not presented (Ausubel, 1963).

Group attention is more likely to be maintained if breaks are scheduled. Teachers know what it is like to sit for longer than 60 minutes without a break. Teaching sessions can also be enhanced by serving nutritious snacks such as apples, fruit juice, or orange and grapefruit slices during a break, rather than the traditional coffee and doughnuts. Physical activity can be promoted by planning a group mini-exercise session. Sometimes simply standing and stretching muscles will help get a group back on target. There are also a number of group games available. Many of these games were designed as ice breakers to facilitate group member participation. Teachers must recognize that successful teaching efforts do not simply happen but that they require meticulous planning. Attention to details such as seating arrangements and equipment is essential. Another key to effective teaching is being knowledgeable in the subject area. Being well prepared builds confidence, puts the nurse–teacher at ease, and allows her to attend to both teaching and leading the group. Personal appearance is also a factor to consider. A neat and well groomed appearance is a confidence booster. Attention to appearance also shows respect for the group and probably adds to the teacher's credibility as well.

Group Assessment

Learner assessment is an essential ingredient of group teaching. This preplanning stage is necessary because groups of individuals differ considerably in age, health knowledge, and attitudes about health. Nurses must assess these key areas before teaching occurs. An assessment provides the foundation for developing a realistic and appropriate teaching plan and lessens the likelihood of encountering the unexpected in the actual teaching situation. Distributing written materials in a health-teaching session for example and then finding that a client cannot read, either from poor vision or illiteracy, is both embarrassing and inconsiderate. The clients and patients to be taught are the best sources of assessment data. Other useful information can be obtained from the health history, the family, significant others, and other health professionals.

Nurses are often responsible for teaching groups who have common health problems such as individuals recovering from a heart attack. In teaching these individuals, the content or subject matter may vary little from one group to another. What *does* change is *how* the content is taught, the process of teaching. The process changes to accommodate differences in age, knowledge, and experience among group members. In planning for several teaching sessions with a group of patients, assessment begins with a review of past and present health histories, including social and demographic data. Current treatment regimens, including diet and activity restrictions are noted. A personal interview with patients and families will provide valuable information that is not available in written records. In personal interviews, attitudes about present health status and treatment regimens, as well as knowledge of illness, are assessed. Interviewing clients before group teaching occurs helps to establish rapport. It also provides the opportunity to assess their knowledge base and how they view their present illness in relation to acceptance, seriousness, and prognosis. Personal interviews are also a time to assess learner readiness.

The public is more health conscious than ever before. Nurses have opportunities to work with groups of well client–consumers who wish to become more informed about health matters. In such groups, nurses function as facilitators and resource persons. Once the group is established and functioning well, there may be only an occasional need for nursing input. An excellent method of assessing the needs and interests of such a group is to administer a health-behavior or risk-appraisal questionnaire. These appraisals include questions about nutrition, exercise and physical fitness, stress management, and the use of tobacco, alcohol, and other drugs. Health appraisals are also useful in assessing the needs and interests in illness settings. Health appraisals can alert patients to risk factors and provide a basis for questions and discussion. Some health appraisals include probability information about the extent to which certain behavior is likely to add to or detract from life expectancy. The appraisals can be used as an ongoing reference. A sample health appraisal developed by the United States Department of Health and Human Services is presented at the end of this chapter.

Health topics for group discussion can be identified by using an interest inventory. The group prioritizes the topics of most interest. In this manner, group members have input into decisions that affect them.

An example of a group teaching project in a cardiac step-down unit is described below:

All patients admitted to the step-down unit were requested to attend two to three teaching sessions covering the topics of nutrition, physical activity, and stress management. No more than six to eight patients per session. Learner assessment included a record review of past and present health history, followed by a 15- to 20-minute interview with each patient. The assessment interview offered the opportunity to meet the patient and family and for them to share concerns and have questions answered. Knowledge deficits and other pertinent data were recorded on an assessment form. An explanation of the teaching session was given to each patient along with a card with the nurse's name, phone number, time and location of the teaching session.

In this simulated situation, the nurse used assessment data to design a teaching plan that included the following activities:

1. An opportunity for the patients to introduce themselves and share some personal interest such as a hobby with other group members. Name cards given to each.
2. Discussion of the benefits of physical activity followed by a 10-minute film on exercises recommended by the cardiac rehabilitation program. Time allotted for discussion and questions.
3. Lecture–discussion and distribution of written materials on food preparation, sodium and cholesterol content in foods, etc. Time allotted for questions and discussion.
4. Ten-minute break—juice refreshment.
5. Group discussion of stress management and how members manage stress. List put on blackboard.
6. Group discussion of what information from the session was most important/relevant and least important/irrelevant.
7. Session brought to a close after summarizing key points and a reminder that the next teaching session was scheduled for the following day.

In evaluating session one, the nurse determined that the content and vocabulary were at the appropriate level for this group of patients. Judging from the discussion, questions, and comments, the class content was interesting and relevant. All of the patients actively participated in class activities and discussion.

Based on the evaluation, the teaching plan for session two included the following activities:

1. Self-introduction by each patient and sharing of personal information with the group.
2. Reinforcement of session one by reviewing key points within each topic.
3. Break-down of the six patients into two groups for a problem-solving discussion of how they planned to adjust their current diets, exercise habits, stress management activities in light of what was recommended to them in class sessions. Allotment of 30 minutes for discussion and report to the total group.
4. Distribution of a one-page evaluation form containing five open-ended questions on the three topics taught in class. Questions four and five related to what the patients liked about the sessions and what they would like changed. The patients were told that the form was not a test but feedback about how to improve the teaching sessions. The nurse requested that the evaluation forms be completed by noon the next day.

DISCUSSION OF TEACHING SESSIONS

The teaching described above reflects the belief that teaching is a systematic process from assessment to evaluation. The probability that these classes were well received is high for the following reasons:

1. Optimal group size, six patients.
2. Homogeneous group in terms of sex and age.
3. Group members shared a common health concern.
4. Illness and hospitalization increased motivation of patients to learn about their condition.
5. The teaching environment was open and supportive.
6. There was adequate space, comfortable chairs, and ample lighting.
7. There was appropriate use of audiovisual aids and equipment was functioning properly.

A key element of the teaching sessions was recognizing the value of each patient to the group. Even if a teaching session is planned for only one or two times, each begins with introductions and a time for sharing. Patients gain identity as individuals rather than as a disease. Group participation can also stimulate interest in learning about health matters. In the second session, the patients met in groups of three to discuss how they planned to implement certain changes in their living patterns. This was an opportunity for them to solve problems and learn from one another. Group involvement can help individuals to draw on their own strengths, to support themselves and one another. In some instances, groups may wish to keep in touch by sharing their addresses or phone numbers, or by forming a support group.

In the teaching sessions described above, activities were planned that enhanced the group experience. Unfortunately, there are many teaching situations in which there may be no opportunity for individuals to become acquainted or share their rich experiences. Groups may meet for extended periods with little attention given to fostering peer support and group interaction.

TEACHING STRATEGIES AND TECHNIQUES

An important aspect of the teacher's role is selecting the appropriate teaching strategies. Nurses must be knowledgeable about different teaching techniques and must practice using them in various teaching situations. Using different teaching strategies provides a change of pace and helps to maintain learner interest and participation. The transition from group discussion to role playing for example helps to keep learners alert and involved in group work. The more commonly used teaching strategies are presented below.

Lecture

The lecture or expository method is a form of direct communication that offers a minimum of verbal exchange between the teacher and learners. The lecture is one of the oldest teaching methods and is probably still used more today than any other method. This method is highly structured and there is usually little input from group members.

Advantages

1. The lecturer's background and experience can add substantially to a better understanding of the subject matter.
2. A lecture is appropriate when important background information is not available to the group, for example, when work is in progress and current research or data sources are scattered.
3. A lecture is cost effective in that a large number of individuals can be reached at the same time.
4. A lecture can be supplemented with handout materials.

Limitations

1. The lecture method implies that all learners need the same information.
2. There is less opportunity for learner involvement.
3. A lecture does not take into account individual differences in background and learning style.
4. Lectures are often longer than the attention span of group members.
5. Lectures provide low-level stimulation.

These points in favor of, and in opposition to, the lecture method are valid, but teachers do not always use the lecture method in the strictest sense of the word. For example, a brief lecture may be used to provide the basis for small group discussion and problem solving. Also, a dynamic and clear lecture presentation can increase student interest and be a meaningful learning experience. The choice of teaching methods is determined from an assessment of the group's learning needs. Group discussion provides opportunities for the exchange of ideas, for learning from the experiences of others and for promoting a sense of belonging (Rankin & Stallings, 1990).

Demonstration

Demonstrations provide an opportunity for the learners to observe and then practice a skill. The demonstration method is important because many clients–patients must learn a psychomotor skill such as injecting insulin or changing a dressing. There is an advantage in being able to practice a skill and receive feedback on the spot. This method also allows for questions and follow-up discussion. A possible limitation is that certain individuals may be self-conscious and not wish to participate in the presence of others.

Field Trips

Field trips provide experiences in new or less familiar settings and situations. In regard to health teaching, a field trip may involve a group of expectant mothers touring the labor and delivery facilities of the hospital in which they plan to deliver their babies. Becoming familiar with the hospital environment and meeting members of the nursing staff will help the mothers to overcome anxiety and fear of the unknown. Field trips are carefully planned as to specific activities or events to be observed, and they should provide a time for questions and follow-up discussion (Bedworth & Bedworth, 1978). An advantage of this method is that information obtained firsthand is likely to be interesting and effective. A limitation is that field trips may be expensive and time consuming to plan and implement

Case Method

The case method involves a description of an event, issue, or problem. The case method may be teacher centered or learner centered. In the former, the teacher uses the case as an example or to support a point. In the latter, learners actively participate in a discussion of the case while the teacher serves as a moderator (Segall et al., 1975). Copies of the case are made available before the group meets so that learners have time for review. The case method may be used to illustrate the management of a particular health problem. The case method can also be used to generate discussion about what to do in certain health emergencies. The advantages and limitations of the case method are listed below.

Advantages

1. Real situations are challenging and interesting.
2. The case method provides practice for future roles or situations.
3. A case provides opportunity for active participation in discussion.

Limitations

1. Some areas of study are not amenable to this form of instruction (for example, physical sciences).
2. There may be a tendency to oversimplify the real world situation.
3. Certain knowledge or skills on the part of the learner are usually required.

Role Playing

In role playing, the participants are actors who portray other characters in an imaginary situation. Role-playing activities are often designed to help students gain empathy for the character they portray and insight into the feelings of others. An advantage of role playing is that other group members who are not participating in the activity observe the behavior of the actors and learn from it as well. A limitation is that some individuals may be uncomfortable playing a role. In health teaching, role playing can be used to help individuals learn how to respond in certain social situations, such as exposure to peer pressure to drink or use drugs. Role playing is useful when a client is confronted with the logical consequences of his actions, for example, a heavy smoker who role plays a patient with lung cancer receiving the news from the physician (Greene & Simons-Morton, 1984).

Advantages

1. Role playing increases learner awareness of the implications of behavior.
2. Learners are actively involved in the role-playing activity.
3. Learner interest and discussion tends to be stimulated.

Limitations

1. Role-playing situation may trigger unpleasant memories of previous life experiences.

2. Role playing requires that participants be spontaneous and creative.

SUMMARY

Nurses use their knowledge of group process to enhance the teaching and learning process. Planned activities that assist group members in feeling they are part of the group and important to its functioning will make the learning experience more meaningful. As health teachers, nurses are involved in a variety of teaching situations. In one teaching session, a nurse may demonstrate a skill, lead a group discussion, and lecture on a health topic. Selecting the appropriate teaching strategy is an important aspect of group teaching. Nurses provide much of the teaching in health-care settings; accepting this responsibility requires that they perform well in this role.

REFERENCES AND READINGS

Anderson, C. *Patient teaching and communicating.* Albany, N.Y.: Delmar Publishers, 1990.

Arnold, E., & Boggs, K. *Interpersonal relationships.* Philadelphia, Pa.: W. B. Saunders Company, 1989.

Ausubel, D. *The psychology of meaningful verbal learning: An introduction to school learning.* New York: Grune & Stratton, 1963.

Bales, R. F. A theoretical framework for interaction process analysis in group dynamics, research and theory. In D. Cartwright, & A. Zander (Eds.), *In-group dynamics research and theory.* Evanston, Il.: Row, Peterson, 1953.

Bedworth, D. A., & Bedworth, A. E. *Health education: A process of human effectiveness.* New York: Harper & Row, 1978.

Department of Health and Human Services. *Health style-a self test.* Washington, D.C.: U.S. Government Printing Office, 1981.

Girdano, D. A., & Dusek, D. E. *Changing health behavior.* Scottsdale, Az.: Gorsuch Scarisbrick Publishers, 1988.

Greene, W. H., & Simons-Morton, B. G. *Introduction to health education.* New York: Macmillan, 1984.

Hayes, E. *Effective teaching styles.* San Francisco, Ca.: Jossey-Bass Publishers, 1989.

Johnson, D. W., & Johnson, R. T. *Learning together and alone* (2nd ed.). Englewood Cliffs, N.J.: Prentice Hall, 1987.

McKeachie, W. J. *Teaching tips* (8th ed.). Lexington, Ma.: D. C. Heath and Company, 1986.

Posthuma, B. W. *Small groups in therapy settings.* Boston, Ma.: Little, Brown and Company, 1989.

Rankin, S. H., & Stallings, K. L. *Patient education: Issues, principles and guidelines* (2nd ed.). Philadelphia, Pa.: Lippincott, 1990.

Sampson, E. E., & Marthas, M. *Group process for the health professionals.* Albany, N.Y.: Delmar Publishers, 1990.

Schmuck, R. A., & Schmuck, P. A. *Group processes in the classroom.* Dubuque, Iowa: William C. Brown Publishers, 1979.

Seaman, D. F. *Working effectively with task oriented groups.* New York: McGraw Hill, 1981.

Segall, A., Vanderschmidt, H., Burglass, R., & Frustman, T. *Systematic course design for the health fields.* New York: Wiley, 1975.

Sharan, S., & Sharan, Y. *Small group teaching.* Englewood Cliffs, N.J.: Educational Technology Publications, 1976.

Smallegan, M. J. Teaching through groups. *Journal of Nursing Education*, January 1982, *21*(1), 23–31.

Tiberius, R. G. *Small group teaching: A trouble-shooting guide.* Toronto, Canada. The Ontario Institute for Studies in Education, 1990.

Van Hoozer, H. L., Bratton, B. D., Ostmoe, P. M., et al. *The teaching process theory and practice in nursing.* Norwalk, Ct.: Appleton-Century-Crofts, 1987.

Wilson, M. *Group theory/process for nursing practice.* Bowie, Md.: Brady Communications, 1985.

HEALTH STYLE *a self test*

How This Booklet Can Help You

All of us want good health. But, many of us do not know how to be as healthy as possible. Good health is not a matter of luck or fate. You have to work at it.

Good health depends on a combination of things . . . the environment in which you live and work . . . the personal traits you have inherited . . . the care you receive from doctors and hospitals . . . and the personal behaviors or habits that you perform daily, usually without much thought. All of these work together to affect your health. Many of us rely too much on doctors to keep us healthy, and we often fail to see the importance of actions we can take ourselves to look and feel healthy. You may be surprised to know that by taking action individually and collectively, you can begin to change parts of your world which may be harmful to your health.

Every day you are exposed to potential risks to good health. Pollution in the air you breathe and unsafe highways are two examples. These are risks that you, as an individual, can't do much about. Improving the quality of the environment usually requires the effort of concerned citizens working together for a healthier community.

There are, however, risks that you can control: risks stemming from your personal behaviors and habits. These behaviors are known as your lifestyle. Health experts now describe lifestyle as one of the most important factors affecting health. In fact, it is estimated that as many as seven of the ten leading causes of death in the United States could be reduced through common sense changes in lifestyle.

That's what the brief test contained in this booklet is all about. The few minutes you take to complete it may actually help you add years to your life! How? Well to start, it will enable you to identify aspects of your present lifestyle that are risky to your health. Then it will encourage you to take steps to eliminate or minimize the risks you identify. All in all, it will help you begin to change your present lifestyle into a new HEALTHSTYLE. If you do, it's possible that you may feel better, look better, and live longer too.

Before You Take the Test

This is not a pass-fail test. Its purpose is simply to tell you how well you are doing to stay healthy. The behaviors covered in the test are recommended for most Americans. Some of them may not apply to persons with certain chronic diseases or handicaps. Such persons may require special instructions from their physician or other health professional.

You will find that the test has six sections: smoking, alcohol and drugs, nutrition, exercise and fitness, stress control, and safety. Complete one section at a time by circling the number corresponding to the answer that best describes your behavior (2 for "Almost Always", 1 for "Sometimes", and 0 for "Almost Never"). Then add the numbers you have circled to determine your score for that section. Write the score on the line provided at the end of each section. The highest score you can get for each section is 10.

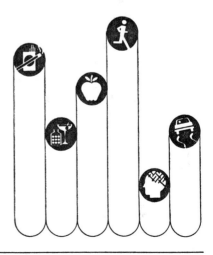

A Test for Better Health

Cigarette Smoking

	Almost Always	Sometimes	Almost Never

If you never smoke, enter a score of 10 for this section and go to the next section on *Alcohol and Drugs*.

	Almost Always	Sometimes	Almost Never
1. I avoid smoking cigarettes.	2	1	0
2. I smoke only low tar and nicotine cigarettes *or* I smoke a pipe or cigars.	2	1	0

Smoking Score: _____

Alcohol and Drugs

	Almost Always	Sometimes	Almost Never
1. I avoid drinking alcoholic beverages *or* I drink no more than 1 or 2 drinks a day.	4	1	0
2. I avoid using alcohol or other drugs (especially illegal drugs) as a way of handling stressful situations or the problems in my life.	2	1	0
3. I am careful not to drink alcohol when taking certain medicines (for example, medicine for sleeping, pain, colds, and allergies), or when pregnant.	2	1	0
4. I read and follow the label directions when using prescribed and over-the-counter drugs.	2	1	0

Alcohol and Drugs Score: _____

Eating Habits

	Almost Always	Sometimes	Almost Never
1. I eat a variety of foods each day, such as fruits and vegetables, whole grain breads and cereals, lean meats, dairy products, dry peas and beans, and nuts and seeds.	4	1	0
2. I limit the amount of fat, saturated fat, and cholesterol I eat (including fat on meats, eggs, butter, cream, shortenings, and organ meats such as liver).	2	1	0
3. I limit the amount of salt I eat by cooking with only small amounts, not adding salt at the table, and avoiding salty snacks.	2	1	0
4. I avoid eating too much sugar (especially frequent snacks of sticky candy or soft drinks).	2	1	0

Eating Habits Score: _____

Exercise/Fitness

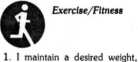

	Almost Always	Sometimes	Almost Never
1. I maintain a desired weight, avoiding overweight and underweight.	3	1	0
2. I do vigorous exercises for 15-30 minutes at least 3 times a week (examples include running, swimming, brisk walking).	3	1	0
3. I do exercises that enhance my muscle tone for 15-30 minutes at least 3 times a week (examples include yoga and calisthenics).	2	1	0
4. I use part of my leisure time participating in individual, family, or team activities that increase my level of fitness (such as gardening, bowling, golf, and baseball).	2	1	0

Exercise/Fitness Score: _____

Stress Control

	Almost Always	Sometimes	Almost Never
1. I have a job or do other work that I enjoy.	2	1	0
2. I find it easy to relax and express my feelings freely.	2	1	0
3. I recognize early, and prepare for, events or situations likely to be stressful for me.	2	1	0
4. I have close friends, relatives, or others whom I can talk to about personal matters and call on for help when needed.	2	1	0
5. I participate in group activities (such as church and community organizations) or hobbies that I enjoy.	2	1	0

Stress Control Score: _____

Safety

	Almost Always	Sometimes	Almost Never
1. I wear a seat belt while riding in a car.	2	1	0
2. I avoid driving while under the influence of alcohol and other drugs.	2	1	0
3. I obey traffic rules and the speed limit when driving.	2	1	0
4. I am careful when using potentially harmful products or substances (such as household cleaners, poisons, and electrical devices).	2	1	0
5. I avoid smoking in bed.	2	1	0

Safety Score: _____

Your HEALTHSTYLE Scores

After you have figured your scores for each of the six sections, circle the number in each column that matches your score for that section of the test.

Cigarette Smoking	Alcohol & Drugs	Eating Habits	Exercise & Fitness	Stress Control	Safety
10	10	10	10	10	10
9	9	9	9	9	9
8	8	8	8	8	8
7	7	7	7	7	7
6	6	6	6	6	6
5	5	5	5	5	5
4	4	4	4	4	4
3	3	3	3	3	3
2	2	2	2	2	2
1	1	1	1	1	1
0	0	0	0	0	0

Remember, there is no total score for this test. Consider each section separately. You are trying to identify aspects of your lifestyle that you can improve in order to be healthier and to reduce the risk of illness. So let's see what your scores reveal.

What Your Scores Mean to YOU

Scores of 9 and 10

Excellent! Your answers show that you are aware of the importance of this area to your health. More importantly, you are putting your knowledge to work for you by practicing good health habits. As long as you continue to do so, this area should not pose a serious health risk. It's likely that you are setting an example for your family and friends to follow. Since you got a very high score on this part of the test, you may want to consider other areas where your scores indicate room for improvement.

Scores of 6 to 8

Your health practices in this area are good, but there is room for improvement. Look again at the items you answered with a "Sometimes" or "Almost Never". What changes can you make to improve your score? Even a small change can often help you achieve better health.

Scores of 3 to 5

Your health risks are showing! Would you like more information about the risks you are facing and about why it is important for you to change these behaviors? Perhaps you need help in deciding how to successfully make the changes you desire. In either case, help is available. See the last page of this booklet.

Scores of 0 to 2

Obviously, you were concerned enough about your health to take the test, but your answers show that you may be taking serious and unnecessary risks with your health. Perhaps you are not aware of the risks and what to do about them. You can easily get the information and help you need to improve, if you wish. A source of contact appears on the last page. The next step is up to you.

YOU Can Start Right Now!

In the test you just completed were numerous suggestions to help you reduce your risk of disease and premature death. Here are some of the most significant:

 Avoid cigarettes. Cigarette smoking is the single most important preventable cause of illness and early death. It is especially risky for pregnant women and their unborn babies. Persons who stop smoking reduce their risk of getting heart disease and cancer. So if you're a cigarette smoker, think twice about lighting that next cigarette. If you choose to continue smoking, try decreasing the number of cigarettes you smoke and switching to a low tar and nicotine brand.

 Follow sensible drinking habits. Alcohol produces changes in mood and behavior. Most people who drink are able to control their intake of alcohol and to avoid undesired, and often harmful, effects. Heavy, regular use of alcohol can lead to cirrhosis of the liver, a leading cause of death. Also, statistics clearly show that mixing drinking and driving is often the cause of fatal or crippling accidents. So if you drink, do it wisely and in moderation.

 Use care in taking drugs. Today's greater use of drugs—both legal and illegal— is one of our most serious health risks.   Even some drugs prescribed by your doctor can be dangerous if taken when drinking alcohol or before driving. Excessive or continued use of tranquilizers (or "pep pills")can cause physical and mental problems. Using or experimenting with illicit drugs such as marijuana, heroin, cocaine, and PCP may lead to a number of damaging effects or even death.

Eat sensibly. Overweight individuals are at greater risk for diabetes, gall bladder disease, and high blood pressure. So it makes good sense to maintain proper weight. But good eating habits also mean holding down the amount of fat (especially saturated fat), cholesterol, sugar and salt in your diet. If you must snack, try nibbling on fresh fruits and vegetables. You'll feel better—and look better, too.

Exercise regularly. Almost everyone can benefit from exercise—and there's some form of exercise almost everyone can do. (If you have any doubt, check first with your doctor.) Usually, as little as 15-30 minutes of vigorous exercise three times a week will help you have a healthier heart, eliminate excess weight, tone up sagging muscles, and sleep better. Think how much difference all these improvements could make in the way you feel!

Learn to handle stress. Stress is a normal part of living; everyone faces it to some degree. The causes of stress can be good or bad, desirable or undesirable (such as a promotion on the job or the loss of a spouse). Properly handled, stress need not be a problem. But unhealthy responses to stress—such as driving too fast or erratically, drinking too much, or prolonged anger or grief—can cause a variety of physical and mental problems. Even on a very busy day, find a few minutes to slow down and relax. Talking over a problem with someone you trust can often help you find a satisfactory solution. Learn to distinguish between things that are "worth fighting about" and things that are less important.

Be safety conscious. Think "safety first" at home, at work, at school, at play, and on the highway. Buckle seat belts and obey traffic rules. Keep poisons and weapons out of the reach of children, and keep emergency numbers by your telephone. When the unexpected happens, you'll be prepared.

Where Do You Go From Here?

Start by asking yourself a few frank questions:
Am I really doing all I can to be as healthy as possible? What steps can I take to feel better? Am I willing to begin now? If you scored low in one or more sections of the test, decide what changes you want to make for improvement. You might pick that aspect of your lifestyle where you feel you have the best chance for success and tackle that one first. Once you have improved your score there, go on to other areas.

If you already have tried to change your health habits (to stop smoking or exercise regularly, for example) don't be discouraged if you haven't yet succeeded. The difficulty you have encountered may be due to influences you've never really thought about—such as advertising—or to a lack of support and encouragement. Understanding these influences is an important step toward changing the way they affect you.

There's Help Available. In addition to personal actions you can take on your own, there are community programs and groups (such as the YMCA or the local chapter of the American Heart Association) that can assist you and your family to make the changes you want to make. If you want to know more about these groups or about health risks contact your local health department. There's a lot you can do to stay healthy or to improve your health—and there are organizations that can help you. Start a new HEALTHSTYLE today!

(From U.S. Department of Health and Human Services, Public Health Service.)

16

Sources of Health Education Materials

Barbara A. Graham

Health educators must know what resources are available and how to access them. The knowledge base for many diseases and conditions is changing rapidly. Keeping abreast of current scientific health information is a professional responsibility. Maintaining an information file on sources of health education materials and community resources is expected practice.

Types of Materials
Health education materials are available in different forms. Some are audio (cassette tapes); others are visual (posters, pamphlets); many have both audio and visual components (films, videocassettes, slide-tape presentations, etc.). Health education materials generally fall into two categories: public information materials and health education materials. While there is some overlap, public information materials are used to reach large audiences with basic factual information that is designed to raise individual awareness about specific health issues. They are also used to increase motivation to learn and stimulate participation in the education program. Health education materials are used to meet the needs of a specific target population. In addition to providing factual information, education materials address attitudes and values as well as the teaching skills necessary to change behavior.

Planning
Preliminary planning is basic to the delivery of health education. Before selecting or evaluating health education materials, the following steps are recommended:

- Assess the characteristics and needs of the target group; this means selecting materials that reflect the values, beliefs, and attitudes of the target audience. The minimal considerations for selecting educational materials should include information about age, sex, ethnicity, cultural values, economic level, residence (urban versus rural), and physical limitations that might affect learning.

- Identify educational goals; selection of appropriate materials is helpful in achieving educational goals. For example, a fact sheet on the prevalence of breast cancer is useful for increasing an individual's awareness of susceptibility to a particular disease, whereas a film is more appropriate for demonstrating breast self-examination.
- Identify the methodology; a variety of methods may be used to communicate health messages and to teach behavior change. Health education methods include lecture, self-instruction, games, demonstrations, and group discussions. If the method of teaching is group discussion, the teacher would select a film that would stimulate discussion, rather than self-instruction materials.
- Consider the setting for health education; the learning environment is an essential consideration in selecting educational materials. For example when constrained by time and space, consider using flip charts and videocassettes.
- Determine available resources; when financial support is limited, it may be more desirable to purchase a few expensive but specialized materials if they are to be used extensively. On the other hand, when trying to reach a large number of individuals, it may be more cost effective to purchase inexpensive materials.
- Decide the medium; being aware of group characteristics can help the teacher to decide on the appropriate medium (audio, poster) to select when preparing to order health education materials. For example, supplementing a family-planning class on diaphragm insertion with a step-by-step booklet that clients can take home is likely to be more effective than a one-time slide show.
- Review current knowledge; it is particularly important that educational materials contain current scientific information and that out-dated, inaccurate information is discarded. (U.S. Department of Health and Human Services, 1982)

The planning process includes appropriate use of resources within one's own agency or institution. There may be a wealth of knowledge and expertise in a single institution yet these resources may be under utilized. Patients and clients benefit from close collaboration among members of the health-care team. A patient who is referred to physical therapy for whirlpool and instruction in crutch walking for example, must have this teaching reinforced on the nursing unit. The patient's progress is closely monitored by both the physical therapist and the nursing staff. Knowing when to teach and when to refer clients to other resources is also important. Referring a patient who has a poor appetite to a nutritionist should be routine practice.

Teaching requires knowledge of community resources as well as knowing how and when to make referrals. A telephone information and referral service and/or a published community directory are also helpful. Basic information about a particular resource in relation to location (directions to), phone number, cost, services provided, and eligibility requirements must be available. In some cases, patients and clients can refer themselves to a source of assistance once they are informed of it. Individuals with a particular health problem can be given written information about resources they might need in the future.

Locating Materials

There is an abundance of educational materials available through a number of different sources, including: federal, state, and local agencies, professional associations, pharmaceutical companies, insurance companies, voluntary agencies, and commercial publishing companies. Many of these materials are available free of charge or at low cost.

There is no one federal agency or department that coordinates the distribution of health education materials. The United States Department of Health and Human Services has made a concerted effort to coordinate the large volume of available materials through its National Health Information Center (NHIC). The NHIC is a central referral source designed to identify organizations and groups that provide health information to the public. The name and address of selected sources can be found at the end of this chapter.

Local and State Resources

Local and state health departments usually stock a wide array of printed materials on such topics as birth control, prenatal care, labor and delivery, infant care, immunizations, nutrition, communicable diseases, chronic diseases, and growth and development. These materials are often free of charge. Local health departments and public school systems have access to films and other materials that they may be willing to share. Voluntary organizations, such as the American Heart Association and the American Cancer Society, are also excellent sources of published materials, films, and speakers. In some states, there are departments of consumer affairs that publish consumer information on a regular basis. These departments may have a toll-free hot line for those seeking specific advice about a consumer health question. Many hospitals broadcast educational programs into patients' rooms over closed-circuit television. Topics may range from how to quit smoking to breast self-examination. Education materials are also developed to meet the needs of individuals with a particular health problem.

Federal Sources

The National Health Information Center
P.O. Box 1133
Washington, DC 20013–1133
(800) 336–4797 Toll free

The Consumer information Center (CIC) is a major federal source that distributes a large number of publications annually. To order the CIC catalog or request information write to:

Consumer Information Center
Pueblo, Colorado 81009

Whenever possible, materials should be ordered from the primary source first. For example, the National Clearinghouse on Alcohol and Drug Information is likely to have the most up to date information on these topics even though other groups promote education in this area. If for any reason materials cannot be obtained from the primary source, write or call:

Superintendent of Documents
U.S. Government Printing Office
Washington, DC 20402
Phone (202) 783–3238

When ordering materials from the Government Printing Office include the GPO stock (publication) numbers. These numbers are listed on each publication. The GPO publishes a free monthly catalog available through any one of the GPO's 27 bookstores around the country.

Other Federal Sources
Arthritis Information Clearinghouse
P.O. Box AMS
Bethesda, MD 20892
(301) 495–4484

Cancer Information Hotline
National Cancer Institute
9000 Rockville Pike
Bethesda, MD 20892
(800) 4CANCER

Centers for Disease Control
Office of Public Inquiries
Atlanta, GA 30333
(404) 639–3534

Centers for Disease Control
Center for Chronic Disease Prevention and Health Promotion (CDPHP)
Division of Adolescent and School Health
Mail Stop K31
1600 Clifton Rd, NE
Atlanta, GA 30333
(404) 488–5372

Centers for Disease Control
National Institute Occupational Safety and Health (NIOSH)
Mail Stop 36
1600 Clifton Rd, NE
Atlanta, GA 30333
(404) 639–3106

Centers for Disease Control—CCDPHP
Office of Smoking and Health
Rhodes Building
1600 Clifton Rd, NE
Atlanta, GA 30333
(404) 488–5701

Clearinghouse on Child Abuse and Neglect Information
P.O. Box 1182
Washington, DC 20013
(703) 821–2086

Consumer Product Safety Commission
Bethesda, MD 20892
(800) 638–2772 (hot line)

Food and Drug Administration
Office of Consumer Inquiries
5600 Fishers Lane, HFE-88, Room 16-63
Rockville, MD 20857
(301) 443–3170

National Clearinghouse on Alcohol and Drug Information (NCAI)
P.O. Box 2345
Rockville, MD 20852
(800) 729–6686

National Institute of Allergy and Infectious Diseases (NIAID)
Building 31
Room 7A32
Bethesda, MD 20892
(301) 496–5717

National Institute of Dental Research (NIDR)
900 Rockville Pike
Bethesda, MD 20892
(301) 496–4261

National Institutes of Health
Division of Public Information
9000 Rockville Pike, Bldg. 1, Room 344
Bethesda, MD 20892
(301) 496–5787

National Institute for Mental Health Information (NIMHI)
Information and Resources Inquiries Branch
5600 Fishers Lane, Room 15C-05
Rockville, MD 20857
(301) 443–4513

National Institute of Neurological and Communicative Disorders and Stroke
(NINCDS)
900 Rockville Pike, Bldg. 31, Room 8A16
Bethesda, MD 20892
(301) 496–5751

National Heart, Lung, and Blood Institute (NHLB) Information Center
4733 Bethesda Avenue, Suite 530
Bethesda, MD 20814–4820
(301) 951–3260

President's Council on Physical Fitness and Sports (PCPFS)
450 Fifth Street, NW
Suite 7103
Washington, DC 20001
(202) 272–3421

Public Health Service (PHS)
Office of the Assistant Secretary for Health
200 Independence Avenue, S.W., Room 717H
Washington, DC 20201

United States Department of Health and Human Services, OIG, Hotline
P.O. Box 17303
Baltimore, MD 21203–7303
(800) 638–3986
(Investigates Complaints)

Violence and Traumatic Stress Research Branch
5600 Fishers Lane, Room 18105
Rockville, MD 20857
(301) 443–3728

Voluntary Organizations
American Association of Retired Persons
1909 K Street, NW
Washington, DC 20049
(202) 872–4700

American Cancer Society
777 3rd Avenue
New York, NY 10017
Contact Local Chapter

American Diabetes Association
1211 Connecticut Avenue, NW
Washington, DC 20036
(202) 331–8303
Contact Local Chapter

American Heart Association
7320 Greenville Avenue
Dallas, TX 75231
Contact Local Chapter

American Lung Association
1740 Broadway
New York, NY 10019
Contact Local Chapter

Arthritis Foundation
1901 Fort Myers Drive, Suite 500
Arlington, VA 22209
(703) 276–7555

National Council on Aging
409 Third Street, SW
Washington, DC 20024
(202) 479–1200

Planned Parenthood (World Population)
810 7th Avenue
New York, NY 10019
(212) 541–7800

AIDS EDUCATION MATERIALS

Books
Learning AIDS
RR Bowker
245 W 17th Street
New York, NY 10011
(800) 521–8110

AIDS Information Source Book
Oryx Press
2214 North Central at Encanto
Phoenix, AZ 85004–1483
(602) 254–6156

AIDS: The Preventable Epidemic
HIV Education Program
Oregon Health Division
P.O. Box 117
Portland, OR 97207

Videotapes
Select Media, Inc.
74 Varick Street, Suite 305
New York, NY 10013
(212) 431–8923

Human Relations Media
Room CC012
175 Tompkins Avenue
Pleasantville, NY 10570–9973
(800) 431–2050 (USA)
(914) 769–7496 (Canada)

NEWIST/CESA #7
IS 1110
University of Wisconsin
Green Bay, WI 54311
(414) 465–2599

Computer Software
STD: A Guide for Today's Young Adults
Georgia State University Foundation
Department of Medical Technology
University Plaza
Atlanta, GA 30303
(404) 651–3034

Understanding AIDS
Substance Abuse Education, Inc.
670 S Fourth Street
Edwardsville, KS 66113
(913) 441–1868

AIDS Education
Health Edco
P.O. Box 21207
Waco, TX 76702
(800) 433–2677

Business and Professional Organizations
American Public Health Association
1015 Fifteenth Street, NW
Washington, DC 20005
(202) 789–5600

Blue Cross Association and Blue Shield Association
550 Twelfth Street, SW
Washington, DC 20065
(202) 479–8000

National Dairy Council (offices also located in states)
6300 North River Road
Rosemont, IL 60018–4233
(708) 696–1860

Group Health Association of America, Inc. (Represents HMOs)
1129 20th Street, NW, Suite 600
Washington, DC 20036
(202) 778–3200

Pharmaceutical Manufacturers' Association (Trade Organization)
Public Relations Division
1100 15th Street, NW
Washington, DC 20005
(202) 835–3400

Sources of Patient Education Materials
Krames Communications
312, 90th Street
1100 Grundy Lane
San Bruno, CA 94066–3030
(415) 742–0400

Pritchett and Hull Associates
Suite 110
3440 Oakcliff, NE
Atlanta, GA 30340
(800) 241–4925

Health Promotion Publications
Business & Health
P.O. Box 1409
Riverton, NJ 08077
(609) 786–0608
(health policy, cost management, benefits, health promotion)

Corporate Fitness
1640 Fifth Street
Santa Monica, CA 90401
(213) 395–0234
(fitness and health promotion planning)

Optimal Health
1842 Hoffman Street
Suite 201
Madison, WI 53704
(608) 249–0186
(health promotion, fitness programming, and marketing in health-care settings)

Promoting Health
840 N Lake Shore Drive
Chicago, IL 60611
(hospital-based health promotion programming)

*References and Readings
Cornacchia, H. J., & Barrett, S. *Consumer health: A guide to intelligent decisions* (4th ed.).
    St. Louis: C. V. Mosby, 1989
U.S. Department of Health and Human Services. *Health information resources.* Washington,
    DC.: U.S. Government Printing Office, 1990.
————. *Source book for health education materials and community resources.* Washington,
    DC.: U.S. Government Printing Office, 1982.
(*Many sources verified through phone calls to various agencies.*)

Index

NOTE: A *t* following a page number indicates tabular material and an *f* following a page number indicates a figure.

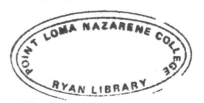

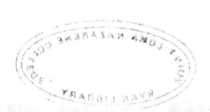